Reducing Mortality in Critically Ill Patients

Giovanni Landoni
Martina Baiardo Redaelli
Chiara Sartini · Alberto Zangrillo
Rinaldo Bellomo
Editors

Reducing Mortality in Critically Ill Patients

Second Edition

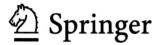 Springer

Editors
Giovanni Landoni
Department of Anesthesia and Intensive Care
IRCCS San Raffaele Scientific Institute and
Vita-Salute San Raffaele University
Milan
Italy

Chiara Sartini
Department of Anesthesia and
Intensive Care
IRCCS San Raffaele Scientific Institute
Milan
Italy

Rinaldo Bellomo
Department of Intensive Care
Austin Hospital
Heidelberg
VIC
Australia

Martina Baiardo Redaelli
Department of Anesthesia and
Intensive Care
IRCCS San Raffaele Scientific Institute
Milan
Italy

Alberto Zangrillo
Department of Anesthesia and
Intensive Care
IRCCS San Raffaele Scientific Institute
and Vita-Salute San Raffaele University
Milan
Italy

ISBN 978-3-030-71916-6   ISBN 978-3-030-71917-3   (eBook)
https://doi.org/10.1007/978-3-030-71917-3

This Springer imprint is published by the registered company Springer Nature Switzerland AG
The registered company address is: Gewerbestrasse 11, 6330 Cham, Switzerland

Preface

Critically ill patients are at high risk of mortality, and each effort is made by clinicians to improve survival. This fragile patient population requires multiple invasive and noninvasive life support interventions that may range from cardiopulmonary resuscitation to the most accurate nutritional support.

Working with such a fragile population is challenging, no critically ill patient is like the other and the vastness of knowledge required in critical care makes this discipline one of the most demanding medical specialties. In this context, evidence-based medicine together with international guidelines is the cornerstone to drive therapeutic choices.

Unfortunately, guidelines cannot cover all the variables met in clinical practice and performing high-quality clinical research is challenging in this specific setting.

However, systematically searching in the scientific literature, we have found more than 300 randomized controlled trials (RCTs) investigating interventions (drug, strategies, or techniques) with a proven statistically significant effect on mortality. The majority of these interventions were found to improve survival, while few of them were found to be detrimental in critically ill patients.

In this textbook, we summarize the available evidence-based interventions, with a significant mortality effect, in critical care medicine. The volume has been crafted to systematically combine the RCTs in dedicated chapters according to the specific topic. Most of them enclose interventions increasing survival, while in three separate chapters the reader will find the summary of the interventions increasing mortality, the interventions with still unclear conflicting evidences, and a last chapter collecting the latest evidences, not matching with the previously treated topics. Although the chapters are arranged in a progressive manner, in order to empower each other, the reader can even choose a single chapter to deepen his specific field of interest.

This volume encloses a fundamental piece of evidence-based medicine. It is addressed to critical care physicians who daily deal with challenging therapeutic choices, to residents and medical students as a base to build their critical care knowledge, and to researcher who wants to understand where the state of the art in critical care evidence is, in order to properly address future studies.

As editors, we are profoundly grateful to all the authors of this book for their excellent contribution and their motivation to help spreading the available knowledge in evidence-based critical care medicine. We must also acknowledge that hundreds of colleagues from all over the world, despite not mentioned as authors of this textbook, gave a significant contribution to this work, spending their time to help us in the consensus building and systematic review process that is beneath this volume and give strength to each chapter.

Milan, Italy	Giovanni Landoni
Milan, Italy	Martina Baiardo Redaelli
Milan, Italy	Chiara Sartini
Milan, Italy	Alberto Zangrillo
Heidelberg, VIC, Australia	Rinaldo Bellomo

Contents

Decision-Making in the Democracy Medicine Era: The Consensus Conference Process

Massimiliano Greco, Maria Luisa Azzolini, and Giacomo Monti

Contents

Randomized controlled trials (RCTs) are the gold standard of evidence-based medicine.

However, their application on the population of critically ill patients acted as a conundrum for researchers in the last decades [1]. A significant number of well-designed, robust, multicenter RCTs failed to find significant effects in this population [2]. This is due to the characteristics of critically ill patients, which have wide variation in mortality risk, according to difference in baseline conditions, ICU admission reason, and previous comorbidities. Lack of external validity, contrasting results between similar trials, and difficulties in interpretation of results led to a blurred picture on the evidence available in critical care.

M. Greco (✉)
Department of Anesthesiology and Intensive Care, IRCCS Humanitas Research Hospital, Rozzano, MI, Italy

Department of Biomedical Sciences, Humanitas University, Pieve Emanuele, MI, Italy
e-mail: massimiliano.greco@hunimed.eu

M. L. Azzolini · G. Monti
Department of Anesthesia and Intensive Care, IRCCS San Raffaele Scientific Institute, Milan, Italy
e-mail: azzolini.marialuisa@hsr.it; monti.giacomo@hsr.it

© Springer Nature Switzerland AG 2021
G. Landoni et al. (eds.), *Reducing Mortality in Critically Ill Patients*,
https://doi.org/10.1007/978-3-030-71917-3_1

Likewise, this condition worsens due to several low-quality non-randomized or observational studies, which should be considered by clinicians as exploratory hypotheses only.

Given these premises, the modern clinicians try to achieve an updated and clear picture of the best evidence available in medical literature. While consensus conferences and guidelines were designed to simplify this task, their approach has been criticized, due to the preeminent role of experts and the possibility of introducing expert-related bias [3, 4].

To overcome these limitations, a third way has been proposed and has already been employed in different medical fields: the democracy-based medicine [5–8].

In this book, we present the result of both an updated democratic consensus conference and the last available randomized evidence influencing mortality in critically ill setting.

The process of consensus building has been described elsewhere [5] and is summarized in this chapter.

1.1   Systematic Review

Authors performed a systematic review on the major scientific databases (MEDLINE/PubMed, Scopus and Embase) to identify all RCTs on any type of intervention influencing mortality in critically ill and perioperative patients, with a statistically significant effect on mortality.

Inclusion criteria were:

- RCT published in a peer-reviewed journal reporting a statistical significant difference in mortality without adjustment for baseline characteristics.
- Involving adult patients in critically ill setting.
- Assessing non-surgical interventions (drugs, strategy, or techniques).

The literature research identified more than 52,255 papers that were screened at title/abstract level, of these 262 were discussed in an in-person meeting, and analyzed by 32 experts. Several papers were excluded because of methodological flaws or exclusion criteria.

1.2   Reaching Consensus in Democracy Medicine

The process of Democracy Medicine was based on an international meeting held at an academic center and on an online surveys/vote. After the systematic review and the experts meeting, interventions reducing and increasing mortality were identified and position statements for the next step generated. Subsequently, an online platform hosted a survey where colleagues could express their agreement on the proposed statements. This second step collected and validated the original statements

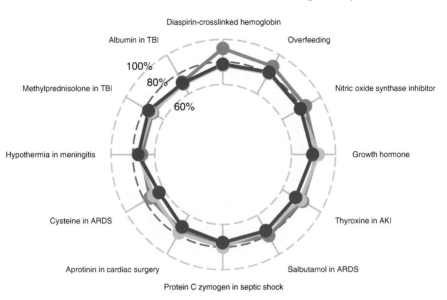

Fig. 1.1   Results of the web-vote on interventions increasing mortality. Abbreviations: AKI = acute kidney injury; ARDS = acute respiratory distress syndrome; TBI = traumatic brain injury

according to the opinions of hundreds of colleagues from 46 countries. Interventions not reaching 67% agreement on their efficacy or on their detrimental effect were excluded.

The results of the web survey for interventions increasing mortality are reported in Fig. 1.1, while results for interventions reducing mortality are reported in Fig. 1.2.

1.3   The Identified Topics, the Book, and the Diffusion of the Evidence to the International Community of Colleagues

Topics reducing mortality [6–71] and increasing mortality [72–83] were thus finally identified and are reported in Table 1.1.

Given the international relevance and the amount of information collected, generated, and organized through the whole process, the authors disseminated consensus results to reach the widest audience of peers. Two main article regarding the consensus were published in the Journal of Cardiothoracic and Vascular Anesthesia [84, 85].

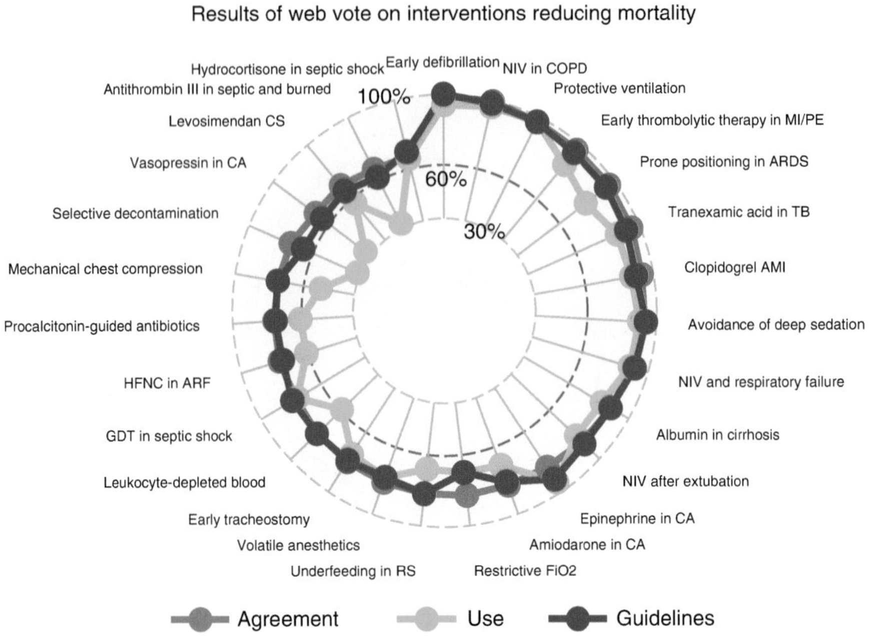

Results of web vote on interventions reducing mortality

Fig. 1.2 Results of the web-vote on interventions reducing mortality. Abbreviations: *NIV* = non-invasive ventilation; *COPD* = chronic obstructive pulmonary disease; *MI* = myocardial infarction; *PE* = pulmonary embolism; *ARDS* = acute distress respiratory syndrome; *AMI* = acute myocardial infarction; *CA* = cardiac arrest; *FiO2* = inspiratory fraction of oxygen; *RS* = refeeding syndrome; *GDT* = goal-directed therapy; *HFNC* = high flow nasal cannula; *ARF* = acute respiratory failure; *CS* = cardiogenic shock

Interventions reducing mortality, with the evidence supporting them, are extensively described in this book. Indeed, the reader will find them along the chapters, included in the appropriate topic. Conversely, the reader will find interventions increasing mortality and those with conflicting evidences (having at the same time RCTs both in favor or against mortality reduction), summarized in two separate chapters.

The last chapter reviews the latest randomized evidences on mortality, published after the consensus conference and dealing with topics not discussed in previous chapters.

1.4   A Common Shell for a Flexible Process

The democratic process has been in place among all the previous consensus conferences [86–92].They focused on critically ill patients [90, 91], on interventions in cardiac anesthesia [88, 92], on the perioperative period of any surgery [86, 87], and on patients with or at risk for acute kidney injury [89].

Table 1.1 The interventions influencing mortality identified by the Consensus Conference

Increasing survival		Increasing mortality
Early defibrillation [26, 27]	Volatile anesthetics in cardiac surgery [8, 65]	Diaspirin cross-linked hemoglobin [82]
NIV in COPD [6, 46]	Early tracheostomy [59, 60]	Overfeeding [76]
Protective ventilation [10, 49, 52]	Leukocyte-depleted blood [32, 33]	NOS inhibitor in septic shock [73]
Early thrombolytic therapy in MI/PE [56–58, 66]	GDT in septic shock [28, 30]	Human growth hormone [78]
Prone positioning in ARDS [9, 12, 50]	HFNC in Respiratory Failure [7]	Thyroxine in AKI [72]
Tranexamic acid in trauma [61]	Procalcitonin-guided antibiotics [70]	IV Salbutamol in ARDS [81]
Clopidogrel in MI [21]	Mechanical chest compression [36–39]	Protein C zymogen [80]
Avoidance of deep sedation [51, 55, 67]	Selective decontamination [11, 22–25]	Aprotinin in noncardiac surgery [79]
NIV and respiratory failure [41–45, 68]	Vasopressin in cardiac arrest [63, 64]	Cysteine prodrug [74]
Albumin in cirrhosis [14]	Levosimendan in cardiogenic shock [34, 35]	Hypothermia in meningitis [77]
Epinephrine in cardiac arrest [71]	Antithrombin III in septic and burned [17, 19, 93]	Methylprednisolone in TBI [75]
Amiodarone in cardiac arrest [15, 16, 62]	Hydrocortisone in septic shock [31]	Albumin in TBI [83]
Restrictive FiO_2 [53, 54]	NIV after extubation [18, 29, 40, 47, 48]	
Underfeeding in refeeding syndrome [69]		

NIV Non-invasive ventilation, *MI* myocardial infarction, *PE* pulmonary embolism, *ARDS* Acute respiratory distress syndrome, *TBI* Traumatic brain injury, *HFNC* High Flow Nasal Cannula, *GDT* Goal Directed Therapy, *NOS* nitric oxide synthase, *COPD* Chronic obstructive pulmonary disease (COPD)

Each time a manuscript with the consensus results was published on an international journal. There were only small differences related to the systematic review (according to the broadness and complexity of the subject), and some variance in the questions posed by the web survey.

The Democratic Consensus process, to our knowledge, is the only method employed to share the evaluation of best medical evidence with a global audience of clinicians and to allow to reach agreement among a large population of colleagues.

This book is a compendium of our last Democracy-Based Medicine process involving critically ill and perioperative patients and comprises RCT-based evidence on highly selected specific topics.

References

1. Vincent JL. We should abandon randomized controlled trials in the intensive care unit. In: Critical care medicine, vol. 38. Baltimore: Lippincott Williams and Wilkins; 2010. https://doi.org/10.1097/CCM.0b013e3181f208ac.
2. Ospina-Tascón GA, Büchele GL, Vincent J-L. Multicenter, randomized, controlled trials evaluating mortality in intensive care: doomed to fail? Crit Care Med. 2008;36(4):1311–22. https://doi.org/10.1097/CCM.0b013e318168ea3e.
3. Bellomo R. The risks and benefits of the consensus process. In: Reducing mortality in the perioperative period. Cham: Springer; 2014. p. 1–7. https://doi.org/10.1007/978-3-319-02186-7_1.
4. Rotondi AJ, Kvetan V, Carlet J, Sibbald WJ. Consensus conferences in critical care medicine. Crit Care Clin. 1997;13(2):417–40. https://doi.org/10.1016/S0749-0704(05)70319-5.
5. Greco M, Zangrillo A, Mucchetti M, et al. Democracy-based consensus in medicine. J Cardiothorac Vasc Anesth. 2015;29(2):506–9. https://doi.org/10.1053/j.jvca.2014.11.005.
6. Plant PK, Owen JL, Elliott MW. Early use of non-invasive ventilation for acute exacerbations of chronic obstructive pulmonary disease on general respiratory wards: a multicentre randomised controlled trial. Lancet. 2000;355(9219):1931–5. https://doi.org/10.1016/S0140-6736(00)02323-0.
7. Frat JP, Thille AW, Mercat A, et al. High-flow oxygen through nasal cannula in acute hypoxemic respiratory failure. N Engl J Med. 2015;372(23):2185–96. https://doi.org/10.1056/NEJMoa1503326.
8. Likhvantsev VV, Landoni G, Levikov DI, Grebenchikov OA, Skripkin YV, Cherpakov RA. Sevoflurane versus Total intravenous anesthesia for isolated coronary artery bypass surgery with cardiopulmonary bypass: a randomized trial. J Cardiothorac Vasc Anesth. 2016;30(5):1221–7. https://doi.org/10.1053/j.jvca.2016.02.030.
9. Guérin C, Reignier J, Richard J-C, et al. Prone positioning in severe acute respiratory distress syndrome. N Engl J Med. 2013;368(23):2159–68. https://doi.org/10.1056/NEJMoa1214103.
10. Brower RG, Matthay MA, Morris A, et al. Ventilation with lower tidal volumes as compared with traditional tidal volumes for acute lung injury and the acute respiratory distress syndrome. N Engl J Med. 2000;342(18):1301–8. https://doi.org/10.1056/NEJM200005043421801.
11. De Jonge E, Schultz MJ, Spanjaard L, et al. Effects of selective decontamination of digestive tract on mortality and acquisition of resistant bacteria in intensive care: a randomised controlled trial. Lancet. 2003;362(9389):1011–6. https://doi.org/10.1016/S0140-6736(03)14409-1.
12. Mancebo J, Fernández R, Blanch L, et al. A multicenter trial of prolonged prone ventilation in severe acute respiratory distress syndrome. Am J Respir Crit Care Med. 2006;173(11):1233–9. https://doi.org/10.1164/rccm.200503-353OC.
13. Lindner KH, Dirks B, Strohmenger HU, Prengel AW, Lindner IM, Lurie KG. Randomised comparison of epinephrine and vasopressin in patients with out-of-hospital ventricular fibrillation. Lancet. 1997;349(9051):535–7. https://doi.org/10.1016/S0140-6736(97)80087-6.
14. Sort P, Navasa M, Arroyo V, et al. Effect of intravenous albumin on renal impairment and mortality in patients with cirrhosis and spontaneous bacterial peritonitis. N Engl J Med. 1999;341(6):403–9. https://doi.org/10.1056/nejm199908053410603.
15. Dorian P, Cass D, Schwartz B, Cooper R, Gelaznikas R, Barr A. Amiodarone as compared with lidocaine for shock-resistant ventricular fibrillation. N Engl J Med. 2002;346(12):884–90. https://doi.org/10.1056/nejmoa013029.
16. Kudenchuk PJ, Cobb LA, Copass MK, et al. Amiodarone for resuscitation after out-of-hospital cardiac arrest due to ventricular fibrillation. N Engl J Med. 1999;341(12):871–8. https://doi.org/10.1056/nejm199909163411203.
17. Baudo F, Caimi TM, de Cataldo F, et al. Antithrombin III (ATILL) replacement therapy in patients with sepsis and/or postsurgical complications: a controlled double-blind, randomized, multicenter study. Intensive Care Med. 1998;24(4):336–42. https://doi.org/10.1007/s001340050576.

18. Ferrer M, Valencia M, Nicolas JM, Bernadich O, Badia JR, Torres A. Early noninvasive ventilation averts extubation failure in patients at risk: a randomized trial. Am J Respir Crit Care Med. 2006;173(2):164–70. https://doi.org/10.1164/rccm.200505-718OC.
19. Lavrentieva A, Bitzani M, Parlapani A, et al. The efficacy of antithrombin administration in the acute phase of burn injury. Thromb Haemost. 2008;100(08):286–90. https://doi.org/10.1160/th07-11-0684.
20. Warren BL, Eid A, Singer P, et al. High-dose Antithrombin III in severe Sepsis. JAMA. 2001;286(15):1869. https://doi.org/10.1001/jama.286.15.1869.
21. Chen ZM, et al. Addition of clopidogrel to aspirin in 45 852 patients with acute myocardial infarction: randomised placebo-controlled trial. Lancet. 2005;366(9497):1607–21. https://doi.org/10.1016/s0140-6736(05)67660-x.
22. de La Cal MA, Cerdá E, García-Hierro P, et al. Survival benefit in critically ill burned patients receiving selective decontamination of the digestive tract. Ann Surg. 2005;241(3):424–30. https://doi.org/10.1097/01.sla.0000154148.58154.d5.
23. Krueger WA, Lenhart F-P, Neeser G, et al. Influence of combined intravenous and topical antibiotic prophylaxis on the incidence of infections, organ dysfunctions, and mortality in critically ill surgical patients. Am J Respir Crit Care Med. 2002;166(8):1029–37. https://doi.org/10.1164/rccm.2105141.
24. Rocha LA, Martín MJ, Pita S, et al. Prevention of nosocomial infection in critically ill patients by selective decontamination of the digestive tract. Intensive Care Med. 1992;18(7):398–404. https://doi.org/10.1007/bf01694341.
25. Ulrich C, Harinck-de Weerd JE, Bakker NC, Jacz K, Doornbos L, de Ridder VA. Selective decontamination of the digestive tract with norfloxacin in the prevention of ICU-acquired infections: a prospective randomized study. Intensive Care Med. 1989;15(7):424–31. https://doi.org/10.1007/bf00255597.
26. Eisenberg MS. Treatment of ventricular fibrillation. JAMA. 1984;251(13):1723. https://doi.org/10.1001/jama.1984.03340370055030.
27. Hallstrom AP, et al. Public-access defibrillation and survival after out-of-hospital cardiac arrest. N Engl J Med. 2004;351(7):637–46. https://doi.org/10.1056/nejmoa040566.
28. Lin S-MM, Da Huang C-D, Lin H-CC, Liu C-YY, Wang C-HH, Kuo H-PP. A modified goal-directed protocol improves clinical outcomes in intensive care unit patients with septic shock. Shock. 2006;26(6):551–7. https://doi.org/10.1097/01.shk.0000232271.09440.8f.
29. Ferrer M, Sellarés J, Valencia M, et al. Non-invasive ventilation after extubation in hypercapnic patients with chronic respiratory disorders: randomised controlled trial. Lancet. 2009;374(9695):1082–8. https://doi.org/10.1016/S0140-6736(09)61038-2.
30. Rivers E, Nguyen B, Havstad S, et al. Early goal-directed therapy in the treatment of severe Sepsis and septic shock. N Engl J Med. 2001;345(19):1368–77. https://doi.org/10.1056/nejmoa010307.
31. Annane D. Effect of treatment with low doses of hydrocortisone and fludrocortisone on mortality in patients with septic shock. JAMA. 2002;288(7):862. https://doi.org/10.1001/jama.288.7.862.
32. Bilgin YM, van de Watering LMG, Eijsman L, et al. Double-blind, randomized controlled trial on the effect of leukocyte-depleted erythrocyte transfusions in cardiac valve surgery. Circulation. 2004;109(22):2755–60. https://doi.org/10.1161/01.cir.0000130162.11925.21.
33. van de Watering LMG, Hermans J, Houbiers JGA, et al. Beneficial effects of leukocyte depletion of transfused blood on postoperative complications in patients undergoing cardiac surgery. Circulation. 1998;97(6):562–8. https://doi.org/10.1161/01.cir.97.6.562.
34. Fuhrmann JT, Schmeisser A, Schulze MR, et al. Levosimendan is superior to enoximone in refractory cardiogenic shock complicating acute myocardial infarction*. Crit Care Med. 2008;36(8):2257–66. https://doi.org/10.1097/ccm.0b013e3181809846.
35. Levin RL, Degrange MA, Porcile R, et al. The calcium sensitizer levosimendan gives superior results to dobutamine in postoperative low cardiac output syndrome. Rev Española Cardiol. 2008;61(5):471–9. https://doi.org/10.1016/s1885-5857(08)60160-7.

36. Cohen TJ, Goldner BG, Maccaro PC, et al. A comparison of active compression-decompression cardiopulmonary resuscitation with standard cardiopulmonary resuscitation for cardiac arrests occurring in the hospital. N Engl J Med. 1993;329(26):1918–21. https://doi.org/10.1056/nejm199312233292603.

37. Gao C, Chen YY, Peng H, Chen YY, Zhuang Y, Zhou S. Clinical evaluation of the AutoPulse automated chest compression device for out-of-hospital cardiac arrest in the northern district of Shanghai, China. Arch Med Sci. 2016;3(3):563–70. https://doi.org/10.5114/aoms.2016.59930.

38. Tucker KJ, Galli F, Savitt MA, Kahsai D, Bresnahan L, Redberg RF. Active compression-decompression resuscitation: effect on resuscitation success after in-hospital cardiac arrest. J Am Coll Cardiol. 1994;24(1):201–9. https://doi.org/10.1016/0735-1097(94)90564-9.

39. Wolcke BB, Mauer DK, Schoefmann MF, et al. Comparison of standard cardiopulmonary resuscitation versus the combination of active compression-decompression cardiopulmonary resuscitation and an inspiratory impedance threshold device for out-of-hospital cardiac arrest. Circulation. 2003;108(18):2201–5. https://doi.org/10.1161/01.cir.0000095787.99180.b5.

40. Nava S, Ambrosino N, Clini E, et al. Noninvasive mechanical ventilation in the weaning of patients with respiratory failure due to chronic obstructive pulmonary disease: a randomized, controlled trial. Ann Intern Med. 1998;128(9):721–8. https://doi.org/10.7326/0003-4819-128-9-199805010-00004.

41. Ferrer M, Esquinas A, Leon M, Gonzalez G, Alarcon A, Torres A. Noninvasive ventilation in severe hypoxemic respiratory failure. Am J Respir Crit Care Med. 2003;168(12):1438–44. https://doi.org/10.1164/rccm.200301-072oc.

42. L'Her E, Duquesne F, Girou E, et al. Noninvasive continuous positive airway pressure in elderly cardiogenic pulmonary edema patients. Intensive Care Med. 2004;30(5):882–8. https://doi.org/10.1007/s00134-004-2183-y.

43. Nava S, Grassi M, Fanfulla F, et al. Non-invasive ventilation in elderly patients with acute hypercapnic respiratory failure: a randomised controlled trial. Age Ageing. 2011;40(4):444–50. https://doi.org/10.1093/ageing/afr003.

44. Park M, Sangean MC, Volpe MS, et al. Randomized, prospective trial of oxygen, continuous positive airway pressure, and bilevel positive airway pressure by face mask in acute cardiogenic pulmonary edema. Crit Care Med. 2004;32(12):2407–15. https://doi.org/10.1097/01.ccm.0000147770.20400.10.

45. Thompson J, Petrie DA, Ackroyd-Stolarz S, Bardua DJ. Out-of-hospital continuous positive airway pressure ventilation versus usual care in acute respiratory failure: a randomized controlled trial. Ann Emerg Med. 2008;52(3):232–241.e1. https://doi.org/10.1016/j.annemergmed.2008.01.006.

46. Brochard L, Mancebo J, Wysocki M, et al. Noninvasive ventilation for acute exacerbations of chronic obstructive pulmonary disease. N Engl J Med. 1995;333(13):817–22. https://doi.org/10.1056/nejm199509283331301.

47. Ferrer M, Esquinas A, Arancibia F, et al. Noninvasive ventilation during persistent weaning failure. Am J Respir Crit Care Med. 2003;168(1):70–6. https://doi.org/10.1164/rccm.200209-1074oc.

48. Ornico SR, Lobo SM, Sanches HS, et al. Noninvasive ventilation immediately after extubation improves weaning outcome after acute respiratory failure: a randomized controlled trial. Crit Care. 2013;17(2):R39. https://doi.org/10.1186/cc12549.

49. Amato MBP, Barbas CSV, Medeiros DM, et al. Effect of a protective-ventilation strategy on mortality in the acute respiratory distress syndrome. N Engl J Med. 1998;338(6):347–54. https://doi.org/10.1056/nejm199802053380602.

50. Gattinoni L, Tognoni G, Pesenti A, et al. Effect of prone positioning on the survival of patients with acute respiratory failure. N Engl J Med. 2001;345(8):568–73. https://doi.org/10.1056/nejmoa010043.

51. Mansouri P, Javadpour S, Zand F, et al. Implementation of a protocol for integrated management of pain, agitation, and delirium can improve clinical outcomes in the intensive care unit: a randomized clinical trial. J Crit Care. 2013;28(6):918–22. https://doi.org/10.1016/j.jcrc.2013.06.019.

52. Villar J, Kacmarek RM, Pérez-Méndez L, Aguirre-Jaime A. A high positive end-expiratory pressure, low tidal volume ventilatory strategy improves outcome in persistent acute respiratory distress syndrome: a randomized, controlled trial. Crit Care Med. 2006;34(5):1311–8. https://doi.org/10.1097/01.ccm.0000215598.84885.01.

53. Girardis M, Busani S, Damiani E, et al. Effect of conservative vs conventional oxygen therapy on mortality among patients in an intensive care unit. JAMA. 2016;316(15):1583. https://doi.org/10.1001/jama.2016.11993.

54. Meyhoff CS, Jorgensen LN, Wetterslev J, Christensen KB, Rasmussen LS. Increased long-term mortality after a high perioperative inspiratory oxygen fraction during abdominal surgery. Anesth Analg. 2012;115(4):849–54. https://doi.org/10.1213/ane.0b013e3182652a51.

55. Brown CH, Azman AS, Gottschalk A, Mears SC, Sieber FE. Sedation depth during spinal anesthesia and survival in elderly patients undergoing hip fracture repair. Anesth Analg. 2014;118(5):977–80. https://doi.org/10.1213/ane.0000000000000157.

56. GREAT Group. Feasibility, safety, and efficacy of domiciliary thrombolysis by general practitioners: Grampian region early anistreplase trial. BMJ. 1992;305(6853):548–53. https://doi.org/10.1136/bmj.305.6853.548.

57. Jerjes-Sanchez C, Ramírez-Rivera A, de Lourdes GM, et al. Streptokinase and heparin versus heparin alone in massive pulmonary embolism: a randomized controlled trial. J Thromb Thrombolysis. 1995;2(3):227–9. https://doi.org/10.1007/bf01062714.

58. Rawles JM. Quantification of the benefit of earlier thrombolytic therapy: five-year results of the Grampian region early anistreplase trial (GREAT). J Am Coll Cardiol. 1997;30(5):1181–6. https://doi.org/10.1016/s0735-1097(97)00299-4.

59. Bösel J, Schiller P, Hook Y, et al. Stroke-related early tracheostomy versus prolonged orotracheal intubation in neurocritical care trial (SETPOINT). Stroke. 2013;44(1):21–8. https://doi.org/10.1161/strokeaha.112.669895.

60. Rumbak MJ, Newton M, Truncale T, Schwartz SW, Adams JW, Hazard PB. A prospective, randomized, study comparing early percutaneous dilational tracheotomy to prolonged translaryngeal intubation (delayed tracheotomy) in critically ill medical patients*. Crit Care Med. 2004;32(8):1689–94. https://doi.org/10.1097/01.ccm.0000134835.05161.b6.

61. CRASH-2 Trial Collaborators. Effects of tranexamic acid on death, vascular occlusive events, and blood transfusion in trauma patients with significant haemorrhage (CRASH-2): a randomised, placebo-controlled trial. Lancet. 2010;376(9734):23–32. https://doi.org/10.1016/s0140-6736(10)60835-5.

62. Kudenchuk PJ, Brown SP, Daya M, et al. Amiodarone, lidocaine, or placebo in out-of-hospital cardiac arrest. N Engl J Med. 2016;374(18):1711–22. https://doi.org/10.1056/NEJMoa1514204.

63. Mentzelopoulos SD, Zakynthinos SG, Tzoufi M, et al. Vasopressin, epinephrine, and corticosteroids for in-hospital cardiac arrest. Arch Intern Med. 2009;169(1):15. https://doi.org/10.1001/archinternmed.2008.509.

64. Mentzelopoulos SD, Malachias S, Chamos C, et al. Vasopressin, steroids, and epinephrine and neurologically favorable survival after in-hospital cardiac arrest. JAMA. 2013;310(3):270. https://doi.org/10.1001/jama.2013.7832.

65. De Hert S, Vlasselaers D, Barbé R, et al. A comparison of volatile and non volatile agents for cardioprotection during on-pump coronary surgery. Anaesthesia. 2009;64(9):953–60. https://doi.org/10.1111/j.1365-2044.2009.06008.x.

66. Sarullo M. Ospedale Buccheri la Ferla F. [The safety and efficacy of systemic salvage thrombolysis in acute myocardial infarct]; 2000. http://www.researchgate.net/publication/12486256. Accessed 20 Aug 2020.

67. Girard TD, Kress JP, Fuchs BD, et al. Efficacy and safety of a paired sedation and ventilator weaning protocol for mechanically ventilated patients in intensive care (awakening and breathing controlled trial): a randomised controlled trial. Lancet. 2008;371(9607):126–34. https://doi.org/10.1016/S0140-6736(08)60105-1.

68. Zhu G, Wang D, Liu S, Jia M, Jia S. Efficacy and safety of noninvasive positive pressure ventilation in the treatment of acute respiratory failure after cardiac surgery. Chin Med J. 2013;126(23):4463–9.

69. Doig GS, Simpson F, Heighes PT, et al. Restricted versus continued standard caloric intake during the management of refeeding syndrome in critically ill adults: a randomised, parallel-group, multicentre, single-blind controlled trial. Lancet Respir Med. 2015;3(12):943–52. https://doi.org/10.1016/S2213-2600(15)00418-X.

70. de Jong E, van Oers JA, Beishuizen A, et al. Efficacy and safety of procalcitonin guidance in reducing the duration of antibiotic treatment in critically ill patients: a randomised, controlled, open-label trial. Lancet Infect Dis. 2016;16(7):819–27. https://doi.org/10.1016/S1473-3099(16)00053-0.

71. Jacobs IG, Finn JC, Jelinek GA, Oxer HF, Thompson PL. Effect of adrenaline on survival in out-of-hospital cardiac arrest: a randomised double-blind placebo-controlled trial. Resuscitation. 2011;82(9):1138–43. https://doi.org/10.1016/j.resuscitation.2011.06.029.

72. Acker CG, Singh AR, Flick RP, Bernardini J, Greenberg A, Johnson JP. A trial of thyroxine in acute renal failure. Kidney Int. 2000;57(1):293–8. https://doi.org/10.1046/j.1523-1755.2000.00827.x.

73. López A, Lorente JA, Steingrub J, et al. Multiple-center, randomized, placebo-controlled, double-blind study of the nitric oxide synthase inhibitor 546C88: effect on survival in patients with septic shock. Crit Care Med. 2004;32(1):21–30. https://doi.org/10.1097/01.CCM.0000105581.01815.C6.

74. Morris PE, Papadakos P, Russell JA, et al. A double-blind placebo-controlled study to evaluate the safety and efficacy of L-2-oxothiazolidine-4-carboxylic acid in the treatment of patients with acute respiratory distress syndrome. Crit Care Med. 2008;36(3):782–8. https://doi.org/10.1097/CCM.0B013E318164E7E4.

75. Olldashi F, Muzha I, Filipi N, et al. Effect of intravenous corticosteroids on death within 14 days in 10008 adults with clinically significant head injury (MRC CRASH trial): randomised placebo-controlled trial. Lancet. 2004;364(9442):1321–8. https://doi.org/10.1016/S0140-6736(04)17188-2.

76. Braunschweig CA, Sheean PM, Peterson SJ, et al. Intensive nutrition in acute lung injury: a clinical trial (INTACT). J Parenter Enter Nutr. 2015;39(1):13–20. https://doi.org/10.1177/0148607114528541.

77. Mourvillier B, Tubach F, Van De Beek D, et al. Induced hypothermia in severe bacterial meningitis: a randomized clinical trial. J Am Med Assoc. 2013;310(20):2174–83. https://doi.org/10.1001/jama.2013.280506.

78. Takala J, Ruokonen E, Webster NR, et al. Increased mortality associated with growth hormone treatment in critically ill adults. N Engl J Med. 1999;341(11):785–92. https://doi.org/10.1056/NEJM199909093411102.

79. Fergusson DA, Hébert PC, Mazer CD, et al. A comparison of aprotinin and lysine analogues in high-risk cardiac surgery. N Engl J Med. 2008;358(22):2319–31. https://doi.org/10.1056/NEJMoa0802395.

80. Pappalardo F, Crivellari M, Di Prima AL, et al. Protein C zymogen in severe sepsis: a double-blinded, placebo-controlled, randomized study. Intensive Care Med. 2016;42(11):1706–14. https://doi.org/10.1007/s00134-016-4405-5.

81. Smith F, Perkins G, Gates S, Young D, Lancet DM-T. Effect of intravenous β-2 agonist treatment on clinical outcomes in acute respiratory distress syndrome (BALTI-2): a multicentre, randomised controlled trial. Lancet. 2012;379:229–35. https://doi.org/10.1016/S0140-6736(11)61623-1.

82. Sloan EP, Koenigsberg M, Gens D, et al. Diaspirin cross-linked hemoglobin (DCLHb) in the treatment of severe traumatic hemorrhagic shock: a randomized controlled efficacy trial. J Am Med Assoc. 1999;282(19):1857–64. https://doi.org/10.1001/jama.282.19.1857.

83. Myburgh J, Cooper DJ, Finfer S, et al. Saline or albumin for fluid resuscitation in patients with traumatic brain injury. N Engl J Med. 2007;357(9):874–84. https://doi.org/10.1056/NEJMoa067514.

84. Sartini C, Lomivorotov V, Pieri M, et al. A systematic review and international web-based survey of randomized controlled trials in the perioperative and critical care setting: interventions reducing mortality. J Cardiothorac Vasc Anesth. 2019;33(5):1430–9. https://doi.org/10.1053/j.jvca.2018.11.026.
85. Sartini C, Lomivorotov V, Pisano A, et al. A systematic review and international web-based survey of randomized controlled trials in the perioperative and critical care setting: interventions increasing mortality. J Cardiothorac Vasc Anesth. 2019;33(10):2685–94. https://doi.org/10.1053/j.jvca.2019.03.022.
86. Landoni G, Rodseth RN, Santini F, et al. Randomized evidence for reduction of perioperative mortality. J Cardiothorac Vasc Anesth. 2012;26(5):764–72. https://doi.org/10.1053/j.jvca.2012.04.018.
87. Landoni G, Pisano A, Lomivorotov V, et al. Randomized evidence for reduction of perioperative mortality: an updated consensus process. J Cardiothorac Vasc Anesth. 2017;31(2):719–30. https://doi.org/10.1053/j.jvca.2016.07.017.
88. Landoni G, Lomivorotov V, Silvietti S, et al. Nonsurgical strategies to reduce mortality in patients undergoing cardiac surgery: an updated consensus process. J Cardiothorac Vasc Anesth. 2018;32(1):225–35. https://doi.org/10.1053/j.jvca.2017.06.017.
89. Landoni G, Bove T, Székely A, et al. Reducing mortality in acute kidney injury patients: systematic review and international web-based surveY. J Cardiothorac Vasc Anesth. 2013;27(6):1384–98. https://doi.org/10.1053/j.jvca.2013.06.028.
90. Pisano A, Landoni G, Lomivorotov V, et al. Worldwide opinion on multicenter randomized interventions showing mortality reduction in critically ill patients: a democracy-based medicine approach. J Cardiothorac Vasc Anesth. 2016;30(5):1386–95. https://doi.org/10.1053/j.jvca.2016.05.005.
91. Landoni G, Comis M, Conte M, et al. Mortality in multicenter critical care trials: an analysis of interventions with a significant effect. Crit Care Med. 2015;43(8):1559–68. https://doi.org/10.1097/CCM.0000000000000974.
92. Landoni G, Augoustides JG, Guarracino F, et al. Mortality reduction in cardiac anesthesia and intensive care: results of the first international consensus conference. Acta Anaesthesiol Scand. 2011;55(3):259–66. https://doi.org/10.1111/j.1399-6576.2010.02381.x.
93. Warren BL, Eid A, Singer P, et al. High-dose antithrombin III in severe sepsis: a randomized controlled trial. J Am Med Assoc. 2001;286(15):1869–78. https://doi.org/10.1001/jama.286.15.1869.

Non-invasive Ventilation

2

Luca Cabrini, Margherita Pintaudi, Nicola Villari, and Dario Winterton

Contents

L. Cabrini (✉)
Intensive Care and Anesthesia Unit, Ospedale di Circolo e Fondazione Macchi, Varese, Italy

Università degli Studi dell'Insubria, Varese, Italy
e-mail: luca.cabrini@uninsubria.it

M. Pintaudi
Anesthesia an Intensive Care, Bassini Hospital, ASST-Nord, Milano, Italy
e-mail: margherita.pintaudi@asst-nordmilano.it

N. Villari
Anesthesia and Intensive Care, Humanitas Gavazzeni Hospital, Bergamo, Italy
e-mail: Nicola.vilari@gavazzeni.it

D. Winterton
Department of Medicine and Surgery, University of Milan-Bicocca, Monza, Italy

© Springer Nature Switzerland AG 2021
G. Landoni et al. (eds.), *Reducing Mortality in Critically Ill Patients*,
https://doi.org/10.1007/978-3-030-71917-3_2

13

2.1 General Principles

Non-invasive ventilation (NIV) refers to the delivery of positive pressure to the airways and lungs in the absence of an intratracheal tube or an extra-glottic device. The term "NIV" includes both continuous positive airway pressure (CPAP) and any form of non-invasive inspiratory positive pressure ventilation (NPPV), in which an expiratory positive airway pressure is almost always present [1].

The main benefits of NIV in the prevention or treatment of acute respiratory failure (ARF) include: conservation or restoration of lung volumes; reduction of the work of breathing; avoidance or reduction of complications associated with tracheal intubation; easier use as compared to invasive mechanical ventilation; application even in patients unfit for tracheal intubation or outside the intensive care unit (ICU) [1, 2]. On the other hand, NIV can be contraindicated in some conditions. Among the possible contraindications only two of them are to be considered absolute: respiratory arrest and the inability to fit the mask. The other contraindications are relative: patient clinically unstable, agitated or uncooperative, the inability to protect airway or to manage excessive secretions, swallowing impairment, multiple (two or more) organ failure, recent upper airway, or upper gastrointestinal surgical procedure [1].

In the last two decades, the use of NIV has continuously increased. A large number of studies evaluated its efficacy and its limits in several acute care settings [3–6]. Notably, among interventions documented by randomized controlled trials (RCTs) that reduce mortality in critically ill adults, NIV was the most extensively studied and documented [7].

2.2 Pathophysiological Principles

Most underlying pathophysiological mechanisms of ARF involve imbalances between respiratory system mechanical work and neuromuscular competence, disorders in gas exchange, and increased cardiac preload and afterload.

By using expiratory and inspiratory positive pressure, NIV allows the respiratory muscles to rest, reduces respiratory work as well as cardiac preload and afterload, and improves alveolar recruitment, thus increasing lung volume. As a consequence, pulmonary compliance and oxygenation are commonly improved [8].

2.3 Main Evidences and Clinical Indications

Eleven multicenter randomized controlled trials (mRCTs) evaluated NIV in different clinical settings so far. The main characteristics of these mRCTs are summarized in Table 2.1.

Table 2.1 Abbreviations: COPD: chronic obstructive pulmonary disease; NIV: non-invasive ventilation; ARF: acute respiratory failure; ARDS: Acute respiratory distress syndrome; CO$_2$:carbon dioxide; mRCT: multicenter randomized controlled trial

First author	Year	No. centers	NIV application	Setting	Mask	Patients in NIV group	Patients in control group	Mortality NIV	Mortality control
Brochard L [5]	1995	5	Hypercapnic	ICU	Face	43	42	4 (hospital)	12 (hospital)
Plant PK [6]	2000	14	Hypercapnic	Ward	Face/full face/nasal	118	118	12 (hospital)	24 (hospital)
Nava S [7]	2011	3	Hypercapnic after t-piece trial failure	Ward	Full face	41	41	16 (1 year)	25 (1 year)
Ferrer M [19]	2003	3	Hypoxemic	ICU	Face/nasal	51	54	10 (90 days)	21 (90 days)
L'Her	2004	4	Hypoxemic	ED	Face	43	46	3 (48-h)	11 (48-h)
Nava S [47]	1998	3	Earlier extubation (failed T-piece trial)	ICU	Face	25	25	18 (90 days)	23 (90 days)
Ferrer M [48]	2003	2	Earlier extubation (failed T-piece trial)	ICU	Face/nasal	21	22	6 (90 days)	13 (90 days)
Collaborating Research Group For Noninvasive Mechanical Ventilation Of Chinese Respiratory Society [49]	2005	11	Earlier extubation (accelerated, in pulmonary infection)	ICU	Face	47	43	1 (hospital)	7 (hospital)
Ferrer M [50]	2009	2	Prevention of postextub. ARF (high risk)	ICU	Face	54	52	6 (hospital)	11 (hospital)
Ferrer M [58]	2006	2	Prevention of postextub. ARF (high risk)	ICU	NA	79	83	13 (hospital)	19 (hospital)
Esteban A [62]	2004	8	Postextubation ARF	ICU	Full face	114	107	28 (90 days)	15 (90 days)

2.3.1 Non-invasive Ventilation in Hypercapnic Patients

Three mRCTs evaluated NIV in the treatment of hypercapnic respiratory failure.

In the earliest one, Brochard et al. enrolled 85 patients with chronic obstructive pulmonary disease (COPD) exacerbation in five hospitals in three countries (France, Italy, and Spain). Patients were randomized to either standard oxygen therapy or NPPV (for at least 6 h/day). Hospital mortality was 29% in the control group vs 9% in the NIV group ($p = 0.02$), thanks to a lower rate of tracheal intubation in the NIV group [9].

Plant et al. conducted an mRCT in 14 UK hospitals, enrolling 236 patients with mild to moderate respiratory acidosis during COPD exacerbations. NPPV was compared to oxygen therapy. Non-invasive ventilation was applied for as long as tolerated on the first day and then progressively discontinued on day 4. In the NIV group, mortality rate was half that of the standard group (12/118 vs 24/118) [10].

More recently, Nava et al. evaluated the efficacy of NIV in patients with chronic pulmonary disease and acute hypercapnic respiratory failure aged over 75 years. These authors enrolled 82 patients in three respiratory ICUs in Italy and Switzerland. Non-invasive ventilation (as NPPV) was compared with standard treatment. Survival was significantly better in the NIV group at hospital discharge (1/41 vs 6/41 deaths) and after 6 and 12 months [11].

Several other single-center RCTs evaluated the efficacy of NIV on mortality in patients with COPD exacerbation [12–20]. Three noteworthy trials were conducted on respiratory or general wards [16, 17, 19]; one trial compared NIV to tracheal intubation in severely ill patients [20]. Two meta-analyses of these studies found a marked beneficial effect of NIV on mortality [4, 21].

State of the Art
Non-invasive ventilation is recommended as a first line intervention for exacerbation of COPD if the patient developed respiratory acidosis [3, 6, 22]. The benefit on survival was demonstrated under various conditions in mRCTs and single-center RCTs. In this setting, NPPV (instead of CPAP) should be adopted, as it supports the increased work of breathing of COPD patients.

2.3.2 Non-invasive Ventilation to Treat Acute Respiratory Failure: Hypoxemic Patients

Two mRCTs evaluated the use of NIV in hypoxemic patients.

Ferrer et al. enrolled 105 patients with severe hypoxemia ($pO2 < 60$ mmHg with Venturi mask at 50% oxygen) in three ICUs in Spain. Non-invasive ventilation (such as NPPV), applied as long as tolerated, was compared to standard oxygen therapy. Both ICU and 90-day mortality were lower in the NIV group (18% vs 39% and 19% vs 41%, respectively); the difference was prominent if pneumonia was the cause of ARF, while the presence of acute respiratory distress syndrome (ARDS) was a predictor of decreased 90-day survival. Only two patients in the standard group received NIV as rescue treatment [23].

L'Her et al. [24] evaluated hypoxemic patients due to cardiogenic pulmonary edema in four French Emergency Departments; patients in the intervention group were treated with CPAP for at least 1 h. The study was stopped after interim analysis showed that 48-h mortality was significantly lower in the intervention group; moreover, the CPAP group had less severe complications.

Hypoxemic ARF has various etiologies, whose responsiveness to NIV can markedly differ [3, 22, 25–27]. Several single-center RCTs [28–42] demonstrated that NIV significantly reduces mortality in cardiogenic pulmonary edema; accordingly, NIV is currently considered as a first-line intervention in this clinical setting [6]. The benefit has been shown for both CPAP and NPPV, and also for pre-hospital use. Non-invasive ventilation proved effective in reducing mortality also in RCTs conducted in immunocompromised patients [43] and chest trauma patients [3, 22, 44] with hypoxemic ARF. On the contrary, the advantage on survival is controversial in the case of pneumonia or ARDS, due to a high failure rate [3, 22, 45]. In this setting, some authors found NIV potentially dangerous (i.e., associated with worse survival) when applied for too long despite its failure, as it delays tracheal intubation [46]. Finally, some single-center RCTs evaluated NIV in asthma and no death was reported in any of these studies [47–49].

State of the Art
Non-invasive ventilation application in hypoxemic patients should be guided by the etiology of ARF. Non-invasive ventilation improves survival in cardiogenic pulmonary edema, chest trauma, and ARF in immunocompromised patients, especially if applied early [4, 6]. When pneumonia or ARDS are present ("de novo" ARF), NIV should be applied cautiously and in highly monitored settings. In the case of NIV failure, tracheal intubation should not be delayed [3, 22, 45]. So far, the effect of NIV on mortality in asthma is unknown and no recommendation or suggestion can be made [6].

2.3.3 Non-invasive Ventilation in the Weaning from Mechanical Ventilation

2.3.3.1 Non-invasive Ventilation in the Weaning of Hypercapnic and Mixed Patients

Multicenter Randomized Evidence
Several mRCTs with different endpoints evaluated the use of NIV for the weaning from mechanical ventilation in hypercapnic patients.

Non-invasive Ventilation in Patients after T-Piece Trial Failure
Nava et al. compared standard weaning to immediate extubation followed by NIV (as NPPV) in 50 patients from three Italian centers intubated because of COPD exacerbations; the authors enrolled only patients suitable for extubation but who

had failed a T-piece weaning trial after 48 h of intubation. Non-invasive ventilation was applied as often as was tolerated during the first 2 days in the intervention group. Mortality at 60 days was significantly higher in the standard group (7/25 vs 2/25 deaths), with four cases of fatal pneumonia (while further three cases of pneumonia were not fatal) in the standard group and no cases of pneumonia in the NIV group [50].

Ferrer et al. [51] compared extubation followed by NIV (as NPPV) to standard weaning in 43 intubated patients, from two Spanish hospitals, who failed a spontaneous breathing trial for three consecutive days. Non-invasive ventilation was applied for at least 4 h continuously. Almost half of the patients had been intubated because of COPD exacerbation. Both ICU and 90-day mortality were significantly reduced in the NIV group; nosocomial pneumonia and septic shock were significantly more common in the control group.

Non-invasive Ventilation to Shorten Standard Weaning

A collaborating research group in 11 Chinese ICUs conducted an mRCT in 90 intubated COPD patients with hypercapnic failure caused by pulmonary infection: the aim was to evaluate NIV as a tool to hasten extubation. Once the patients reached the "pulmonary infection control (PIC) window," defined by several criteria suggesting infection control, they were randomized to either standard weaning or extubation (without a preliminary weaning trial) immediately followed by NIV (such as NPPV). Mortality rate (1/47 vs 7/43) and incidence of pneumonia were significantly lower in the NIV group [52].

Non-invasive Ventilation to Prevent Post-Extubation Failure

Ferrer et al. evaluated NIV in preventing ARF after tracheal extubation. This mRCT enrolled 106 patients with chronic respiratory disorders in two Spanish hospitals: patients were randomized to either NIV (as NPPV, applied for a maximum of 24 h after extubation) or oxygen therapy after a standard weaning if they passed a T-piece weaning trial but were hypercapnic on spontaneous breathing. The trial had been preceded by a previous study from the same authors (see below) suggesting a potential benefit of NIV in this population. In the NIV group, 90-day mortality (but not hospital and ICU mortality) was significantly lower (6/54 vs 16/52); a trend towards lower incidence of pneumonia was also present (6% vs 17%, $p = 0.12$). It should be noted that 20 out of the 25 patients who developed post-extubation ARF in the control group received rescue NIV, and rescue NIV was also applied to 7 of the 8 patients developing post-extubation ARF in the NIV group [53].

State of the Art

When compared to standard weaning, NIV used in the weaning process significantly decreases mortality rates; the benefit seems to be maximal in COPD patients

[54]. Hypercapnic patients are among the most responsive to NIV in most conditions. Early extubation followed by NIV seems to be a promising strategy for hypercapnic patients even after a failed T-piece trial and could be attempted in ICUs with experienced staff [4, 6]. Little data is available about the role of NIV to facilitate weaning from mechanical ventilation in hypoxemic patients.

The routine use of NIV to prevent post-extubation ARF in unselected patients who passed a T-piece trial is still controversial.

2.3.3.2 Non-invasive Ventilation in the Weaning of Patients at Risk for Post-Extubation ARF

Ferrer et al. evaluated the use of NIV in preventing post-extubation ARF in patients at higher risk for this complication, defined by at least one of the following criteria: age >65years, cardiac failure as the cause of intubation, or increased illness severity (APACHE score >12 the day of extubation). The authors enrolled 162 patients in two Spanish hospitals. Patients were extubated after they had passed a T-piece trial and were randomized to either standard oxygen therapy or NIV (as NPPV, applied for a maximum of 24 h after extubation). Reintubation rate and ICU mortality were lower in the NIV group (2/79 vs 12/83 deaths); neither hospital mortality nor 90-day mortality were different, except for patients who were hypercapnic during spontaneous breathing by T-piece, in which both survival rates were better in the NIV group. Rescue NIV was applied to 19 out of the 27 patients who developed post-extubation ARF in the control group and in 4 out of 13 in the NIV group [55].

State of the Art

Non-invasive ventilation (as NPPV) should be considered after planned extubation in patients at high risk of post-extubation ARF [3–4, 6, 56, 57].

2.3.4 Non-invasive Ventilation to Treat Post-Extubation Respiratory Failure: Evidence of Increased Mortality

Esteban et al. conducted a multicenter trial in 37 centers in eight countries (mainly in Europe, North and South America). The authors enrolled 221 patients who were electively extubated after at least 48 h of mechanical ventilation and who developed ARF within the subsequent 48 h. Non-invasive ventilation (as NPPV, applied continuously for at least 4 h) was compared to standard therapy, which included supplemental oxygen, bronchodilators, respiratory physiotherapy, and any other indicated therapy. Rescue NIV was applied in 28 patients in the control group (three died). ICU mortality rate was higher in the NIV group (25% vs 14%). The difference appeared to be due to a different rate of death (38% in the NIV group vs 22%) among reintubated patients (whose rate was not different between the two groups);

moreover, the interval between the development of ARF and reintubation was significantly longer in the NIV group. A potential logical explanation for these results proposed by the authors was that the delay in reintubation negatively affected survival, through various mechanisms like cardiac ischemia, muscle fatigue, aspiration pneumonia, and complications of emergency reintubation. A trend towards better outcomes was observed for COPD patients treated with NIV [58].

One further single-center RCT evaluated NIV in this setting reporting data on mortality. Keenan et al. [59] compared NIV (as NPPV) with standard oxygen treatment in 81 patients, only a low percentage of whom had COPD. The authors did not find any difference in ICU and hospital survival.

State of the Art
NIV use to treat post-extubation ARF is commonly discouraged [4, 6]. At a minimum, NIV failure should be promptly recognized and intubation not delayed. Patients affected by hypercapnic disorders might be more responsive to NIV [56, 57, 60].

2.4   Three Issues To Be Considered

First, even though many mRCTs on NIV are available, some important application fields of NIV lack mRCTs in support: in particular, no mRCT so far evaluated the efficacy of NIV in one of the most promising fields, that is the prevention and treatment of postoperative ARF [57, 61, 62].

Second, the large majority of mRCTs took place in a few European countries: Italy, France, and Spain. Moreover, most evidence on this topic comes from very few highly experienced centers and authors. In other words, the generalizability of the findings of these mRCTs could be questionable, despite the fact that mRCTs are usually considered to offer the best generalizable data.

Finally, given its beneficial impact in many areas, investigation should go into why NIV is still underused and which educational and organizational interventions would be most effective in bringing NIV (safely, effectively, and containing costs) to all the patients who could benefit from it.

2.5   Conclusions

Several mRCTs showed that NIV could have a beneficial effect on survival. Non-invasive ventilation should be considered to treat ARF, mainly in hypercapnic patients and at an early stage. Non-invasive ventilation could also reduce mortality when applied in the weaning process, particularly in hypercapnic patients after a failed T-piece trial or after control of pulmonary infection. Non-invasive ventilation can improve survival when applied to patients at high risk of post-extubation respiratory failure. On the contrary, NIV could be harmful if applied to treat an established post-extubation ARF.

More research is warranted to evaluate NIV in other fields and in controversial areas; furthermore, authors should evaluate the best way to offer safe and cost-effective NIV to all those who could benefit.

Clinical summary

Intervention	Indication	Cautions	Side-effects	Way of delivery	Notes
Non-invasive ventilation	Hypercapnic respiratory failure (e.g., exacerbation of COPD) Hypoxemic respiratory failure (cardiogenic pulmonary edema, chest trauma) Accelerate weaning in hypercapnic intubated patients	NIV should be avoided in post-extubation ARF Close monitoring is needed in pneumonia, early ARDS, invasive ventilation should not be delayed Effect on asthma and to prevent post-extubation ARF is unclear	CO_2 rebreathing, noise, patient-ventilator dyssynchrony, skin lesion, discomfort, claustrophobia, failure, aspiration pneumonia, barotrauma, hypotension	Continuous positive airway pressure Non-invasive inspiratory positive pressure ventilation (usually with an expiratory airway pressure) The optimal settings have not been defined yet	mRCT to evaluate the effect of NIV in pulmonary edema and to prevent postoperative ARF are needed The possibility to generalize mRCT results out of highly specialized centers is questionable

References

1. Nava S, Hill N. Non-invasive ventilation in acute respiratory failure. Lancet. 2009;374(9685):250–9.
2. Cabrini L, Idone C, Colombo S, Monti G, Bergonzi PC, Landoni G, et al. Medical emergency team and non-invasive ventilation outside ICU for acute respiratory failure. Intensive Care Med. 2009;35(2):339–43.
3. Keenan SP, Sinuff T, Burns KE, Muscedere J, Kutsogiannis J, Mehta S, et al. Clinical practice guidelines for the use of noninvasive positive-pressure ventilation and noninvasive continuous positive airway pressure in the acute care setting. CMAJ. 2011;183(3):E195–214.
4. Cabrini L, Landoni G, Oriani A, Plumari VP, Nobile L, Greco M, Pasin L, Beretta L, Zangrillo A. Noninvasive ventilation and survival in acute care settings: a comprehensive systematic review and metaanalysis of randomized controlled trials. Crit Care Med. 2015;43(4):880–8.
5. Cabrini L, Landoni G, Bocchino S, Lembo R, Monti G, Greco M, Zambon M, Colombo S, Pasin L, Beretta L, Zangrillo A. Long-term survival rate in patients with acute respiratory failure treated with noninvasive ventilation in ordinary wards. Crit Care Med. 2016;44(12):2139–44.
6. Rochwerg B, Brochard L, Elliott MW, Hess D, Hill NS, Nava S, Navalesi P Members Of The Steering Committee, Antonelli M, Brozek J, Conti G, Ferrer M, Guntupalli K, Jaber S, Keenan S, Mancebo J, Mehta S, Raoof S Members Of The Task Force. Official ERS/ATS clinical practice guidelines: noninvasive ventilation for acute respiratory failure. Eur Respir J. 2017;50(2):pii: 1602426. https://doi.org/10.1183/13993003.02426-2016.

7. Sartini C, Lomivorotov V, Pieri M, Lopez-Delgado JC, Baiardo Redaelli M, Hajjar L, et al. A systematic review and international web-based survey of randomized controlled trials in the perioperative and critical care setting: interventions reducing mortality. J Cardiothorac Vasc Anesth. 2019;33(5):1430–9.

8. Cabrini L, Plumari VP, Nobile L, Olper L, Pasin L, Bocchino S, et al. Non-invasive ventilation in cardiac surgery: a concise review. Heart Lung Vessel. 2013;5(3):137–41.

9. Brochard L, Mancebo J, Wysocki M, Lofaso F, Conti G, Rauss A, et al. Noninvasive ventilation for acute exacerbations of chronic obstructive pulmonary disease. N Engl J Med. 1995;333(13):817–22.

10. Plant PK, Owen JL, Elliott MW. Early use of non-invasive ventilation for acute exacerbations of chronic obstructive pulmonary disease on general respiratory wards: a multicentre randomised controlled trial. Lancet. 2000;355(9219):1931–5.

11. Nava S, Grassi M, Fanfulla F, Domenighetti G, Carlucci A, Perren A, et al. Non-invasive ventilation in elderly patients with acute hypercapnic respiratory failure: a randomised controlled trial. Age Ageing. 2011;40(4):444–50.

12. Angus RM, Ahmed AA, Fenwick LJ, Peacock AJ. Comparison of the acute effects on gas exchange of nasal ventilation and doxapram in exacerbations of chronic obstructive pulmonary disease. Thorax. 1996;51(10):1048–50.

13. Barbe F, Togores B, Rubi M, Pons S, Maimo A, Agusti AG. Noninvasive ventilatory support does not facilitate recovery from acute respiratory failure in chronic obstructive pulmonary disease. Eur Respir J. 1996;9(6):1240–5.

14. Celikel T, Sungur M, Ceyhan B, Karakurt S. Comparison of noninvasive positive pressure ventilation with standard medical therapy in hypercapnic acute respiratory failure. Chest. 1998;114(6):1636–42.

15. Dhamija A, Tyagi P, Caroli R, Ur Rahman M, Vijayan VK. Noninvasive ventilation in mild to moderate cases of respiratory failure due to acute exacerbation of chronic obstructive pulmonary disease. Saudi Med J. 2005;26(5):887–90.

16. Dikensoy O, Ikidag B, Filiz A, Bayram N. Comparison of non-invasive ventilation and standard medical therapy in acute hypercapnic respiratory failure: a randomised controlled study at a tertiary health centre in SE Turkey. Int J Clin Pract. 2002;56(2):85–8.

17. Keenan SP, Powers CE, McCormack DG. Noninvasive positive-pressure ventilation in patients with milder chronic obstructive pulmonary disease exacerbations: a randomized controlled trial. Respir Care. 2005;50(5):610–6.

18. Khilnani GC, Saikia N, Banga A, Sharma SK. Non-invasive ventilation for acute exacerbation of COPD with very high PaCO(2): a randomized controlled trial. Lung India. 2010;27(3):125–30.

19. Pastaka C, Kostikas K, Karetsi E, Tsolaki V, Antoniadou I, Gourgoulianis KI. Non-invasive ventilation in chronic hypercapnic COPD patients with exacerbation and a pH of 7.35 or higher. Eur J Intern Med. 2007;18(7):524–30.

20. Conti G, Antonelli M, Navalesi P, Rocco M, Bufi M, Spadetta G, et al. Noninvasive vs. conventional mechanical ventilation in patients with chronic obstructive pulmonary disease after failure of medical treatment in the ward: a randomized trial. Intensive Care Med. 2002;28(12):1701–7.

21. Ram FS, Picot J, Lightowler J, Wedzicha JA. Non-invasive positive pressure ventilation for treatment of respiratory failure due to exacerbations of chronic obstructive pulmonary disease. Cochrane Database Syst Rev. 2004;3(3):CD004104.

22. Hess DR. Noninvasive ventilation for acute respiratory failure. Respir Care. 2013;58(6):950–72.

23. Ferrer M, Esquinas A, Leon M, Gonzalez G, Alarcon A, Torres A. Noninvasive ventilation in severe hypoxemic respiratory failure: a randomized clinical trial. Am J Respir Crit Care Med. 2003;168(12):1438–44.

24. L'Her E, Duquesne F, Girou E, de Rosiere XD, Le Conte P, Renault S, Allamy JP, Boles JM. Noninvasive continuous positive airway pressure in elderly cardiogenic pulmonary edema patients. Intensive Care Med. 2004;30(5):882–8.

25. Mehta S, Al-Hashim AH, Keenan SP. Noninvasive ventilation in patients with acute cardiogenic pulmonary edema. Respir Care. 2009;54(2):186–95. discussion 195–7

26. Weng CL, Zhao YT, Liu QH, Fu CJ, Sun F, Ma YL, et al. Meta-analysis: noninvasive ventilation in acute cardiogenic pulmonary edema. Ann Intern Med. 2010;152(9):590–600.
27. Potts JM. Noninvasive positive pressure ventilation: effect on mortality in acute cardiogenic pulmonary edema: a pragmatic meta-analysis. Pol Arch Med Wewn. 2009;119(6):349–53.
28. Park M, Lorenzi-Filho G, Feltrim MI, Viecili PR, Sangean MC, Volpe M, et al. Oxygen therapy, continuous positive airway pressure, or noninvasive bilevel positive pressure ventilation in the treatment of acute cardiogenic pulmonary edema. Arq Bras Cardiol. 2001;76(3):221–30.
29. Gray A, Goodacre S, Newby DE, Masson M, Sampson F, Nicholl J, et al. Noninvasive ventilation in acute cardiogenic pulmonary edema. N Engl J Med. 2008;359(2):142–51.
30. Kelly CA, Newby DE, McDonagh TA, Mackay TW, Barr J, Boon NA, et al. Randomised controlled trial of continuous positive airway pressure and standard oxygen therapy in acute pulmonary oedema; effects on plasma brain natriuretic peptide concentrations. Eur Heart J. 2002;23(17):1379–86.
31. Lin M, Yang YF, Chiang HT, Chang MS, Chiang BN, Cheitlin MD. Reappraisal of continuous positive airway pressure therapy in acute cardiogenic pulmonary edema. Short-term results and long-term follow-up. Chest. 1995;107(5):1379–86.
32. Levitt MA. A prospective, randomized trial of BiPAP in severe acute congestive heart failure. J Emerg Med. 2001;21(4):363–9.
33. Masip J, Betbese AJ, Paez J, Vecilla F, Canizares R, Padro J, et al. Non-invasive pressure support ventilation versus conventional oxygen therapy in acute cardiogenic pulmonary oedema: a randomised trial. Lancet. 2000;356(9248):2126–32.
34. Nava S, Carbone G, DiBattista N, Bellone A, Baiardi P, Cosentini R, et al. Noninvasive ventilation in cardiogenic pulmonary edema: a multicenter randomized trial. Am J Respir Crit Care Med. 2003;168(12):1432–7.
35. Park M, Sangean MC, Volpe Mde S, Feltrim MI, Nozawa E, Leite PF, et al. Randomized, prospective trial of oxygen, continuous positive airway pressure, and bilevel positive airway pressure by face mask in acute cardiogenic pulmonary edema. Crit Care Med. 2004;32(12):2407–15.
36. Sharon A, Shpirer I, Kaluski E, Moshkovitz Y, Milovanov O, Polak R, et al. High-dose intravenous isosorbide-dinitrate is safer and better than Bi-PAP ventilation combined with conventional treatment for severe pulmonary edema. J Am Coll Cardiol. 2000;36(3):832–7.
37. Takeda S, Takano T, Ogawa R. The effect of nasal continuous positive airway pressure on plasma endothelin-1 concentrations in patients with severe cardiogenic pulmonary edema. Anesth Analg. 1997;84(5):1091–6.
38. Schmidbauer W, Ahlers O, Spies C, Dreyer A, Mager G, Kerner T. Early prehospital use of non-invasive ventilation improves acute respiratory failure in acute exacerbation of chronic obstructive pulmonary disease. Emerg Med J. 2011;28(7):626–7.
39. Ducros L, Logeart D, Vicaut E, Henry P, Plaisance P, Collet JP, et al. CPAP for acute cardiogenic pulmonary oedema from out-of-hospital to cardiac intensive care unit: a randomised multicentre study. Intensive Care Med. 2011;37(9):1501–9.
40. Frontin P, Bounes V, Houze-Cerfon CH, Charpentier S, Houze-Cerfon V, Ducasse JL. Continuous positive airway pressure for cardiogenic pulmonary edema: a randomized study. Am J Emerg Med. 2011;29(7):775–81.
41. Weitz G, Struck J, Zonak A, Balnus S, Perras B, Dodt C. Prehospital noninvasive pressure support ventilation for acute cardiogenic pulmonary edema. Eur J Emerg Med. 2007;14(5):276–9.
42. Takeda S, Nejima J, Takano T, Nakanishi K, Takayama M, Sakamoto A, et al. Effect of nasal continuous positive airway pressure on pulmonary edema complicating acute myocardial infarction. Jpn Circ J. 1998;62(8):553–8.
43. Hilbert G, Gruson D, Vargas F, Valentino R, Gbikpi-Benissan G, Dupon M, et al. Noninvasive ventilation in immunosuppressed patients with pulmonary infiltrates, fever, and acute respiratory failure. N Engl J Med. 2001;344(7):481–7.
44. Hernandez G, Fernandez R, Lopez-Reina P, Cuena R, Pedrosa A, Ortiz R, et al. Noninvasive ventilation reduces intubation in chest trauma-related hypoxemia: a randomized clinical trial. Chest. 2010;137(1):74–80.

45. Agarwal R, Aggarwal AN, Gupta D. Role of noninvasive ventilation in acute lung injury/acute respiratory distress syndrome: a proportion meta-analysis. Respir Care. 2010;55(12):1653–60.
46. Wood KA, Lewis L, Von Harz B, Kollef MH. The use of noninvasive positive pressure ventilation in the emergency department: results of a randomized clinical trial. Chest. 1998;113(5):1339–46.
47. Gupta D, Nath A, Agarwal R, Behera D. A prospective randomized controlled trial on the efficacy of noninvasive ventilation in severe acute asthma. Respir Care. 2010;55(5):536–43.
48. Soroksky A, Stav D, Shpirer I. A pilot prospective, randomized, placebo-controlled trial of bilevel positive airway pressure in acute asthmatic attack. Chest. 2003;123(4):1018–25.
49. Soma T, Hino M, Kida K, Kudoh S. A prospective and randomized study for improvement of acute asthma by non-invasive positive pressure ventilation (NPPV). Intern Med. 2008;47(6):493–501.
50. Nava S, Ambrosino N, Clini E, Prato M, Orlando G, Vitacca M, et al. Noninvasive mechanical ventilation in the weaning of patients with respiratory failure due to chronic obstructive pulmonary disease. A randomized, controlled trial. Ann Intern Med. 1998;128(9):721–8.
51. Ferrer M, Esquinas A, Arancibia F, Bauer TT, Gonzalez G, Carrillo A, et al. Noninvasive ventilation during persistent weaning failure: a randomized controlled trial. Am J Respir Crit Care Med. 2003;168(1):70–6.
52. Collaborating Research Group for Noninvasive Mechanical Ventilation of Chinese Respiratory Society. Pulmonary infection control window in treatment of severe respiratory failure of chronic obstructive pulmonary diseases: a prospective, randomized controlled, multi-centred study. Chin Med J. 2005;118(19):1589–94.
53. Ferrer M, Sellares J, Valencia M, Carrillo A, Gonzalez G, Badia JR, et al. Non-invasive ventilation after extubation in hypercapnic patients with chronic respiratory disorders: randomised controlled trial. Lancet. 2009 Sep 26;374(9695):1082–8.
54. Burns KE, Meade MO, Premji A, Adhikari NK. Noninvasive ventilation as a weaning strategy for mechanical ventilation in adults with respiratory failure: a Cochrane systematic review. CMAJ. 2014;186(3):E112–22.
55. Ferrer M, Valencia M, Nicolas JM, Bernadich O, Badia JR, Torres A. Early noninvasive ventilation averts extubation failure in patients at risk: a randomized trial. Am J Respir Crit Care Med. 2006;173(2):164–70.
56. Hess DR. The role of noninvasive ventilation in the ventilator discontinuation process. Respir Care. 2012;57(10):1619–25.
57. Glossop AJ, Shephard N, Bryden DC, Mills GH. Non-invasive ventilation for weaning, avoiding reintubation after extubation and in the postoperative period: a meta-analysis. Br J Anaesth. 2012;109(3):305–14.
58. Esteban A, Frutos-Vivar F, Ferguson ND, Arabi Y, Apezteguia C, Gonzalez M, et al. Noninvasive positive-pressure ventilation for respiratory failure after extubation. N Engl J Med. 2004;350(24):2452–60.
59. Keenan SP, Powers C, McCormack DG, Block G. Noninvasive positive-pressure ventilation for postextubation respiratory distress: a randomized controlled trial. JAMA. 2002;287(24):3238–44.
60. Agarwal R, Aggarwal AN, Gupta D, Jindal SK. Role of noninvasive positive-pressure ventilation in postextubation respiratory failure: a meta-analysis. Respir Care. 2007;52(11):1472–9.
61. Landoni G, Rodseth RN, Santini F, Ponschab M, Ruggeri L, Szekely A, et al. Randomized evidence for reduction of perioperative mortality. J Cardiothorac Vasc Anesth. 2012;26(5):764–72.
62. Cabrini L, Nobile L, Plumari VP, Landoni G, Borghi G, Mucchetti M, et al. Intraoperative prophylactic and therapeutic non-invasive ventilation: a systematic review. Br J Anaesth. 2014;112(4):638–47.

High-Flow Nasal Cannulae

3

Carolina Soledad Romero Garcia, Esther Romero,
and Joaquín Moreno

Contents

3.1 General Principles

Acute respiratory failure is one of the common causes of admission to the intensive care units (ICUs), both as a primary cause and as a complication during the hospital stay [1, 2]. Traditionally, patients with respiratory failure have been treated with three different strategies depending on the severity of the pathology: conventional oxygen therapy (COT), non-invasive ventilation options (NIV), and mechanical ventilation (MV).

C. S. Romero Garcia (✉)
Critical Care and Anesthesia Department, Hospital General Universitario, Universidad Europea de Valencia, Valencia, Spain
e-mail: romero_carolinasol@gva.es

E. Romero
Critical Care and Anesthesia Department, Hospital Clínico Universitario, Valencia, Spain

J. Moreno
Critical Care and Anesthesia Department, Hospital General Universitario, Valencia, Spain

© Springer Nature Switzerland AG 2021
G. Landoni et al. (eds.), *Reducing Mortality in Critically Ill Patients*,
https://doi.org/10.1007/978-3-030-71917-3_3

The high-flow nasal cannulae therapy (HFNC) was first intended for use in neonates. They were originally manufactured with the aim of maintaining the benefit of high oxygen flows (and therefore, the increase in end-expiratory pulmonary pressures) without interfering with the blood flow to skin areas vulnerable to pressure sore. Over the last decade, HFNC have also been extended to the adult population. The possibility that one may provide non-invasive ventilation with less discomfort and easier clearance of airway secretions is conceptually appealing [2–4].

Nowadays, the success and broad utilisation of HFNC is in consonance to its relative simplicity of use, the better patient comfort, and the advantages shown versus classical oxygen therapy in some cases [5]. Still, there is much debate regarding the role of the HFNC, and recently, high-quality studies have been published on this topic, mainly in the management of critically ill patients.

3.2   Pathophysiological Principles

HFNC administer high flows (10–60 L/min) of a mixture of humidified air and oxygen via wide-bore nasal cannulae specially designed. There are only two parameters than can be adjusted on the device: the fraction of inspired oxygen and the gas flow rate. The fraction of inspired oxygen ranges between 0.21 and 1, and the gas flow rate that can be administered between 10 and 60 L/min.

The benefits of high-flow nasal oxygen (HFNO) are described below:

1. Constant oxygen flow regardless of changes in respiratory dynamics [6].

   Measured FiO_2 in different breathing situations is stable when the gas flow administered is greater than 40 L/min. This flow could be up to 60 L/min to assure a constant high FiO_2 but it is usually more difficult to achieve with this device.

2. Generation of a Positive End-expiratory pressure (PEEP) [7].

   High flows administered through HFNC can generate a PEEP of 4–5 cm H_2O in the nasopharynx. Although this pressure is comparatively low, it could theoretically suffice to avoid alveolar closure. The main concern is whether a patient can constantly keep this pressure when the mouth is open, that is, with a leak in the system. The presence of a permanent leak is detrimental but could be overpassed with higher flow rates.

3. Reduction in the anatomical dead space [4, 8].

   An increase in the flow rate administered by the HFNC wash the expired volume of carbon dioxide (CO_2) from the airway, and it will be replaced with oxygen-enriched gas. Once more, if the patient opens the mouth creating a leak in the circuit, it will alter the CO_2 washout, even though the effect remains unclear.

4. Decreased work of breathing [6].

   The tracheal insufflation originated during the inspiratory pause via the HFNC concedes an improvement in the tidal volume. It reduces the resistance in the superior airway and increases the end-expiratory lung impedance. All these circumstances combined allow a reduction in the respiratory rate.

5. Improved mucociliary clearance [8, 9].

The humidified gas is delivered generally at 37 °C avoiding upper airway dryness and prevents an excessive accumulation of respiratory secretions. The heated flow improves the cilia function and helps coughing.

The disadvantages and limitations of HFNO are not numerous when applied in the correct setting. The first one could be the potential toxicity due to the high FiO_2 used [5]. In addition, the delay in intubation that occurs after the improvement in respiratory mechanics and the arterial gasometry parameters could mask an acute respiratory failure. The delay in diagnosing conditions requiring mechanical ventilation might increase morbidity, mortality, and hospital costs [3].

Contrary to NIV, HFNC settings do not incorporate inspiratory positive airway pressure (IPAP) and expiratory positive airway pressure (EPAP). Other missing parameters when using HFNC are the backup respiratory rate and the backup inspiratory time. Data of respiratory therapy is also not available when using this device. HFNC should not be administered as an alternative in pathologies where NIV has strong indications such as respiratory failure due to chronic obstructive pulmonary disease (COPD) exacerbation and cardiogenic pulmonary oedema [3].

3.3 Main Evidence and Clinical Use

HFNC offer some immediate physiological benefits in patients requiring respiratory support [2, 7, 10]. It remains to be determined whether HFNC provide any clinically important advantage and improvement in patient outcomes, such as by preventing the need for invasive mechanical ventilation and by mortality rate reduction.

Most randomised controlled trials (RCT) conducted in the last 15 years showed significantly amelioration in symptoms like dyspnoea, improved oxygenation, and reduced the usage of NIV in patients with mild hypoxemia [11–13] and respiratory failure. In the FLORALI trial [14], HFNC demonstrated lower intubation rates and overall mortality in patients with acute respiratory failure with $PaO_2/FiO_2 < 200$ mmHg when compared to COT and NIV.

Hypercapnic failure represents another indication of HFNC therapy. Some recent RCTs have suggested that at a gas flow of 30 L/min for a brief duration of time, the inspiratory pressure decreases in comparison to 10 and 20 L/min flow rate [11, 15]. HFNC have shown similar effects than NIV delivered at discreet levels of pressure support in hypercapnic COPD associated with mild to moderate exacerbation.

In the post-extubation setting, most RCTs describe a potential benefit of HFNC, not only in terms of mortality but also lowering treatment failure rates in patients at high risk of reintubation compared to COT. Hernández et al. [16] studied post-extubation respiratory failure after HFNC or NIV in high-risk patients. The results suggested that HFNC were not inferior to NIV avoiding reintubation and post-extubation respiratory failure. In this study, the outcome time to reintubation was similar in both groups, probably because NIV and HFNC were switched to COT after 32 h. The group receiving HFNC in the following 32 h after extubation presented an augmentation in the reintubation rate. Besides, a significant decrease in the risk of reintubation compared with HFNO alone was evidenced in patients with low-risk of intubation [12]. The use of HFNC compared with COT has also reduced the risk of reintubation within 72 h [17].

There are some systematic reviews and meta-analysis [18–25] that have assessed the use of HFNC compared to COT or NIV. Most of the evidence is focus on the hypoxemic respiratory failure in different areas like the ICUs, wards and in the emergency departments (EDs). Nevertheless, an important amount of heterogeneity is evident between different populations amongst studies, making the analysis of the true effect uncertain. Evidence regarding this issue might change the estimate of the effect described previously.

3.4   Therapeutic Use

One of the most important clinical goals in the ICU is minimising the duration of invasive mechanical ventilation by allowing the rapid safe extubation [1–3, 5]. Prolonged intubation increases the risk of ventilator-induced lung injury, ventilator-induced diaphragmatic dysfunction, infections, and myopathy [26].

Main indications of HFNC are:

1. Acute respiratory distress syndrome (ARDS) and acute hypoxemic respiratory failure.

   ARDS and hypoxemic failure are a common indication of HFNC and might increase post-extubation success [2–6]. It has been described previously the benefit [7, 12–14] of HFNC compared with COT to avoid the need of reintubation. HFNC are also indicated in low to moderate respiratory failure [11]. An inappropriate use and prescription will inevitably result in deleterious treatment leading to increased morbidity and mortality.

2. Post-extubation failure [11].

   Regardless of a successful extubation, in the 15–30% of cases, patients develop acute respiratory distress and require reintroduction of invasive mechanical ventilation during the first 48 h. In the post-extubation period, it is absolutely crucial to prevent and identify early clinical deterioration. This will restrain the development of respiratory failure and will decrease the morbimortality rates.

3. Other uses of HFNC

   Hypoxemia caused by severe heart failure.

   In congestive heart failure (CHF) patients might benefit from HFNC by reducing the preload though these results are inconclusive and need further analysis (Fig. 3.1) [27].

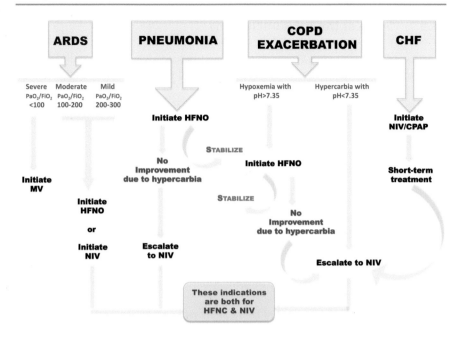

Fig. 3.1 Suggested therapeutic algorithm. Abbreviations: ARDS: acute respiratory distress syndrome; COPD: chronic obstructive pulmonary disease; CHF: congestive heart failure; MV: mechanical ventilation; NIV: non-invasive ventilation; CPAP: continues positive airway pressure; HFNC: high-flow nasal cannulae; HFNO: high-flow nasal oxygen

Airway Instrumentation Management Preoxygenation is a key component of tracheal intubation technique in order to store oxygen to increase the functional residual capacity (FRC) volume. This represents the main oxygen reservoir prolonging the duration of apnoea, until hypoxemia occurs, during the induction of general anaesthesia. In critically ill patients, an adequate preoxygenation could be compromised in several pathological conditions. Preoxygenation with the standard bag-valve mask might be difficult to perform in these patients so HFNC might be a reasonable and a beneficial alternative. Guitton et al. [28] have compared the preoxygenation desaturation in rapid sequence intubation manoeuvres with HFNC finding no differences between groups and obtaining similar results that Frat et al. [14].

Immunocompromised Patients This frailty population has morbimortality that would potentially be as high as 70% when intubation is required [29]. Although there is an important heterogeneity amongst different studies that do not include all the immunocompromised patients, HFNC represent some benefits and it is a well-tolerated therapy [30] with better outcomes in terms of morbidity and mortality.

Care at the End of Life In the particular case of patients with do-not-intubation or do-not-resuscitate orders, HFNC may be beneficial. HFNC improve not only patient's dyspnoea but also reduce costs when comparing this treatment with conventional therapies [31].

3.5   State of the Art/Conclusions

The use of HFNC in critical care units has been extended due to the feasibility of the system, the easy to implement monitorisation, and the patient's good tolerance and comfort.

Other clinical settings to treat patients with HFNC therapy are being investigated. Clinical data is scarce, but they might have a promising role in different conditions.

HFNC seem more effective than COT and non-inferior to NIV in most studies, and they should be considered as part of the therapeutic arsenal available to treat mild hypercapnic conditions or hypoxemic respiratory failure disease.

Other indications of HFNC that have demonstrated a reduction in mortality are in the post-extubation failure and in the congestive heart failure.

HFNC could delay desaturation and potentially reduce morbidity although it has not yet been proved in medical techniques that require airway instrumentation.

Special populations like immunocompromised patients with acute respiratory failure may benefit from HFNC treatment with lower mortality rates compared with standard care.

The inappropriate indication of HFNC may induce a delay in intubation that will increase the morbimortality by masking clinical deterioration.

References

1. Telias I, Fergusson D. Added benefit of noninvasive ventilation to high-flow nasal oxygen to prevent reintubation in higher-risk patients. JAMA. 2019;322(15):1455–7.
2. Nishimura M. High-flow nasal cannula oxygen therapy in adults: physiological benefits, indication, clinical benefits, and adverse effects. Respir Care. 2016;61(4):529–41.
3. Helviz, Einav. A systematic review of the high-flow nasal cannula for adult patients. Crit Care. 2018;22:71.
4. Vella MA, Pascual-Lopez J, Kaplan LJ. High-flow nasal cannula system not just another nasal cannula. JAMA Surg. 2018;153(9):854–5.
5. Rochwerg B, Brochard L, Elliott MW, Hess D, Hill NS, Nava S, et al. Official ERS/ATS clinical practice guidelines: non-invasive ventilation for acute respiratory failure. Eur Respir J. 2017;50(2):1602426.
6. Chikata Y, Onodera M, Oto J, Nishimura M. FIO2 in an adult model simulating high-flow nasal cannula therapy. Respir Care. 2016;62(2):193–8.
7. Mauri T, Turrini C, Eronia N, Grasselli G, Volta CA, Bellani G, Pesenti A. Physiologic effects of high-flow nasal cannula in acute hypoxemic respiratory failure. AJRCCM. 2016;195(9):1207–15.
8. Onodera Y, Akimoto R, Suzuki H, Okada M, Nakane M, Kawamae K. A high-flow nasal cannula system set at relatively low flow effectively washes out CO2 from the anatomical dead space of a respiratory system. Intensive Care Med Exp. 2018;6(1):7.
9. Parke R, McGuinness S, Eccleston M. Nasal high-flow therapy delivers low level positive airway pressure. Br J Anaesth. 2009;103(6):886–90.
10. Möller W, Feng S, Domanski U, Franke KJ, Celik G, Bartenstein P, Becker S, Meyer G, Schmid O, Eickelberg O, Tatkov S, Nilius G. Nasal high flow reduces dead space. Appl Physiol. 2017;122(1):191–7.

11. Fernandez R, Subira C, Frutos-Vivar F, Rialp G, Laborda C, Masclans JR, Lesmes A, Panadero L, Hernandez G. High-flow nasal cannula to prevent postextubation respiratory failure in high-risk on-hypercapnic patients: a randomised multicenter trial. Intensive Care. 2017;7:47.

12. Hernandez G, Vaquero C, Gonzalez P, Subira C, Frutos-Vivar F, Rialp G, et al. Effect of post extubation high-flow nasal cannula vs conventional oxygen therapy on reintubation in low-risk patients. JAMA. 2016;315(13):1354–61.

13. Sun J, et al. High flow nasal cannula oxygen therapy versus non-invasive ventilation for chronic obstructive pulmonary disease with acute-moderate hypercapnic respiratory failure: an observational cohort study. Int J Chron Obstruct Pulmon Dis. 2019;14:1229–37.

14. Frat JP, Thille AW, Mercat A, et al. High-flow oxygen through nasal cannula in acute hypoxemic respiratory failure. N Engl J Med. 2015;372:2185–96.

15. Rittayamai, et al. Effects of high-flow nasal cannula and non-invasive ventilation on inspiratory effort in hypercapnic patients with chronic obstructive pulmonary disease: a preliminary study. Ann Intensive Care. 2019;9:122.

16. Hernandez G, Vaquero C, Colinas L, Cuena R, Gonzalez P, Canabal A, et al. Effect of post extubation high-flow nasal cannula vs non invasive ventilation on reintubation and post extubation respiratory failure in high-risk patients. JAMA. 2017;316(19):2047–8.

17. Thille A, Muller G, Gacouin A, Coudroy R, Decavele M, Sonneville R, et al. Effect of post extubation high-flow nasal oxygen with non invasive ventilation vs high-flow nasal oxygen alone on reintubation among patients at high risk of extubation failure. JAMA. 2019;322(15):1465–75.

18. Monro-Somerville T, Sim M, Ruddy J, Vilas M, Gillies MA. The effect of high-flow nasal cannula oxygen therapy on mortality and intubation rate in acute respiratory failure: a systematic review and meta-analysis. Crit Care Med. 2017;45(4):e449–56.

19. Doshi P, Whittle JS, Bublewicz M, et al. Insufflation in the treatment of respiratory failure: a randomised clinical trial. Ann Emerg Med. 2017;72(1):73–83.e5.

20. Zhu Y, Yin H, Zhang R, Wei J. High-flow nasal cannula oxygen therapy versus conventional oxygen therapy in patients with acute respiratory failure: a systematic review and meta-analysis of randomised controlled trials. BMC Pulm Med. 2017;17:201.

21. Rochwerg, et al. High flow nasal cannula compared with conventional oxygen therapy for acute hypoxemic respiratory failure: a systematic review and meta-analysis. Intensive Care Med. 2019;45(5):563–72.

22. Leeies M, Flynn E, Turgeon AF, et al. High-flow oxygen via nasal cannulae in patients with acute hypoxemic respiratory failure: a systematic review and meta-analysis. Syst Rev. 2017;6:202.

23. Ou X, Hua Y, Liu J, Gong C, Zhao W. Effect of high-flow nasal cannula oxygen therapy in adults with acute hypoxemic respiratory failure: a meta-analysis of randomised controlled trials. CMAJ. 2017;189:E260–7.

24. Tinelli V, Cabrini L, Fominskiy E, Franchini S, Ferrante L, Ball L, Pelosi P, Landoni G, Zangrillo A, Secchi A. High flow nasal cannula oxygen vs. conventional oxygen therapy and noninvasive ventilation in emergency department patients: a systematic review and meta-analysis. J Emerg Med. 2019;57(3):322–8.

25. Bocchile RLR, Cazati DC, Timenetsky KT, SerpaNeto A. The effects of high-flow nasal cannula on intubation and re-intubation in critically ill patients: a systematic review, meta-analysis and trial sequential analysis. Efeitos do uso de cateter nasal de alto fluxo na intubação e na reintubação de pacientes críticos: revisão sistemática, metanálise e análise de sequência de ensaios. Rev Bras Ter Intensiva. 2018;30(4):487–95.

26. Petezuno T, Fan E. 2016 year in review: mechanical ventilation. Respir Care. 2017;62(5):629–35.

27. Doshi P, Whittle JS, Bublewicz M, Kearney J, Ashe T, Graham R, et al. High-velocity nasal insufflation in the treatment of respiratory failure: a randomised clinical trial. Annals Emerg Med. 2018;72(1):73–83.e5.

28. Guitton C, Ehrmann S, Volteau C, Colin G, Maamar A, Jean-Michel V, Mahe PJ, Landais M, Brule N, Bretonnière C, Zambon O, Vourc'h M. Nasal high-flow preoxygenation for endotra-

cheal intubation in the critically ill patient: a randomised clinical trial. Intensive Care Med. 2019;45(4):447–58.

29. Coudry R, Frat J, Ehrmann S, The REVA Network, et al. High-flow nasal oxygen therapy alone or with non-invasive ventilation in immunocompromised patients admitted to ICU for acute hypoxemic respiratory failure: the randomised multicentre controlled FLORALI-IM protocol. BMJ Open. 2019;9(8):e029798.

30. Lemaile V, et al. High-flow nasal cannula oxygenation in immunocompromised patients with acute hypoxemic respiratory failure: a groupe de recherche respiratoireenréanimation onco-hématologique study. Crit Care Med. 2017;45(3):e274–80.

31. Mittal A, Mazjoub A, Gajic O, Murad H, Wilson M. Palliative high-flow nasal cannula in acute respiratory failure: systematic review and meta-analysis. Crit Care Med. 2018;46(1):530.

Restrictive Inspiratory Oxygen Fraction

4

Antonio Pisano, Maria Venditto, and Luigi Verniero

Contents

4.1 General Principles

Administration of supplemental oxygen is a very common practice in critically ill patients and during surgery. In particular, in both the intensive care unit (ICU) and the perioperative settings, patients needing tracheal intubation and mechanical ventilation are often exposed to high inspiratory oxygen fractions (FiO_2) and, consequently, to supranormal levels of arterial oxygen partial pressure (PaO_2) [1–6]. In the last few years, according to the well-known toxicity of oxygen [5–9] and to the findings of two randomized controlled trials (RCTs) which reported a lower ICU mortality with a "conservative" FiO_2 approach in critically ill patients [10] and an increased long-term mortality in surgical patients receiving high intraoperative FiO_2 [11], respectively, limiting FiO_2 in mechanically ventilated patients has been suggested as a possible strategy to reduce mortality in both the ICU and the surgical settings [12, 13]. However, just 6 years ago the first book of the series "Reducing mortality in..." (which also includes the present updated book) included a chapter

A. Pisano (✉) · M. Venditto · L. Verniero
Cardiac Anesthesia and Intensive Care Unit, A.O.R.N. "Dei Colli", Monaldi Hospital, Naples, Italy
e-mail: antonio.pisano@ospedalideicolli.it; maria.venditto@live.it

© Springer Nature Switzerland AG 2021
G. Landoni et al. (eds.), *Reducing Mortality in Critically Ill Patients*,
https://doi.org/10.1007/978-3-030-71917-3_4

discussing, although with some skepticism and only based on meta-analytic data, an opposite (i.e., favorable) role of perioperative supplemental oxygen on survival, possibly due to a reduction in surgical site infection (SSI) rates [7, 14]. Moreover, the favorable effect of a conservative FiO_2 strategy on survival in mechanically ventilated ICU patients was not confirmed by a recent large multicenter RCT [15], while an even more recent relatively large RCT did not find neither beneficial effects (on SSI rate) nor harmful pulmonary or cardiac complications with high perioperative FiO_2 in patients undergoing abdominal surgery [16]. Finally, several meta-analyses published between 2018 and 2020 compared the use of "low" vs. "high" FiO_2 in both surgical and ICU patients, without providing overall robust evidence in neither direction [6, 17–19]. In the next sections, we discuss the key features and findings of the abovementioned investigations, the possible mechanisms of the association between FiO_2 and mortality, and to what extent all this may be currently translated into clinical practice.

4.2   Main Evidences

In the recently updated international "democracy-based" consensus conference aimed at identifying all nonsurgical strategies which have been shown by sufficiently strong randomized evidence (see Chap. 1) to affect mortality in the perioperative and critical care setting [12, 20], restrictive FiO_2 was included among interventions reducing mortality according to the findings of two RCTs published in 2016 [10] and 2012 [11], respectively.

The oxygen-ICU trial [10] included 434 patients with an ICU length of stay (LOS) of at least 72 h randomized to either a conservative group, in which FiO_2 was set to maintain PaO_2 between 70 and 100 mmHg (with an arterial oxygen saturation [SaO_2] of 94–98%), or a conventional group in which a PaO_2 of up to 150 mmHg (with an SaO_2 of 97–100%) was allowed. The primary outcome (ICU mortality) was significantly lower in the conservative group as compared with the conventional group (11.6 vs 20.2%, relative risk [RR] 0.57, 95% confidence interval [CI] 0.37–0.90; $p = 0.01$). Patients in the conservative group had a significantly lower incidence of shock (3.7 vs 10.6%, RR 0.35, 95% CI 0.16–0.75; $p = 0.006$), liver failure (1.9 vs 6.4%, RR 0.29, 95% CI 0.10–0.82; $p = 0.02$), and bloodstream infection (5.1 vs 10.1%, RR 0.50, 95% CI 0.25–0.998; $p = 0.049$). Moreover, median mechanical ventilation-free hours were 72 (interquartile range [IQR] 35–110) in the conservative group and 48 (IQR 24–96) in the conventional group (median difference 24 h, IQR 0–46; $p = 0.02$). No statistically significant differences in other secondary outcomes (including respiratory failure, renal failure, new infections, surgical revision, and ICU and hospital LOS) were found.

The PROXI trial, one of the largest RCTs investigating the impact of high perioperative FiO_2 on the incidence of SSI, failed to show any difference in SSI rate among 1400 patients randomized to receive either 80 or 30% oxygen during and for 2 h after elective or emergency laparotomy [21]. Moreover, a post hoc analysis including 1382 out of the 1400 original patients found a significantly increased mortality after a median follow-up of 2.3 years (range 1.3–3.4 years) in patients receiving 80% oxygen as compared with those receiving 30% oxygen (23.2 vs 18.3%, hazards ratio [HR] 1.3, 95% CI 1.03–1.64; $p = 0.03$) [11]. Of note, a statistically significant difference between the two groups in long-term mortality was found among patients undergoing cancer surgery but not among non-cancer patients.

The recent "Improving Oxygen Therapy in Acute-illness" (IOTA) meta-analysis [6], which included data from the oxygen-ICU trial [10] (but not from the PROXI trial [11, 21]), investigated the impact of conservative as compared with liberal oxygen therapy on morbidity and mortality in different settings of acute illness (including sepsis, stroke, trauma, myocardial infarction, cardiac arrest, ICU, and emergency surgery) and found that liberal oxygen therapy leading to SaO_2 values above 94–96% was associated with significantly higher in-hospital, 30-day, and long-term mortality (see Table 4.1). Although these findings seem to confirm the potential benefits of a restrictive FiO_2 strategy in acutely ill patients, subsequent investigations involving only ICU patients have yielded conflicting results. In particular, the lately published ICU-ROX trial [15] included 965 mechanically ventilated patients from 21 ICUs randomized to either a conservative oxygen therapy ($SaO_2 < 97\%$ with FiO_2 gradually decreased up to 0.21 if SaO_2 was above the acceptable lower limit, usually 90%) or a conventional oxygen therapy (any SaO_2 above the acceptable lower limit, usually $FiO_2 \geq 0.3$). The authors found no significant differences in either the primary endpoint (number of ventilator-free days by day 28) or any of the key secondary endpoints: among the latter, 90-day mortality was 34.7% in the conservative group vs 32.5% in the conventional group (unadjusted odds ratio [OR] 1.1, 95% CI 0.84–1.44), while 180-day mortality was 35.7% in the conservative group vs 34.5% in the conventional group (unadjusted OR 1.05, 95% CI 0.81–1.37). Consistently, according to a Cochrane systematic review published in 2019 (and not including the large ICU-ROX trial), there is very high uncertainty about the evidence of an impact of higher versus lower FiO_2 on mortality, major complications, and lung injury among ICU patients [18] (see Table 4.1).

As mentioned, newest meta-analyses of RCTs comparing perioperative administration of 80% vs either 30 or 30–35% oxygen in adult surgical patients also yielded conflicting results (both among themselves and as compared with the PROXI trial and its follow-up [11, 21]): as detailed in Table 4.1, in fact, Smith et al. [19] found no difference in the rate of SSI or mortality, while de Jonge et al. [17] found a reduction in SSI rates only in patients undergoing general anesthesia with tracheal intubation. Finally, in a subsequent multicenter RCT, Ferrando et al. [16] randomized 740 patients undergoing abdominal surgery to a FiO_2 of either 0.8 or 0.3 intraoperatively and for the first 3 postoperative hours and found no difference in the SSI rate during the first postoperative week (RR 0.94, 95% CI 0.59–1.50; $p = 0.9$) or in any of the secondary composite endpoints, including (among others) adverse events and 6-month mortality.

4.3 Pathophysiological Principles: Possible Mechanisms of Reduced Mortality

Exposure to high oxygen concentrations has been shown to have several possible adverse effects (listed in Table 4.2) [6–8, 18, 22, 23] which may theoretically lead (or contribute) to increased mortality in surgical or critically ill patients. For

Table 4.1 Main features and findings of recent meta-analyses comparing lower versus higher inspiratory oxygen fractions in the perioperative and acute/critical illness settings

First author, year of publication	Setting	No of patients (RCTs)	Comparators	Main findings
Chu, 2018 [6]	Acutely ill adults (sepsis, stroke, trauma, MI, cardiac arrest, ICU, emergency surgery)	16,037 (25 RCTs)	Conservative oxygen therapy (median FiO_2 0.21, IQR 0.21–0.25) vs Liberal oxygen therapy (median FiO_2 0.52, IQR 0.39–0.85)	Increased mortality in the liberal oxygen therapy group: • In-hospital (RR 1.21, 95% CI 1.03–1.43, $I^2 = 0\%$, high quality) • 30-day (RR 1.14, 95% CI 1.01–1.29, $I^2 = 0\%$, high quality) • At the longest follow-up (RR 1.10, 95% CI 1.0–1.2, $I^2 = 0\%$, high quality) No significant differences in disability at longest follow-up, risk of hospital-acquired pneumonia, any hospital-acquired infection, and hospital LOS
Barbateskovic, 2019 [18]	ICU	1285 (7 RCTs)	Lower vs higher FiO_2 (or PaO_2 targets)	In the higher $FiO_2(PaO_2)$ group: • Increased mortality at the time point closest to 3 months (RR 1.18, 95% CI 1.01–1.37, $I^2 = 0\%$, very low-certainty evidence) • Increased risk of serious adverse events at the time point closest to 3 months (RR 1.13, 95% CI 1.04–1.23, $I^2 = 0\%$, very low-certainty evidence) No difference between groups in lung injury at the time point closest to 3 months (RR 1.03, 95% CI 0.78–1.36; $I^2 = 0\%$; very low-certainty evidence)

Table 4.1 (continued)

First author, year of publication	Setting	No of patients (RCTs)	Comparators	Main findings
de Jonge, 2019 [17]	Surgical patients	7817 (17 RCTs)	0.8 vs 0.3–0.35 FiO_2	No difference between groups in SSI rate (RR0.89, 95% CI0.73–1.07; $I^2 = 45.4\%$) No difference between groups in SSI rate among non-intubated patients (RR 1.2, 95% CI 0.91–1.58) Reduced SSI rate in the 0.8 FiO_2 group among intubated patients (RR 0.8, 95% CI 0.64–0.99)
Smith, 2020 [19]	Adult surgical patients	10,212 (12 RCTs)	0.8 vs 0.3 FiO_2	No statistically significant differences between groups in: • Mortality up to 30 days (RR 1.12, 95% CI 0.56–2.22, $p = 0.76$) • SSI rate at 15 days (RR 1.41, 95% CI 1.0–2.01, $p = 0.05$) • SSI rate at the longest follow-up (RR 1.23, 95% CI 1.0–1.51, $p = 0.05$)

RCT Randomized controlled trial, *MI* Myocardial infarction, *ICU* Intensive care unit, *FiO_2* Inspiratory oxygen fraction, *IQR* Interquartile range, *RR* Relative risk, *I^2* Heterogeneity, *LOS* Length of stay, *PaO_2* Arterial oxygen partial pressure, *SSI* Surgical site infection

Table 4.2 Possible adverse effects of hyperoxia

Reduced vital capacity (mainly due to absorption atelectasis)
Impaired ventilation/perfusion ratio
Increased alveolar-capillary permeability
Enhanced pulmonary and airway inflammation
Acute lung injury and pulmonary fibrosis
Increased ROS formation (possibly leading to cell apoptosis and tissue/DNA damage)
Systemic and coronary vasoconstriction
Reduced coronary blood flow and cardiac output
Central nervous system toxicity (e.g., seizures)
Cerebral vasoconstriction
Enhanced cancer recurrence/dissemination?

ROS Reactive Oxygen Species

example, administration of high FiO_2 during general anesthesia promotes atelectasis formation (primarily because oxygen is absorbed much faster than nitrogen in lungs due to the high alveolar-capillary gradient) and may accordingly increase the risk of pneumonia and other postoperative pulmonary complications [8, 23]. Moreover, hyperoxic coronary and systemic vasoconstriction, as well as the oxidative stress due to increased formation of reactive oxygen species (ROS), may worsen myocardial injury in patients with myocardial ischemia/infarction [7, 8]. Enhancement of oxidative stress and inflammation leading to clinical deterioration and increased mortality has also been found in patients with chronic obstructive pulmonary disease (COPD) receiving high-flow oxygen [7]. Finally, oxygen promotes neovascularization [7] which, together with ROS overproduction, has been involved in cancer progression [8] and might explain (at least in part) the findings of the PROXI trial showing an increased long-term mortality with higher FiO_2 only among cancer patients [11]. However, there is no doubt that hypoxia is a rather frequent occurrence and is also harmful in these clinical settings. In addition, the role of perioperative supplemental oxygen in preventing SSI (and associated mortality) has a plausible rationale which is based in part on the same effects of oxygen which may lead (or contribute) to serious complications and increased mortality: in fact, through increased ROS production, supplemental oxygen may promote oxidative killing of bacteria by neutrophils; moreover, hyperoxia promotes tissue healing (also enhancing neovascularization) and may activate immune response [7]. Of note, oxygen seems to play an ambivalent (and conflicting) role also in cancer patients since tumor hypoxia has been associated to treatment failure [24].

4.4   Implications for Clinical Practice

The clinical relevance of the above discussed effects of oxygen is not clear: for example, in addition to fail to show any difference in SSI rates, relatively large RCTs such as the PROXI trial [21] and the latest investigation by Ferrando et al. [16] found no difference in the incidence of atelectasis among patients randomized to a perioperative FiO_2 of either 0.3 or 0.8. It is possible that beneficial or detrimental effects of either a restrictive or liberal FiO_2 strategy may prevail according to the clinical context (e.g., type and severity of patient illness and comorbidities), so that different subgroups of patients may have different susceptibility to the effects of hyperoxia and, accordingly, some subgroups of patients may benefit, in terms of survival, from a restrictive FiO_2 strategy while others may not. A recent meta-analysis showed that acute hyperoxia significantly reduced cardiac output (CO) in healthy volunteers and in patients with either coronary artery disease (CAD) or heart failure (HF) but not in patients with sepsis or in those undergoing coronary artery bypass graft (CABG) surgery, while the increase in systemic vascular resistances was substantial in HF patients, less pronounced in healthy volunteers and in CAD and CABG patients, and negligible in septic patients [22]. Consistently, a post hoc analysis of the ICU-ROX trial lately suggested a possible increase in mortality with a conservative oxygen strategy in patients with sepsis although with the limitations of an unplanned analysis which was underpowered for this purpose [25]. Moreover, "restrictive" vs "liberal" FiO_2 is only apparently a dichotomous choice, which conversely comprises a continuous wide range of possible settings which should take into account the individual patient: "high FiO_2" may not necessarily mean deliberate hyperoxia but maybe prevention of inadvertent hypoxia [7, 14], while a conservative FiO_2 approach may imply avoidance of useless (and potentially harmful) hyperoxia but can also increase the risk of hypoxemia [26]. A thorough discussion about the complexity (and current uncertainty) of the relationship between FiO_2 and mortality in the ICU setting can be found in an editorial by Young and Bellomo [26]. In the light of latest available evidence and waiting for new possible insights from ongoing investigations [27, 28], both the 2016 WHO guidelines (which, rather surprisingly, only on the basis of a meta-analysis recommend a FiO_2 of 0.8 intraoperatively and for the 2–6 immediate postoperatively hours in *all* surgical patients undergoing general anesthesia with tracheal intubation [17]) and, at the opposite, the growing enthusiasm for a restrictive oxygen therapy approach in *any* acute and critical illness setting should be regarded with caution. Avoiding useless hyperoxia while adopting adequate monitoring to prevent harms from hypoxia, as suggested by Young and Bellomo [26], is probably the wisest strategy in both the ICU and perioperative settings.

Clinical summary

Drug/technique	Setting	Cautions	Dose	Notes
Restrictive inspiratory oxygen fraction (FiO_2)	Surgical patients Mechanically ventilated intensive care unit (ICU) patients Acute illness	Inadvertent hypoxia Possibly harmful in some subgroups of patients (sepsis?) Possible increase in surgical site infection (SSI) rates in the perioperative setting	A perioperative FiO_2 of 0.8 as compared with 0.3 increased long-term mortality in surgical patients FiO_2 set to maintain an oxygen partial pressure (PaO_2) of 70–100 mmHg reduced ICU mortality as compared with a conventional group (PaO_2 up to 150 mmHg)	Current guidelines are conflicting (e.g., WHO recommends a perioperative FiO_2 of 0.8 in order to reduce SSI) Latest investigations (including randomized controlled trials and meta-analyses) are inconclusive or uncertain about any impact of FiO_2 on mortality, SSI rates, and other adverse effects Avoiding useless hyperoxia while adopting adequate monitoring to prevent harms from hypoxia is probably the most reasonable approach currently

References

1. Young PJ, Beasley RW, Capellier G, et al. Oxygenation targets, monitoring in the critically ill: a point prevalence study of clinical practice in Australia and New Zealand. Crit Care Resusc. 2015;17:202–7.
2. Kraft F, Andel H, Gamper J, et al. Incidence of hyperoxia and related in-hospital mortality in critically ill patients: a retrospective data analysis. Acta Anaesthesiol Scand. 2018;62(3):347–56.
3. Palmer E, Post B, Klapaukh R, et al. The association between supraphysiologic arterial oxygen levels and mortality in critically ill patients: a multicenter observational cohort study. Am J Respir Crit Care Med. 2019;200:1373–80.
4. Blum JM, Fetterman DM, Park PK, et al. A description of intraoperative ventilator management and ventilation strategies in hypoxic patients. Anesth Analg. 2010;110:1616–22.
5. Staehr-Rye AK, Meyhoff CS, Scheffenbichler FT, et al. High intraoperative inspiratory oxygen fraction and risk of major respiratory complications. Br J Anaesth. 2017;119(1):140–9.
6. Chu DK, Kim LH, Young PJ, et al. Mortality and morbidity in acutely ill adults treated with liberal versus conservative oxygen therapy (IOTA): a systematic review and meta-analysis. Lancet. 2018;391(10131):1693–705.
7. Pisano A, Capasso A. Perioperative supplemental oxygen to reduce perioperative mortality. In: Landoni G, Ruggeri L, Zangrillo A, editors. Reducing mortality in the perioperative period. Cham: Springer; 2014. p. 77–83.
8. Hedenstierna G, Meyhoff CS. Oxygen toxicity in major emergency surgery-anything new? Intensive Care Med. 2019;45(12):1802–5.
9. O'Driscoll BR, Howard LS, Earis J, Mak V, British Thoracic Society Emergency Oxygen Guideline Group. BTS guideline for oxygen use in adults in healthcare and emergency settings. Thorax. 2017;72(suppl 1):ii1–ii90.
10. Girardis M, Busani S, Damiani E, et al. Effect of conservative vs conventional oxygen therapy on mortality among patients in an intensive care unit: the oxygen-ICU randomized clinical trial. JAMA. 2016;316(15):1583–9.
11. Meyhoff CS, Jorgensen LN, Wetterslev J, et al; PROXI Trial Group. Increased long-term mortality after a high perioperative inspiratory oxygen fraction during abdominal surgery: follow-up of a randomized clinical trial. Anesth Analg. 2012;115(4):849–54.
12. Sartini C, Lomivorotov V, Pieri M, et al. A systematic review and international web-based survey of randomized controlled trials in the perioperative and critical care setting: interventions reducing mortality. J Cardiothorac Vasc Anesth. 2019;33(5):1430–9.
13. Pisano A, Oppizzi M, Turi S, Landoni G. Reducing major adverse cardiac events and all-cause mortality in noncardiac surgery: perioperative strategies. In: Kaplan JA, Cronin B, Maus TM, editors. Kaplan's essentials of cardiac anesthesia for noncardiac surgery. Philadelphia, PA: Elsevier; 2019. p. 538–77.
14. Pisano A. Perioperative supplemental oxygen to reduce surgical site infection: too easy to be true. J Trauma Acute Care Surg. 2014;76(5):1332.
15. ICU-ROX Investigators and The Australian and New Zealand Intensive Care Society Clinical Trials Group, Mackle D, Bellomo R, Bailey M, et al. Conservative oxygen therapy during mechanical ventilation in the ICU. N Engl J Med. 2019; https://doi.org/10.1056/NEJMoa1903297. [Epub ahead of print]
16. Ferrando C, Aldecoa C, Unzueta C, et al. Effects of oxygen on post-surgical infections during an individualised perioperative open-lung ventilatory strategy: a randomised controlled trial. Br J Anaesth. 2020;124(1):110–20.
17. de Jonge S, Egger M, Latif A, et al. Effectiveness of 80% vs 30–35% fraction of inspired oxygen in patients undergoing surgery: an updated systematic review and meta-analysis. Br J Anaesth. 2019;122(3):325–34.
18. Barbateskovic M, Schjørring OL, Russo Krauss S, et al. Higher versus lower fraction of inspired oxygen or targets of arterial oxygenation for adults admitted to the intensive care unit. Cochrane Database Syst Rev. 2019;2019(11):8.

19. Smith BK, Roberts RH, Frizelle FA. O_2 no longer the Go_2: a systematic review and meta-analysis comparing the effects of giving perioperative oxygen therapy of 30% FiO_2 to 80% FiO_2 on surgical site infection and mortality. World J Surg. 2020;44(1):69–77.
20. Sartini C, Lomivorotov V, Pisano A, et al. A systematic review and international web-based survey of randomized controlled trials in the perioperative and critical care setting: interventions increasing mortality. J Cardiothorac Vasc Anesth. 2019;33(10):2685–94.
21. Meyhoff CS, Wetterslev J, Jorgensen LN, PROXI Trial Group, et al. Effect of high perioperative oxygen fraction on surgical site infection and pulmonary complications after abdominal surgery: the PROXI randomized clinical trial. JAMA. 2009;302:1543–50.
22. Smit B, Smulders YM, van der Wouden JC, et al. Hemodynamic effects of acute hyperoxia: systematic review and meta-analysis. Crit Care. 2018;22(1):45.
23. Hedenstierna G, Edmark L. Mechanisms of atelectasis in the perioperative period. Best Pract Res Clin Anaesthesiol. 2010;24(2):157–69.
24. Graham K, Unger E. Overcoming tumor hypoxia as a barrier to radiotherapy, chemotherapy and immunotherapy in cancer treatment. Int J Nanomedicine. 2018;13:6049–58.
25. Young P, Mackle D, Bellomo R, ICU-ROX Investigators the Australian New Zealand Intensive Care Society Clinical Trials Group, et al. Conservative oxygen therapy for mechanically ventilated adults with sepsis: a post hoc analysis of data from the intensive care unit randomized trial comparing two approaches to oxygen therapy (ICU-ROX). Intensive Care Med. 2020;46(1):17–26.
26. Young PJ, Bellomo R. The risk of hyperoxemia in ICU patients. Much ado about O_2. Am J Respir Crit Care Med. 2019;200(11):1333–5.
27. Schjørring OL, Perner A, Wetterslev J, HOT-ICU Investigators, et al. Handling oxygenation targets in the intensive care unit (HOT-ICU)-protocol for a randomised clinical trial comparing a lower vs a higher oxygenation target in adults with acute hypoxaemic respiratory failure. Acta Anaesthesiol Scand. 2019;63:956–65.
28. Li XF, Jiang D, Jiang YL, et al. PROtective ventilation with a low versus high inspiratory oxygen fraction (PROVIO) and its effects on postoperative pulmonary complications: protocol for a randomized controlled trial. Trials. 2019;20(1):619.

Mechanical Ventilation in ARDS

5

Antonio Pisano, Rosanna Buonomo, Teresa P. Iovino,
Roberta Maj, Federico Masserini, and Luigi Verniero

Contents

5.1   General Principles

Since its first description in 1967, many aspects of acute respiratory distress syndrome (ARDS) have changed, including understanding of its pathophysiology,
diagnostic criteria and definitions (see Table 5.1), therapeutic strategies, and even
the meaning of the "A" within the acronym "ARDS" (which initially stood for

A. Pisano (✉) · L. Verniero
Cardiac Anesthesia and Intensive Care Unit, A.O.R.N. "Dei Colli", Monaldi Hospital,
Naples, Italy
e-mail: antonio.pisano@ospedaleicolli.it

R. Buonomo
Postgraduate school of Anesthesia and Critical Care, University of Campania "Luigi
Vanvitelli", Naples, Italy

T. P. Iovino
II Anesthesia and Critical Care Unit, A.O.R.N. "Cardarelli", Naples, Italy

R. Maj · F. Masserini
U.O. Anestesia e Rianimazione San Raffaele, IRCCS San Raffaele, Milan, Italy
e-mail: rmazzani@ao.pr.it; federico.masserini@unimi.it

© Springer Nature Switzerland AG 2021   43
G. Landoni et al. (eds.), *Reducing Mortality in Critically Ill Patients*,
https://doi.org/10.1007/978-3-030-71917-3_5

Table 5.1 Acute Respiratory Distress Syndrome (ARDS) diagnostic criteria according to the current (Berlin) definition [4] and to the early American-European Consensus Conference [5]. *PaO₂* Arterial oxygen partial pressure, *FiO₂* Inspiratory oxygen fraction, *PEEP* Positive end-expiratory pressure, *CPAP* Continuous positive airway pressure, *ALI* Acute Lung Injury

Berlin ARDS definition (2012)	American-European Consensus Conference ARDS definition (1994)
Impaired oxygenation:[a] • *Mild ARDS.* $PaO_2/FiO_2 \leq 300$ (but >200) mmHg with PEEP/CPAP ≥ 5 cm H_2O • *Moderate ARDS.* $PaO_2/FiO_2 \leq 200$ (but >100) mmHg with PEEP ≥ 5 cm H_2O • *Severe ARDS.* $PaO_2/FiO_2 \leq 100$, with PEEP ≥ 5 cm H_2O	Impaired oxygenation:[a] • *ALI.* $PaO_2/FiO_2 \leq 300$ (but >200) mmHg • *ARDS.* $PaO_2/FiO_2 \leq 200$ mmHg

[a]In association (in summary) with acute onset, bilateral pulmonary infiltrates at chest imaging, and no cardiac disease as the leading cause

"adult") [1–6]. However, ARDS remains a major critical care issue, accounting for about 10% of intensive care unit (ICU) admissions, with an in-hospital/ICU mortality still around 40% [2, 6].

Both pathophysiology and clinical management of ARDS are linked to the mechanisms of ventilator-induced lung injury (VILI), firstly, because the risk of VILI is increased in ARDS patients due to a disruption of lung architecture, which leads to poorly compliant and heterogeneously aerated lungs [2, 3, 7], and, secondly, because mechanical ventilation itself may act as a second "hit" that causes ARDS in the presence of pulmonary (e.g., pneumonia, aspiration of gastric content, toxic inhalation, lung contusion, near-drowning) or extra-pulmonary (e.g., sepsis, trauma, burns, pancreatitis, blood transfusion, cardiopulmonary bypass) predisposing inflammatory insults [8, 9].

Lung-protective ventilation (LPV) and prone positioning (PP) are currently the two cornerstones of ARDS treatment. LPV with low tidal volumes (V_T), moderate-to-high levels of positive end-expiratory pressure (PEEP) and, possibly, recruitment maneuvers (i.e., a transitory increase in transpulmonary pressure aimed at opening atelectatic alveoli) may prevent or attenuate VILI [2, 7, 8] and has been widely shown in randomized controlled trials (RCTs) to reduce mortality in ARDS patients [10–13]. However, evidence about the favorable effects in terms of survival of PEEP and recruitment maneuvers is not as conclusive as that about low V_T [14, 15]; on the contrary, a recent investigation suggested possible harm from lung recruitment and PEEP titration strategies [16].

Mechanical ventilation in the prone position has been shown for over 40 years to improve oxygenation in ARDS patients [17, 18], but only in recent years a large multicenter RCT [19] (as well as several meta-analyses [20–22]) succeeded in demonstrating a reduced mortality with this intervention.

In this chapter, we discuss the main evidences about the role of LPV and PP in reducing mortality among ARDS patients, the pathophysiological mechanisms through which these interventions are believed to improve survival, and their use in clinical practice. Moreover, other therapeutic strategies related to mechanical venti-lation which have been investigated for a possible role in improving outcomes (including mortality) in ARDS patients, such as pressure-controlled ventilation as compared with volume-controlled ventilation, high-frequency oscillatory ventila-tion (HFOV), use of esophageal pressure for PEEP titration, and targeting mechani-cal ventilation according to driving pressure, are briefly discussed.

5.2   Main Evidences

5.2.1   Lung-Protective Ventilation

LPV is one of the interventions best proven to affect mortality in critically ill patients [23]. In fact, as many as three multicenter RCTs found a significant reduction in mortality with LPV in ARDS patients [11–13].

In 1998, Amato et al. [11] randomly assigned 53 patients with early ARDS to receive conventional ventilation or LPV. Conventional ventilation consisted in $V_T = 12$ mL/kg of body weight with a target arterial partial pressure of carbon diox-ide (P_aCO_2) of 35–38 mmHg and the lowest PEEP allowing acceptable oxygenation while LPV was intended as $V_T < 6$ mL/kg with permissive hypercapnia (P_aCO_2 up to 80 mmHg) and PEEP above the lower inflection point (P_{flex}) on the static pressure-volume curve. A dramatic reduction in 28-day mortality in the latter group (38 vs 71%, $p < 0.001$) was reported, together with significantly lower rates of barotrauma (7 vs 42%, $p = 0.02$).

The ARDS Network trial [12], published 2 years later, enrolled 861 patients (from ten ICUs) with acute lung injury (ALI) or ARDS (according to the definitions at that time, see Table 5.1). Patients were randomized to receive either low-V_T ven-tilation or "traditional" ventilation. In the former group, V_T was initially set at 6 mL/kg of predicted body weight (PBW) (Fig. 5.1) [2, 12, 13] and was subse-quently reduced, if necessary, in order to maintain a plateau pressure (P_{PLAT}; i.e., the airway pressure measured after a 0.5 s inspiratory pause) ≤ 30 cm H_2O. The control

Fig. 5.1 Calculation of predicted body weight (PBW). *Cm* Centimeters, *in* Inches. Modified from Silversides and Ferguson [2] Copyright © 2013 BioMed Central Ltd.

$$\text{Males}$$

$$PBW\ (Kg) = \begin{cases} 50 + 0.91\ (\text{height}\ (cm) - 152.4) \\ \quad\quad\quad\quad or \\ 50 + 2.3\ (\text{height}\ (in) - 60) \end{cases}$$

$$\text{Females}$$

$$PBW\ (Kg) = \begin{cases} 45.5 + 0.91\ (\text{height}\ (cm) - 152.4) \\ \quad\quad\quad\quad or \\ 45.5 + 2.3\ (\text{height}\ (in) - 60) \end{cases}$$

group received an initial V_T of 12 mL/kg PBW, subsequently reduced if necessary, to maintain a $P_{PLAT} \leq 50$ cm H_2O. Unlike the previous study, PEEP was similar in the two groups. Mortality before home discharge without ventilatory assistance was significantly less in the low-V_T group (31 vs 39.8%, $p = 0.007$). No differences in the incidence of barotrauma were found.

Finally, Villar and colleagues [13] enrolled 103 ARDS patients (from eight ICUs) and showed a significant reduction in mortality (32 vs 53.3%, $p = 0.04$) among patients ventilated with $V_T = 5–8$ mL/kg PBW and initial PEEP 2 cm H_2O above P_{flex} as compared with those ventilated with higher V_T (9–11 mL/kg PBW) and lower PEEP (≥ 5 cmH_2O). No difference in the incidence of barotrauma was found in this study as well.

Although two of the three above-mentioned investigations included higher levels of PEEP as part of an LPV strategy, two subsequent meta-analyses of multicenter RCTs comparing higher PEEP (with or without recruitment maneuvers) versus lower PEEP, with similar (low) V_T between groups, failed to show a clear benefit of higher PEEP on survival in ARDS patients [14, 15]. Most remarkably, the recent Alveolar Recruitment for ARDS (ART) trial [16] randomized 1010 patients with moderate-to-severe ARDS (see Table 5.1) from 120 ICUs to either an open lung strategy involving recruitment maneuvers and PEEP titration according to the best respiratory system compliance or to a conventional low-PEEP strategy: both 28-day and 6-month mortality were higher in the experimental group as compared with the conventional control group (55.3 vs 49.3%, hazard ratio [HR] 1.20, 95% confidence interval [CI] 1.01–1.42, $p = 0.04$ and 65.3 vs 59.9%, HR1.18, 95%CI 1.01–1.38, $p = 0.04$, respectively). Moreover, patients in the experimental group had significantly fewer mean ventilator-free days and an increased risk of barotrauma and pneumothorax requiring drainage, while no differences were found in ICU and hospital length of stay (LOS) as well as in ICU and in-hospital mortality.

5.2.2   Prone Positioning

After a series of major investigations yielding neutral results with regard to a possible role of PP in reducing mortality among ARDS patients [24–27], the PROSEVA trial by Guérin et al. [19] was the first (and it remains the only) RCT which reported a significant reduction in mortality with PP in ARDS patients. Nonetheless, the evidence provided acquires strength when considering the progressive refinements that the study design has undergone over time, especially as compared with the earliest large RCTs. In particular, the duration of PP was far higher (17–18 h per day, on average) in the newer studies [26, 27] than in the two older studies (<10 h per day) [24, 25]. Moreover, only the most recent of the previous RCTs [27] limited enrollment to the most severe ARDS patients ($PaO_2/FiO_2 \leq 200$ mmHg with PEEP ≥ 5 cm H_2O) and employed a strict LPV protocol. Finally, the PROSEVA trial [19] featured a more homogeneous population, in terms of ARDS severity, and a longer duration of PP, which can both explain the differences in the results compared to the older trials [28–30].

The PROSEVA trial [19] included 466 patients (from 27 ICUs) with "severe" ARDS, defined as $PaO_2/FiO_2 < 150$ mmHg in patients receiving LPV with $V_T \approx 6$ mL/kg PBW, PEEP ≥ 5 cm H_2O and $FiO_2 \geq 0.6$ (with these criteria persisting after a stabilization period of 12–24 h, in order to select the most severe cases) [30]. Patients were randomized to either undergo early PP (within 1 h after randomization) or to be left supine. Additionally, the study included, among others [30] PP sessions of at least 16 h per day with prefixed criteria to stop them (on average, 17 h per day for 4 days), an experience >5 years with PP management in all centers involved, a minimized crossover between the two groups and more time spent on prone position, as compared with the investigation by Taccone et al. [27]. Mortality at 28 days was 16% in the prone group and 32.8% in the supine group ($p < 0.001$). A significant reduction in 90-day mortality (23.6 vs 41%, $p < 0.001$) was also found in the prone group.

These results are consistent with those of both patient-level [20] and study-level [21] meta-analyses of the previous RCTs. In addition, all the updated meta-analyses which included the PROSEVA trial have confirmed these findings [17, 29, 31].

5.2.3   Other Mechanical Ventilation Strategies

There is currently no clear evidence that pressure-controlled ventilation (PCV) may provide advantages in terms of survival over volume-controlled ventilation (VCV) in ARDS patients [32]. In the only RCT showing a significantly increased in-hospital mortality with VCV as compared with PCV, multivariate analysis suggested that such difference could not be attributable to the ventilatory mode [33].

High-frequency oscillatory ventilation (HFOV), consisting in delivering very low V_T at very high rates, is theoretically the perfect LPV strategy and has been suggested to provide potential benefits in ARDS patients [6]. However, the large multi-center OSCILLATE trial [34], which was stopped after randomization of 548 patients due to safety concerns, found a significantly increased in-hospital mortality in patients with moderate-to-severe ARDS randomized to early HFOV as compared with those receiving conventional LPV with low V_T and high PEEP (47 vs 35%, relative risk [RR] 1.33, 95% CI 1.09–1.64, $p = 0.005$). Routine use of HFOV is currently strongly discouraged [6].

The use of esophageal pressure (P_{ES}) to titrate PEEP in ARDS patients seemed to be a promising approach until recently [35], but the lately published EPVent-2 study [36], which included 200 patients (from 14 ICUs) with moderate-to-severe ARDS randomized to either P_{ES}-guided PEEP titration or empirical PEEP-FiO_2 setting, failed to show any difference between groups in 28-day mortality, days free from mechanical ventilation, or any other planned clinical endpoint.

Finally, a recent multilevel mediation analysis of nine previous RCTs suggested that driving pressure (i.e., the difference between P_{PLAT} and PEEP) rather than other ventilatory parameters is strongly associated with mortality in ARDS patients [37]. However, currently available evidence does not support targeting driving pressure when setting mechanical ventilation in ARDS patients, particularly if this means increasing PEEP [6, 38].

5.3   Pathophysiological Principles: Mechanisms of Reduced Mortality

ARDS is characterized by diffuse alveolar-capillary membrane disruption that results in increased permeability and subsequent pulmonary edema and atelectasis. Alveolar damage however is not homogeneously distributed, as atelectasis mainly affects the dependent lung regions (namely, those most subjected to hydrostatic pressure) while non-dependent regions remain better aerated [2, 3, 7]. For these reasons, also the volume that needs to be ventilated decreases (hence the term "baby lung") [3].

Although barotrauma (e.g., pneumothorax) may occur as a consequence of mechanical ventilation with high volumes, the main determinant of VILI is thought to be alveolar overdistension (volutrauma) rather than airway pressure [7]. Therefore, it is reasonable that low-V_T ventilation prevents or minimizes VILI in ARDS patients, by avoiding overinflation of the decreased normally aerated regions. However, VILI can occur even during a low-V_T ventilation, due to cyclic alveolar opening and closure (atelectrauma), which leads to epithelial sloughing, hyaline membranes, and pulmonary edema [2, 7]. Since atelectrauma is intensified in the presence of broad heterogeneities in ventilation [7], as in ARDS, higher levels of PEEP may contribute to minimize VILI by reducing alveolar collapse during expiration [2, 7].

Prone positioning improves oxygenation, often considerably, due to a reduction in intrapulmonary shunt: while blood flow distribution remains essentially unchanged (thus prevailing into dorsal regions), the conversion from the supine to prone position induces an increase in aeration in dorsal regions that exceeds ventral derecruitment [18, 28, 30]. As a consequence, in addition to lung ventilation and ventilation-to-perfusion ratio [39], also transpulmonary pressure and lung densities are more homogeneously distributed along the ventral-to-dorsal axis.

The primary determinant of these effects is the shape matching between the conically shaped lungs and the cylindrically shaped chest wall (see Fig. 5.2) [28] that implies a greater distention in the ventral lung regions [18]. Since the hydrostatic pressure (i.e., the forces due to gravity) is always greater in the regions that lie below (the so-called dependent regions), in the prone position it mainly acts on ventral regions, where it is counteracted by regional expansion. In other words, there is a larger volume of dependent lung in supine position as compared to prone [39]. Other factors, such as the reduced compression of lung tissue by the heart, contribute to the more homogeneous distribution of lung density/inflation in the prone position [18, 28, 39].

Improvement in oxygenation however does not seem to be the primary mechanism of mortality reduction by PP. Indeed, a retrospective analysis of data from the PROSEVA trial showed that the reduction in mortality observed in ARDS patients receiving prone ventilation was not dependent on whether PP improved gas exchange [40].

Fig. 5.2 The greater lung expansion in ventral regions, due to shape matching between lung and thorax, counteracts hydrostatic pressure, which acts mostly on those ventral regions in the prone position. This leads to a more homogeneous inflation of alveoli along the ventral-to-dorsal axis in the prone position, as compared to supine. Adapted from Gattinoni et al. [18] with permission

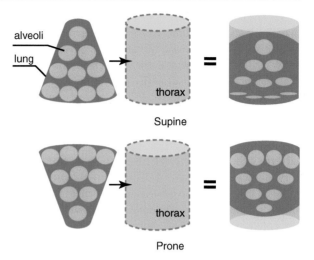

The survival benefit may be rather attributed, also for PP, to the prevention of VILI [18, 28, 30, 40, 41], whose major determinants are, as mentioned, volutrauma (pertaining to lung stress, namely the increase in transpulmonary pressure), and atelectrauma [2, 30]. The more uniform distribution of the gravitational transpulmonary pressure gradient, as well as of both V_T and end-expiratory lung volume, results in a homogenization of the strain (i.e., the V_T to end-expiratory lung volume ratio) imposed by mechanical ventilation and, consequently, in a reduction of the resulting stress [18, 28, 30]. Finally, a more uniformly distributed V_T translates into a reduced atelectrauma [40], and improvements in PaO_2/FiO_2 ratio resulting from PP may itself indirectly contribute to the prevention of VILI by reducing the need for iatrogenic interventions to sustain oxygenation [18].

5.4 Therapeutic Use

Low-V_T ventilation (with $P_{PLAT} \leq 30$ cm H_2O) is indicated in patients with ARDS of any severity [42, 43]. However, probably not all ARDS patients (e.g., those with stiff chest wall and, consequently, high pleural pressure) really need a so low P_{PLAT} (and V_T) in order to avoid alveolar overdistension [7].

Low-V_T ventilation often results in hypercapnia and acidosis, with possible metabolic complications such as acute hyperkalemia [2, 9]. These abnormalities can be counteracted by increasing respiratory rate (RR), but it should be considered that high RR (usually >30 breaths/min) may lead to dynamic hyperinflation and auto-PEEP [9]. However, since low-V_T ventilation was shown to reduce mortality despite hypercapnia [11, 12], it may be speculated that the latter itself may be beneficial due to rightward shift of the oxy-hemoglobin dissociation curve, systemic and microcirculatory vasodilation, and inhibitory effects on inflammatory cells. Moreover, mean

pCO_2 levels of 66.5 mmHg or higher and a pH up to 7.15 can be tolerated unless specific contraindications exist, such as increased intracranial pressure [2].

A discussion of the use of "ultraprotective" ventilator strategies ($V_T \approx 3$ mL/kg PBW) in association with extracorporeal arteriovenous CO_2 removal or extracorporeal membrane oxygenation (ECMO) is beyond the scope of this chapter.

As mentioned, the role of PEEP and recruitment maneuvers in the treatment of ARDS is not as definite as that of low V_T. Higher levels of PEEP should be reserved for moderate-to-severe forms of ARDS [43]. Maybe, in patients with mild ARDS (and possibly in a proportion of patients with a more severe disease), the potential adverse effects of higher PEEP levels (e.g., impairment of venous return, circulatory depression, lung overdistension) may overcome the advantages [7, 14]. Clinical trials could have failed to show clear benefits of high PEEP levels [14, 15], or even highlighted possible harms [16], due to the difficult in tailoring PEEP on the single patient. In fact, lung inflation is strictly dependent on transpulmonary pressure (P_{TP}), that is the difference between alveolar and pleural pressure: since pleural pressure is broadly and unpredictably variable among ARDS patients, it is difficult to determine which level of PEEP is needed to prevent alveolar collapse and, therefore, atelectrauma in the individual patient [7]. Finally, some concerns exist about the possible complications of recruitment maneuvers, including transient desaturation, hemodynamic impairment, pneumothorax, and even worsening of VILI [2, 7].

Prone positioning is strongly recommended in patients with severe ARDS [43]. In order to be effective in reducing mortality, PP should be initiated early and maintained for at least 12 h per day (even if maybe >16 is better) until stable improvement in oxygenation is achieved (optimal duration of PP has yet to be established [29]). Contraindications are few and not well defined: conditions such as pelvic/spinal instability, severe facial or neck trauma, open wounds/burns on the ventral body surface, non-stabilized fractures, increased intracranial pressure, hemodynamic instability, serious cardiac arrhythmias and pregnancy should preclude PP or, at least, impose a careful evaluation of the risks/benefits balance [18, 41, 44].

A skilled and well-coordinated team is pivotal in order to avoid potentially serious complications, including endotracheal tube displacement, kinking or obstruction, and vascular lines kinking/removal [17–19, 29, 41, 44]. Finally, although a higher risk of pressure ulcers was reported by previous trials and meta-analyses [17, 29], and also confirmed in an ancillary study of the PROSEVA trial [45], it is not clear whether such findings are related to PP itself or to the greater survival which results from it [30, 45].

Clinical summary

Technique	Indications	Cautions	Side-Effects	Dose	Notes
Protective ventilation (low tidal volume with or without high PEEP and recruitment maneuvers)	All ARDS patients (low V_T) Moderate-to-severe ARDS patients (low V_T + high PEEP)	Hypercapnia may be hazardous in patients with increased intracranial pressure Excessive respiratory rate may lead to dynamic hyperinflation and auto-PEEP	Low V_T: • hypercapnia • acidemia • acute hyperkalemia High PEEP and recruitment maneuvers: • hemodynamic impairment • lung overdistension • pneumothorax • possible increase in mortality	Initial V_T of 6 mL/kg of predicted body weight (adjusted to maintain $P_{PLAT} \leq 30$ cm H_2O) Initial PEEP 2 cm H_2O above P_{flex} (adjusted according to oxygenation)	The role of PEEP and recruitment maneuvers has to be further clarified PEEP titration guided by esophageal pressure does not seem to affect outcomes High-frequency oscillatory ventilation may increase mortality No clear differences between volume-controlled and pressure-controlled ventilation
Prone positioning	Severe ARDS Moderate-to-severe ARDS (PaO_2/FiO_2 < 150 mmHg)	Possible contraindications: • pelvic/spinal instability • severe facial or neck trauma • increased intracranial pressure • open wounds/burns on the ventral body surface • non-stabilized fractures • hemodynamic instability/ serious arrhythmias • pregnancy	Major airway problems: • endotracheal tube kinking/obstruction • endotracheal tube displacement (unplanned extubation or selective main stem bronchus intubation) Pressure ulcers (debated)	At least 12 h per day (maybe >16 h/day could be better, but the optimal daily duration is unknown)	Must be associated with protective ventilatory strategies Requires high experience and specifically trained personnel Feasible during ECMO

References

1. Walkey AJ, Summer R, Ho V, et al. Acute respiratory distress syndrome: epidemiology and management approaches. Clin Epidemiol. 2012;4:159–69.
2. Silversides JA, Ferguson ND. Clinical review: acute respiratory distress syndrome - clinical ventilator management and adjunct therapy. Crit Care. 2013;17(2):225.
3. Gattinoni L, Tonetti T, Quintel M. Regional physiology of ARDS. Crit Care. 2017;21(Suppl 3):312.
4. ARDS Definition Task Force, Ranieri VM, Rubenfeld GD, Thompson BT, et al. Acute respiratory distress syndrome: the Berlin definition. JAMA. 2012;307:2526–33.
5. Bernard GR, Artigas A, Brigham KL, et al. The American–European consensus conference on ARDS. Definitions, mechanisms, relevant outcomes, and clinical trial coordination. Am J Respir Crit Care Med. 1994;149:818–24.
6. Fan E, Brodie D, Slutsky AS. Acute respiratory distress syndrome: advances in diagnosis and treatment. JAMA. 2018;319(7):698–710.
7. Slutsky AS, Ranieri VM. Ventilator-induced lung injury. N Engl J Med. 2013;369(22):2126–36.
8. Sutherasan Y, Vargas M, Pelosi P. Protective mechanical ventilation in the non-injured lung: review and meta-analysis. Crit Care. 2014;18(2):211.
9. Lellouche F, Lipes J. Prophylactic protective ventilation: lower tidal volumes for all critically ill patients? Intensive Care Med. 2013;39(1):6–15.
10. Hickling KG, Henderson SJ, Jackson R. Low mortality associated with low volume pressure limited ventilation with permissive hypercapnia in severe adult respiratory distress syndrome. Intensive Care Med. 1990;16:372–7.
11. Amato MB, Barbas CS, Medeiros DM, et al. Effect of a protective-ventilation strategy on mortality in the acute respiratory distress syndrome. N Engl J Med. 1998;338:347–54.
12. The Acute Respiratory Distress Syndrome Network. Ventilation with lower tidal volumes as compared with traditional tidal volumes for acute lung injury and the acute respiratory distress syndrome. N Engl J Med. 2000;342:1301–8.
13. Villar J, Kacmarek RM, Pérez-Méndez L, et al. A high positive end-expiratory pressure, low tidal volume ventilatory strategy improves outcome in persistent acute respiratory distress syndrome: a randomized, controlled trial. Crit Care Med. 2006;34(5):1311–8.
14. Briel M, Meade M, Mercat A, et al. Higher vs lower positive end-expiratory pressure in patients with acute lung injury and acute respiratory distress syndrome: systematic review and meta-analysis. JAMA. 2010;303(9):865–73.
15. Santa Cruz R, Rojas JI, Nervi R, et al. High versus low positive end-expiratory pressure (PEEP) levels for mechanically ventilated adult patients with acute lung injury and acute respiratory distress syndrome. Cochrane Database Syst Rev. 2013;6:CD009098.
16. Writing Group for the Alveolar Recruitment for Acute Respiratory Distress Syndrome Trial (ART) Investigators, Cavalcanti AB, Suzumura ÉA, Laranjeira LN, et al. Effect of lung recruitment and titrated positive end-expiratory pressure (PEEP) vs low PEEP on mortality in patients with acute respiratory distress syndrome: a randomized clinical trial. JAMA. 2017;318(14):1335–45.
17. Sud S, Friedrich JO, Adhikari NK, et al. Effect of prone positioning during mechanical ventilation on mortality among patients with acute respiratory distress syndrome: a systematic review and meta-analysis. CMAJ. 2014;186(10):E381–90.
18. Gattinoni L, Taccone P, Carlesso E, et al. Prone position in acute respiratory distress syndrome. Rationale, indications, and limits. Am J Respir Crit Care Med. 2013;188(11):1286–93.
19. Guérin C, Reignier J, Richard JC, et al. Prone positioning in severe acute respiratory distress syndrome. N Engl J Med. 2013;368(23):2159–68.
20. Gattinoni L, Carlesso E, Taccone P, et al. Prone positioning improves survival in severe ARDS: a pathophysiologic review and individual patient meta-analysis. Minerva Anestesiol. 2010;76:448–54.

21. Sud S, Friedrich JO, Taccone P, et al. Prone ventilation reduces mortality in patients with acute respiratory failure and severe hypoxemia: systematic review and meta-analysis. Intensive Care Med. 2010;36:585–99.
22. Munshi L, Del Sorbo L, Adhikari NKJ, et al. Prone position for acute respiratory distress syndrome. A systematic review and meta-analysis. Ann Am Thorac Soc. 2017;14(Supplement 4): S280–8.
23. Sartini C, Lomivorotov V, Pieri M, et al. A systematic review and international web-based survey of randomized controlled trials in the perioperative and critical care setting: interventions reducing mortality. J Cardiothorac Vasc Anesth. 2019;33(5):1430–9.
24. Gattinoni L, Tognoni G, Pesenti A, et al. Effect of prone positioning on the survival of patients with acute respiratory failure. N Engl J Med. 2001;345:568–73.
25. Guérin C, Gaillard S, Lemasson S, et al. Effects of systematic prone positioning in hypoxemic acute respiratory failure: a randomized controlled trial. JAMA. 2004;292:2379–87.
26. Mancebo J, Fernández R, Blanch L, et al. A multicenter trial of prolonged prone ventilation in severe acute respiratory distress syndrome. Am J Respir Crit Care Med. 2006;173:1233–9.
27. Taccone P, Pesenti A, Latini R, et al. Prone positioning in patients with moderate and severe acute respiratory distress syndrome: a randomized controlled trial. JAMA. 2009;302:1977–84.
28. Guerin C, Baboi L, Richard JC. Mechanisms of the effects of prone positioning in acute respiratory distress syndrome. Intensive Care Med. 2014;40(11):1634–42.
29. Lee JM, Bae W, Lee YJ, et al. The efficacy and safety of prone positional ventilation in acute respiratory distress syndrome: updated study-level meta-analysis of 11 randomized controlled trials. Crit Care Med. 2014;42(5):1252–62.
30. Guérin C. Prone ventilation in acute respiratory distress syndrome. Eur Respir Rev. 2014;23(132):249–57.
31. Hu SL, He HL, Pan C, et al. The effect of prone positioning on mortality in patients with acute respiratory distress syndrome: a meta-analysis of randomized controlled trials. Crit Care. 2014;18(3):R109.
32. Chacko B, Peter JV, Tharyan P, et al. Pressure-controlled versus volume-controlled ventilation for acute respiratory failure due to acute lung injury (ALI) or acute respiratory distress syndrome (ARDS). Cochrane Database Syst Rev. 2015;1:CD008807.
33. Esteban A, Alía I, Gordo F, et al. Prospective randomized trial comparing pressure-controlled ventilation and volume-controlled ventilation in ARDS. For the Spanish lung failure collaborative group. Chest. 2000;117(6):1690–6.
34. Ferguson ND, Cook DJ, Guyatt GH, OSCILLATE Trial Investigators; Canadian Critical Care Trials Group, et al. High-frequency oscillation in early acute respiratory distress syndrome. N Engl J Med. 2013;368(9):795–805.
35. Pisano A, Iovino TP, Maj R. Lung-protective ventilation and mortality in acute respiratory distress syndrome. In: Landoni G, Mucchetti M, Zangrillo A, Bellomo R, editors. Reducing mortality in critically ill patients. Cham: Springer; 2015. p. 23–9.
36. Beitler JR, Sarge T, Banner-Goodspeed VM, EPVent-2 Study Group, et al. Effect of titrating positive end-expiratory pressure (PEEP) with an esophageal pressure-guided strategy vs an empirical high PEEP-FiO$_2$ strategy on death and days free from mechanical ventilation among patients with acute respiratory distress syndrome: a randomized clinical trial. JAMA. 2019;321(9):846–57.
37. Amato MBP, Meade MO, Slutsky AS, et al. Driving pressure and survival in the acute respiratory distress syndrome. N Engl J Med. 2015;372(8):747–55.
38. Pelosi P, Ball L. Should we titrate ventilation based on driving pressure? Maybe not in the way we would expect. Ann Transl Med. 2018;6(19):389.
39. Henderson AC, Sá RC, Theilmann RJ, et al. The gravitational distribution of ventilation-perfusion ratio is more uniform in prone than supine posture in the normal human lung. J Appl Physiol. 2013;115(3):313–24.

40. Albert RK, Keniston A, Baboi L, et al. Prone position-induced improvement in gas exchange does not predict improved survival in the acute respiratory distress syndrome. Am J Respir Crit Care Med. 2014;189(4):494–6.
41. Messerole E, Peine P, Wittkopp S, et al. The pragmatics of prone positioning. Am J Respir Crit Care Med. 2002;165(10):1359–63.
42. Ferguson ND, Fan E, Camporota L, et al. The Berlin definition of ARDS: an expanded rationale, justification, and supplementary material. Intensive Care Med. 2012;38(10):1573–82.
43. Fan E, Del Sorbo L, Goligher EC, American Thoracic Society, European Society of Intensive Care Medicine, and Society of Critical Care Medicine, et al. An Official American Thoracic Society/European Society of Intensive Care Medicine/Society of Critical Care Medicine clinical practice guideline: mechanical ventilation in adult patients with acute respiratory distress syndrome. Am J Respir Crit Care Med. 2017;195(9):1253–63.
44. Scholten EL, Beitler JR, Prisk GK, Malhotra A. Treatment of ARDS with prone positioning. Chest. 2017;151(1):215–24.
45. Girard R, Baboi L, Ayzac L, et al. The impact of patient positioning on pressure ulcers in patients with severe ARDS: results from a multicentre randomised controlled trial on prone positioning. Intensive Care Med. 2014;40(3):397–403.

Early Tracheostomy

6

Federico Longhini, Eugenio Garofalo, and Andrea Bruni

Contents

6.1 General Principles

Mechanical ventilation is required in nearly 40% of critically ill patients admitted to an Intensive Care Unit (ICU). Although a little of these patients may benefit of non-invasive ventilation (NIV), the vast majority required invasive mechanical ventilation (iMV), which is usually delivered through and endotracheal tube.

When endotracheal intubation is protracted, the risk for development of Ventilator-Associated Pneumonia (VAP) increases, leading to a worsened outcome. Furthermore, endotracheal intubation can also produce laryngeal injury and sinusitis [1], when nasal intubation is performed.

F. Longhini (✉)
Anesthesia and Intensive Care Unit, "Mater Domini" University Hospital, "Magna Graecia" University, Catanzaro, Italy

Department of Medical and Surgical Sciences, Magna Graecia University, Catanzaro, Italy
e-mail: flonghini@unicz.it

E. Garofalo · A. Bruni
Anesthesia and Intensive Care Unit, "Mater Domini" University Hospital, "Magna Graecia" University, Catanzaro, Italy
e-mail: eugenio.garofalo@unicz.it; andreabruni@unicz.it

© Springer Nature Switzerland AG 2021
G. Landoni et al. (eds.), *Reducing Mortality in Critically Ill Patients*,
https://doi.org/10.1007/978-3-030-71917-3_6

The conversion of endotracheal intubation to tracheotomy is a common and accepted practice, especially in case of prolonged iMV since it reduces the complications related to endotracheal intubation. Furthermore, tracheotomy has other advantages, such as reduced need for sedation, improved patient's comfort, better airway hygiene and decreased airway resistances [2].

The first reports of technique similar to tracheostomy can be found in books older than 4000 years, with the aim of relieving upper-airway obstruction [3]. However, its use for airway management during iMV became more common during the epidemic of polio in 1950s [4]. From polio epidemic, the development of new tubes and dilatational technique made this procedure more and more popular, simpler, and feasible at the bedside. Despite their interchangeable use, the terms *tracheostomy* and *tracheotomy* refer to an opening in the trachea with or without a surgical attachment to the skin, respectively.

6.2   Physiological Advantages

Besides benefits above mentioned, tracheotomy presents further physiological advantages.

First of all, there is a reduction of the natural dead space. In fact, when patient breaths through a tracheal cannula, the airflow is diverted from the upper native airway directly into the trachea and bronchial tree. It should be noted, however, that, although the dead space is reduced by 80–100 ml, the inspired air bypasses the upper airway, which is fundamental for conditioning and humidification. Therefore, active humidification and warming is necessary to avoid complications such as chronic inflammation of the bronchial tree and the dehydration and retention of secretions.

Second, a tracheal cannula is definitely shorted than any other trans-laryngeal tube, reducing the resistances generated by the prothesis. Therefore, the patient has to cope with lower respiratory resistances workload. Furthermore, some technical advances and features (such as the presence of fenestration, the removal of the inner cannula, and the deflation of the cuff) may further reduce the airflow resistances and inspiratory work of breathing [5–7].

Third, although the presence of a tracheotomy tube may impair the swallowing [8], oral feeding may be resumed after a proper clinical assessment including the evaluation of the tongue and oral muscle strength, the presence of gag reflex, the presence and efficiency of volitional and reflex cough, and the performance of a modified Evans blue test [9].

Fourth, the placement of a speaking valve on the tracheotomy tube provides the possibility to preserve the speech and leave the patient to communicate with the caregivers while spontaneously breathing. This is also possible in mechanically ventilated patients with a fenestrated cuffed cannula or, in alternative, with cuffless tubes during the so-called trans-tracheal open ventilation [10, 11].

6.3   Indications

In critically ill patients, indications for placement of a tracheal cannula may be either temporary or definitive tracheotomy. The most important and common indications for tracheotomy are:

- the presence of the upper-airway/laryngeal obstruction [12]
- the difficulty or failure to cough, presence of copious secretions not adequately cleared, and, more generally, failure to protect lower respiratory tract
- the presence of a chronic respiratory failure deeming necessary prolonged (>16 h/day) mechanical ventilation, such as in patients with neuromuscular diseases [13]
- presence of difficult or prolonged weaning [14], in patients with the perspective of a successful weaning after correction of the causes for failure and clinical stabilization.

6.4   Timing

Besides correct indications, it is also important to choose the right timing to perform a tracheotomy.

In the past, a great challenge has been to assess the effectiveness and safety of early versus late tracheotomy in critically ill adults with different clinical conditions, with respect to their clinical outcomes. Early tracheotomy is defined as a procedure performed within the first 10 days from tracheal intubation, while late tracheotomy if occurring later than 10 days [15].

A certain number of clinical trials have been conducted to investigate and compare these different strategies with respect to mortality, duration of mechanical ventilation, occurrence of VAP, ICU length of stay, and other potentially relevant outcomes, such as recannulation, reintubation, nutrition, self-extubation, successful weaning, bed-to-chair transfer, cannula displacement, and duration of sedation [15].

6.5   Main Evidences on Mortality

In the literature, some randomized controlled trials have compared early and late tracheotomy, to assess if one strategy would improve survival rate, as compared to the other one.

In 2004, Rumbak and colleagues published the first randomized controlled trial comparing early versus late tracheotomy [16]. One-hundred twenty patients, projected to need ventilation support for more than 14 days, received percutaneous dilational tracheotomy within 48 h from intubation (early group) or 14–16 days after (late group). The mortality rate was significantly lower in the early tracheotomy group (31.6%), as opposed to the delayed group (61.7%).Of note, early tracheotomy was characterized by a reduced rate of patients developing VAP, shorter ICU length of stay and time spent under mechanical ventilation and sedation [16].

Two years later, Barquist and colleagues randomized 60 trauma patients to receive early (before day 8) or late (after day 28) tracheotomy [17]. The trial was halted after the first interim analysis (50% of the recruitment) due to lack of differences in all assessed outcomes. In particular, mortality rate was 6.9% and 16.1% in early and late tracheotomy group, respectively [17].

In 2008, another study by Blot and colleagues randomized 123 patients, with an expected duration of iMV longer than 7 days, to receive early (within 48 h) or late (after 14 days) tracheotomy. In this trial, the mortality rate was similar between the two populations (20 vs. 24%, respectively); furthermore, also the incidence of VAP was similar between groups [18].

In 2010, a large Italian multicenter trial has randomized 419 critically ill patients with acute respiratory failure and mechanically ventilated for 24 h, to receive early (6–8 days) or late (13–15 days) tracheotomy [19]. The first clinical outcome was the rate of VAP that tended to reduction in early tracheotomy (14%), as compared to late group (21%, $p = 0.07$), with a 33% risk reduction [19]. Survivals at 28 days and 1 year were not different between the two tracheotomy timing strategies [19].

Following, another French trial randomized 216 adults requiring mechanical ventilation 4 or more days after cardiac surgery to receive early (immediate at day 4) or late (after day 15) tracheotomy [20] Also, in this trial, the mortality rates at 28, 60, and 90 days, and the incidence of VAP and infections were similar between groups [20].

Yue et al. enrolled 495 patients receiving iMV with an acute respiratory failure characterized by an arterial partial pressure to inspired fraction of oxygen ratio <200 mmHg. Patients were randomized to undergo or an early (day 3) tracheotomy or a late (day 15) strategy [21]. Early tracheotomy resulted in more ventilator-free, sedation-free, and ICU-free days, higher successful weaning and ICU discharge rate, and lower incidence of VAP; however, the 28-day mortalities (14 vs 10%, respectively) and cumulative 60-day incidence of death, were similar between early and late tracheotomy [21].

In 2012, 60 patients with severe ischemic or hemorrhagic stroke and an estimated need for at least 2 weeks of ventilation were randomized by Bosel and colleagues to either early tracheostomy (within day 1–3 from intubation) or to standard tracheostomy (between day 7 and 14 from intubation if extubation could not be achieved or was not feasible) [22]. ICU mortality (10 versus 47%; $p < 0.01$) and 6-month mortality (27 versus 60%; $p = 0.02$) were lower in the early group than in the standard group, respectively. On the opposite, no differences were observed with regard to the ICU length of stay or to most secondary outcomes, including adverse effects [22].

In the end, Young et al. randomized 990 patients, requiring at least 7 days of ventilatory support, to receive early (within 4 days) or late (after day 10) tracheotomy. The all-cause mortality 30 days from randomization was not statistically different in the two groups (30.8 versus 31.5%). The 1- and 2-year survival also showed no statistically significant differences [23].

Therefore, results from the literature are quite contradictory. A systematic review and meta-analysis published by Andriolo and colleagues reported a moderate quality of evidence for a lower mortality rate at the longest follow-up time in the group receiving early tracheostomy, than late tracheotomy (47.1% versus 53.2%, respectively), with a statistically significant risk ratio of 0.83 (95% confidence interval 0.70–0.98; $p = 0.03$) [15].

6.6 Conclusions

Considering the uneven evidences from the literature and trials, the procedure of tracheostomy should not follow strict rules regarding time, but should be tailored to the individual patient. In particular, healthcare providers should consider the underlying cause of respiratory failure and the clinical course. As a general consideration and suggestion, it is reasonable that physicians should wait at least 10 days before deciding to perform tracheostomy, if prolonged iMV cannot be predicted.

References

1. Holzapfel L, Chevret S, Madinier G, Ohen F, Demingeon G, Coupry A, Chaudet M. Influence of long-term oro- or nasotracheal intubation on nosocomial maxillary sinusitis and pneumonia: results of a prospective, randomized, clinical trial. Crit Care Med. 1993;21:1132–8.
2. Nieszkowska A, Combes A, Luyt CE, Ksibi H, Trouillet JL, Gibert C, Chastre J. Impact of tracheotomy on sedative administration, sedation level, and comfort of mechanically ventilated intensive care unit patients. Crit Care Med. 2005;33:2527–33.
3. Lassen HC. A preliminary report on the 1952 epidemic of poliomyelitis in Copenhagen with special reference to the treatment of acute respiratory insufficiency. Lancet. 1953;1:37–41.
4. Szmuk P, Ezri T, Evron S, Roth Y, Katz J. A brief history of tracheostomy and tracheal intubation, from the bronze age to the space age. Intensive Care Med. 2008;34:222–8.
5. Hussey JD, Bishop MJ. Pressures required to move gas through the native airway in the presence of a fenestrated vs a nonfenestrated tracheostomy tube. Chest. 1996;110:494–7.
6. Cowan T, Op't Holt TB, Gegenheimer C, Izenberg S, Kulkarni P. Effect of inner cannula removal on the work of breathing imposed by tracheostomy tubes: a bench study. Respir Care. 2001;46:460–5.
7. Ceriana P, Carlucci A, Navalesi P, Prinianakis G, Fanfulla F, Delmastro M, Nava S. Physiological responses during a T-piece weaning trial with a deflated tube. Intensive Care Med. 2006;32:1399–403.
8. Shaker R, Dodds WJ, Dantas RO, Hogan WJ, Arndorfer RC. Coordination of deglutitive glottic closure with oropharyngeal swallowing. Gastroenterology. 1990;98:1478–84.
9. Thompson-Henry S, Braddock B. The modified Evan's blue dye procedure fails to detect aspiration in the tracheostomized patient: five case reports. Dysphagia. 1995;10:172–4.
10. Gregoretti C, Squadrone V, Fogliati C, Olivieri C, Navalesi P. Transtracheal open ventilation in acute respiratory failure secondary to severe chronic obstructive pulmonary disease exacerbation. Am J Respir Crit Care Med. 2006;173:877–81.
11. Gregoretti C, Olivieri C, Navalesi P. Physiologic comparison between conventional mechanical ventilation and transtracheal open ventilation in acute traumatic quadriplegic patients. Crit Care Med. 2005;33:1114–8.
12. De Leyn P, Bedert L, Delcroix M, Depuydt P, Lauwers G, Sokolov Y, Van Meerhaeghe A, Van Schil P. Tracheotomy: clinical review and guidelines. Eur J Cardiothorac Surg. 2007;32:412–21.

13. Ergan B, Oczkowski S, Rochwerg B, Carlucci A, Chatwin M, Clini E, Elliott M, Gonzalez-Bermejo J, Hart N, Lujan M, Nasilowski J, Nava S, Pepin JL, Pisani L, Storre JH, Wijkstra P, Tonia T, Boyd J, Scala R, Windisch W. European Respiratory Society guidelines on long-term home non-invasive ventilation for management of COPD. Eur Respir J. 2019;54:1901003.
14. Boles JM, Bion J, Connors A, Herridge M, Marsh B, Melot C, Pearl R, Silverman H, Stanchina M, Vieillard-Baron A, Welte T. Weaning from mechanical ventilation. Eur Respir J. 2007;29:1033–56.
15. Andriolo BN, Andriolo RB, Saconato H, Atallah AN, Valente O. Early versus late tracheostomy for critically ill patients. Cochrane Database Syst Rev. 2015;1:CD007271.
16. Rumbak MJ, Newton M, Truncale T, Schwartz SW, Adams JW, Hazard PB. A prospective, randomized, study comparing early percutaneous dilational tracheotomy to prolonged translaryngeal intubation (delayed tracheotomy) in critically ill medical patients. Crit Care Med. 2004;32:1689–94.
17. Barquist ES, Amortegui J, Hallal A, Giannotti G, Whinney R, Alzamel H, MacLeod J. Tracheostomy in ventilator dependent trauma patients: a prospective, randomized intention-to-treat study. J Trauma. 2006;60:91–7.
18. Blot F, Similowski T, Trouillet JL, Chardon P, Korach JM, Costa MA, Journois D, Thiery G, Fartoukh M, Pipien I, Bruder N, Orlikowski D, Tankere F, Durand-Zaleski I, Auboyer C, Nitenberg G, Holzapfel L, Tenaillon A, Chastre J, Laplanche A. Early tracheotomy versus prolonged endotracheal intubation in unselected severely ill ICU patients. Intensive Care Med. 2008;34:1779–87.
19. Terragni PP, Antonelli M, Fumagalli R, Faggiano C, Berardino M, Pallavicini FB, Miletto A, Mangione S, Sinardi AU, Pastorelli M, Vivaldi N, Pasetto A, Della Rocca G, Urbino R, Filippini C, Pagano E, Evangelista A, Ciccone G, Mascia L, Ranieri VM. Early vs late tracheotomy for prevention of pneumonia in mechanically ventilated adult ICU patients: a randomized controlled trial. JAMA. 2010;303:1483–9.
20. Trouillet JL, Luyt CE, Guiguet M, Ouattara A, Vaissier E, Makri R, Nieszkowska A, Leprince P, Pavie A, Chastre J, Combes A. Early percutaneous tracheotomy versus prolonged intubation of mechanically ventilated patients after cardiac surgery: a randomized trial. Ann Intern Med. 2011;154:373–83.
21. Zheng Y, Sui F, Chen XK, Zhang GC, Wang XW, Zhao S, Song Y, Liu W, Xin X, Li WX. Early versus late percutaneous dilational tracheostomy in critically ill patients anticipated requiring prolonged mechanical ventilation. Chin Med J. 2012;125:1925–30.
22. Bosel J, Schiller P, Hook Y, Andes M, Neumann JO, Poli S, Amiri H, Schonenberger S, Peng Z, Unterberg A, Hacke W, Steiner T. Stroke-related early tracheostomy versus prolonged orotracheal intubation in neurocritical care trial (SETPOINT): a randomized pilot trial. Stroke. 2013;44:21–8.
23. Young D, Harrison DA, Cuthbertson BH, Rowan K. Effect of early vs late tracheostomy placement on survival in patients receiving mechanical ventilation: the TracMan randomized trial. JAMA. 2013;309:2121–9.

Pharmacological Management of Cardiac Arrest

7

Vladimir Lomivorotov, Martina Baiardo Redaelli, and Vladimir Boboshko

Contents

V. Lomivorotov (✉)
Department of Anesthesiology and Intensive Care, E. Meshalkin National Medical Research Center, Novosibirsk, Russia

Department of Anaesthesiology and Intensive Care, Novosibirsk State University, Novosibirsk, Russia
e-mail: vvlom@mail.ru

M. Baiardo Redaelli
Department of Anesthesia and Intensive Care, IRCCS San Raffaele Scientific Institute, Milan, Italy
e-mail: baiardoredaelli.martina@hsr.it

V. Boboshko
Department of Anesthesiology and Intensive Care, E. Meshalkin National Medical Research Center, Novosibirsk, Russia

© Springer Nature Switzerland AG 2021
G. Landoni et al. (eds.), *Reducing Mortality in Critically Ill Patients*,
https://doi.org/10.1007/978-3-030-71917-3_7

7.1   General Principles

Cardiac arrest (CA) is defined as the abrupt loss of blood flow due to sudden interruption of heart function. Cardiac arrest is associated with the loss of breathing and consciousness, and it is primarily due to a disturbance in the electrical activity of heart [1]. The etiology of CA is multifactorial and includes cardiac and non-cardiac causes [2]. The exact incidence of CA incidence is difficult to estimate, as epidemiologic reports often include CA subtypes according to location of occurrence. The management of out-of-hospital cardiac arrest (OHCA) is different from that of in-hospital cardiac arrest (IHCA) for several aspects, including longer times for trained personnel to attend, limited equipment and availability of drugs on scene, and several challenges to implementation of treatment guidelines [3].

In the United States, OHCA is responsible for over 350,000 deaths in every year [4] and is still the major public health challenge worldwide. The global incidence of IHCA in adults has not been well described, it has been estimated for the United States to be around 292,000 events annually, or 9–10 IHCA per 1000 admissions [5].

Despite advances in resuscitation and critical care medicine, the rates of survival after CA are largely variable at global level [6] and still remain as low as 11% at hospital discharge [4].

Shockable rhythms (ventricular fibrillation (VF) and pulseless ventricular tachycardia (pVT)) are associated with better clinical outcomes if promptly treated with defibrillation, when compared with non-shockable rhythms [7]. Early initiation of cardiopulmonary resuscitation (CPR) is associated with improved outcomes for both OHCA [8] and IHCA [9].

Chest compressions, ventilation, and early defibrillation, when applicable, are the cornerstones of CA treatment [10].

However, drugs are universally employed in cardiac arrest as a resuscitative measure to enhance coronary perfusion pressure (CPP) and peripheral blood flow and to further improve defibrillation success. Many drugs have been tested in this setting to improve outcomes after OHCA and IHCA. Most of existing evidences concerns the use of antiarrhythmic drugs and vasopressors (epinephrine, vasopressin) and comes from trials conducted in the OHCA setting. Other medications that are used in the treatment of CA, with possible favorable effects on survival, include steroids, magnesium sulfate, bretylium tosylate, and sodium bicarbonate.

7.2   Pathophysiologic Principles

Weisfeldt and Becker described the resuscitation after CA from primary cardiac causes as a time-sensitive three-phase model [11]. This model for CA suggests that the optimal treatment is phase-specific and identify *the electrical phase,* which start at the time of CA and last approximately 4 min following the arrest; *the circulatory phase,* between 4 and 10 min; and *the metabolic phase*, that starts 10 min after CA. In the electrical phase, immediate defibrillation leads to 50% survival [12].

Antiarrhythmic drugs possibly plays a role in reducing the maintenance or recurrence of arrhythmia the return of spontaneous circulation occurs (ROSC) [13].

In the circulatory phase, the accumulation of metabolites and tissue hypoxia reduce the chance of effective defibrillation, thus restoration of CPP is pivotal. Study in humans showed a positive correlation between initial and maximum CPP and ROSC. Furthermore, initial CPP was a stronger predictor for ROSC than the time of no-flow [14]. The importance of hemodynamic optimization during the circulatory phase provides the rationale for the use of vasopressor agents during CPR.

During the metabolic phase, the ischemia and reperfusion mechanism may result in circulating metabolic factors that cause additional injury and the efficacy of circulatory supportive measures are reduced [15]. Vasopressors, helpful during the previous phase, may however contribute to complementary organ ischemia and may lead to reduced survival during the metabolic phase. Identifying drugs with positive effects in this phase is very challenging, due to the extremely low survival rates in patients with prolonged CA.

7.3   Main Evidences

7.3.1   Advanced Cardiac Life Support with/without Drugs

Placing an intravenous (iv) access for drug administration is a mandatory part of advanced cardiac life support (ACLS). The administration of iv drugs in CA was assessed in a prospective, randomized controlled trial (RCT) during OHCA: the authors compared the clinical outcomes of patients receiving standard ACLS with iv drug administration (418 patients) versus ACLS maneuvers without iv drug (433 patients) [16]. The rate of survival to hospital discharge was 10.5% for the iv drug group and 9.2% for the no iv drug group ($p = 0.61$) and 32% vs 21%, respectively, in patients admitted to hospital after ROSC ($p < 0.001$). As compared with the no iv drug group, in the iv drug group survival with favorable neurological outcome was 9.8% vs 8.1% ($p = 0.45$), and 1-year survival was 10% vs 8% ($p = 0.53$). Compared with patients who didn't received iv drugs during ACLS following OHCA, patients who received drug administration through an iv access had higher rates of short-term survival without statistically significant differences in survival at hospital discharge or long-term survival.

7.3.2   Antiarrhythmics

Lidocaine and amiodarone are commonly used to improve the successful of defibrillation in shock-refractory VF or pVT and to prevent arrhythmic recurrences. Amiodarone belongs to class III antiarrhythmic drug and acts by blocking potassium rectifier currents that drives the repolarization of the heart during the phase 3 of the cardiac action potential.

In a double-blind RCT by Kudenchuk and colleagues, patients with OHCA from VF or pVT who were still in cardiac arrest after the third precordial shock were assigned to receive either 300 mg of iv amiodarone (246 patients) or placebo (258 patients) [17]. Patients treated with amiodarone had more possibilities to achieve ROSC and to survive at admission (risk ratio [RR], 1.27; 95% confidence interval [CI], 1.02–1.59); however, when comparing survival rate at discharge there was no significant difference between the two groups (RR, 1.02; 95% CI, 0.65–1.59). Amiodarone compared with placebo significantly improved the outcome for initial resuscitation, according to survival to hospital admission.

The effects of amiodarone versus lidocaine during CPR were assessed in two studies. Dorian and colleagues [18] randomized 247 OHCA patients with VF/pVT refractory to defibrillation to receive (double-blind) either amiodarone 5 mg/kg or lidocaine 1.5 mg/kg. If VF persisted after a further shock, a second dose was administered (1.5 mg/kg lidocaine or 2.5 mg/kg amiodarone) and resuscitation continued. Patients that were treated with amiodarone had a significantly higher rate of survival to admission compared with the lidocaine group (RR, 1.90; 95% CI, 1.16–3.11). However, no statistically significant difference was found in the survival rates between the two groups at discharge (RR, 1.67; 95% CI, 0.57–4.88). In another double-blinded, parallel designed trial, Somberg and colleagues showed superiority of amiodarone compared with lidocaine for the treatment of shock-refractory VT [19]. These authors randomized 29 patients to receive either up to two boluses 150 mg iv amiodarone (18 patients) or 100 mg lidocaine (11 patients) followed by infusion for 24 h. If the first assigned medication failed to cease VT, the patient was crossed over to the alternative medication. The 24-h survival was 39% in the amiodarone group and 9% in the lidocaine group ($p < 0.01$). This study found that amiodarone is more effective in the treatment of shock-resistant VT than lidocaine.

In contrast with the above-discussed trials, a recent large RCT showed that the treatment with neither amiodarone nor lidocaine resulted in a significantly higher rate of survival to hospital discharge compared with placebo after OHCA caused by shock-refractory VF or pVT [20]. In this study, 3026 patients were randomized to amiodarone (974), lidocaine (993), or placebo (1059); the rates of survival at hospital discharge were 24.4%, 23.7%, and 21.0%, respectively. The survival rate differences were of 3.2 percentage points for amiodarone versus placebo (95% CI, −0.4 to 7.0; $p = 0.08$); 2.6 percentage points for lidocaine versus placebo (95% CI, −1.0 to 6.3; $p = 0.16$); and 0.7 percentage points for amiodarone versus lidocaine (95% CI, −3.2 to 4.7; $p = 0.70$). ROSC rate was higher in patients receiving lidocaine compared with those receiving placebo, but there was no significant difference between patients receiving amiodarone compared with those receiving placebo. There was heterogeneity of treatment effect with respect to whether the arrest was witnessed or not ($p = 0.05$); the administration of active drugs was associated with a significantly higher survival rate compared to the placebo group among patients with bystander-witnessed arrest but not among those with unwitnessed arrest.

Bretylium tosylate is an antiarrhythmic drug [21]. It blocks the release of noradrenaline at nerve terminals, thus decreasing the output from the sympathetic nervous system. Furthermore, it blocks K+ channels and is considered a class III antiarrhythmic. Nowak et al. evaluated the effectiveness of intravenous bretylium tosylate as a first-line drug for patients in CA [22]. Fifty nine patients with CA due to VF or asystole initially received a rapid intravenous bolus of either bretylium (10 mg/kg) or placebo. If VF or asystole persisted, a second bolus of bretylium or normal saline was given after 20 min. 35% of patients who received bretylium was successfully resuscitated, whereas survival was only 6% in placebo group ($p < 0.05$). Two trials by Haynes et al. [23] and Olson et al. [24], respectively, compared the efficacy of lidocaine and bretylium in CA. There was no difference in survival to hospital discharge or ROSC occurrence [23, 24]. Bretylium is not commercially available anymore.

7.3.3 Inotropic/Vasopressor Drugs

Vasopressors are widely used during CA to increase CPP and cerebral perfusion pressure and, accordingly, improve the chance of ROSC. The rationale for vasopressor use during CA was described in the above-mentioned time-sensitive three-phase model by Weisfeldt and Becker [11]. Evidences proved that the use of vasopressors is associated with increased rate of ROSC. Epinephrine and vasopressin are the most frequently studied vasopressors in CA.

7.3.3.1 Epinephrine

Epinephrine is an α- and β-adrenergic agonist and its main cardiovascular effects include arterial and venous vasoconstriction together with increased inotropy and chronotropy [25]. Clinical effects of epinephrine in animal studies include increased rate of ROSC and short-term survival [26], but also postresuscitative myocardial dysfunction [27].

Despite epinephrine being universally considered "standard of care" in the treatment of CA, there were no well-designed RCTs to establish its efficacy until 2011, when Jacobs et al. published a double-blind, randomized, placebo-controlled trial of epinephrine use in OHCA which included 534 patients [28]. ROSC occurred in 22 out of 262 patients (8.4%) who received placebo and in 64 out of 272 patients (23.5%) who received epinephrine (odds ratio [OR], 3.4; 95% CI 2.0–5.6). Survival to hospital discharge occurred in 5 (1.9%) for patients who received placebo and 11 (4.0%) for patients epinephrine (OR, 2.2; 95% CI 0.7–6.3). Patients randomized to epinephrine during CA had no statistically significant improvement in survival to hospital discharge although there was a significantly improved likelihood of achieving ROSC.

In a randomized, double-blind trial that involved 8014 patients with OHCA in the United Kingdom, patients received either parenteral epinephrine (4015 patients) or saline (3999 patients), along with standard care [29]. The primary outcome (30-day survival) occurred in 130/4015 patients (3.2%) in the epinephrine group and in 94/3999 patients (2.4%) in the placebo group (unadjusted OR for survival, 1.39; 95% CI, 1.06–1.82; $p = 0.02$). However, there was no significant between-group difference in the rate of a favorable neurologic outcome.

For several years, clinicians have also wondered about the optimal dose of epinephrine to be used in CA. The "standard" epinephrine dose (1.0 mg) is not based on body weight. A large multicenter RCT failed to show any benefit from repeated high doses of epinephrine as compared with repeated standard doses in OHCA patients [30]. In this study, 3327 patients were randomly assigned to receive up to 15 doses of epinephrine either high doses (5 mg each) or standard doses (1 mg each) according to the current protocol for ACLS. Among the high-dose group of patients, the 26.5% survived to hospital admission, compared to the 23.6% of those in the standard-dose group ($p = 0.05$); at hospital discharge the 2.3% of patients in the high-dose group and 2.8% in the standard-dose group were alive ($p = 0.34$). Repeated high doses of epinephrine improved the rate of ROSC, but did not improve the long-term survival after OHCA compared with repeated standard doses.

7.3.3.2 Vasopressin

Vasopressin was been recommended as an alternative vasopressor to replace the first or second dose of epinephrine in CA [31]. It exerts his activity via specific G-protein-coupled receptors. Three specific vasopressin receptors (V1, V2, V3) are responsible for the pharmacological effects of vasopressin. Animal studies found improved CPP, ROSC, and myocardial blood flow for vasopressin compared with epinephrine [32]. Endogenous vasopressin levels are significantly higher in survivors to CPR than in patients who do not have ROSC [33]. However, human studies comparing vasopressin with epinephrine yielded mixed results. In the first RCT of epinephrine vs vasopressin in CA, Lindner and colleagues [34] randomly assigned 40 patients with VF resistant to defibrillation to either 1 mg iv epinephrine ($n = 20$) or 40 U iv vasopressin ($n = 20$) as primary drug therapy for CA. Seven patients (35%) in the epinephrine group and 14 patients (70%) in the vasopressin group survived to hospital admission ($p = 0.06$). At 24 h, 4 patients (20%) in the epinephrine group and 12 patients (60%) in the vasopressin group were alive ($p = 0.02$). 3 out of the 20 patients (15%) who received epinephrine and 8 out of the 20 patients (40%) who received vasopressin survived to hospital discharge ($p = 0.16$). In this small study, therefore, although a significantly larger proportion of patients who were treated with vasopressin was resuscitated successfully from out-of-hospital VF and survived for 24 h as compared with those treated with epinephrine, and no difference between groups was found in survival to hospital discharge.

Wenzel et al. compared the administration two doses of 40 IU of vasopressin or 1 mg of epinephrine randomizing 1219 OHCA patients, and additional treatment with epinephrine was added if needed [35]. No statistically significant difference in survival was found at discharge. However, in asystolic patients, vasopressin achieved a significantly higher rate of ROSC and survival to hospital discharge (29 vs. 20%, p 1/4 0.02, and 4.7 vs. 1.5%, p 1/4 0.04, respectively). Finally, a randomized controlled study from Ong et al. compared a single administration of either epinephrine (1 mg) or vasopressin (40 IU) at the admission in the emergency department in 727 OHCA patients [36]. This study did not found significant survival difference at hospital discharge although there was a trend towards improved survival in the subgroup of patients with shockable rhythm treated with vasopressin.

7.3.4   Steroids

Adrenal insufficiency is associated with poor outcome and is common both in critically ill and post-cardiac arrest patients [37]. The reason of these hormonal changes relies in multiple pathophysiological mechanisms including increased metabolic demand, ischemia/reperfusion injury of the adrenal glands, and the ongoing systemic inflammatory response after CA [38]. Steroids administration in this setting could work via both hemodynamic and immunologic mechanisms. However, despite the possible pathophysiological rationale, there is lack of evidence that corticosteroid therapy could exert beneficial effects in the setting of CA [39].

In a placebo-controlled trial published in 2009, Mentzelopoulos et al. randomized patients with IHCA to multiple doses of epinephrine (1 mg) plus placebo or a combination of vasopressin (20 IU) and epinephrine every for the five first resuscitation cycles [40]. Parallel with the first injection (on the first resuscitation cycle), a dose of methylprednisolone (40 mg) was given to the intervention group. Additionally, in patients with hemodynamic instability after resuscitation, hydrocortisone (300 mg) was administered daily in the intervention group. Among the 99 enrolled patients, a statistically significant benefit was found in the treatment group with regard to the primary endpoints of ROSC (81 vs. 52%, p 1/4 0.003) and survival at hospital discharge (19 vs. 4%, p 1/4 0.02).

In a subsequent larger trial by the same research group, in which some limitations of the 2009 study were addressed, patients were randomized according to the same study protocol (vasopressin, steroids, epinephrine [VSE], or control group) [41]. Unlike the previous study, this was multicenter (including 268 IHCA patients) and, accordingly, better powered. As compared with the control group, patients randomized to the VSE group had better probability of an ROSC of at least 20 min (83.9%[109/130] vs 65.9%[91/138]; OR, 2.98; 95% CI, 1.39–6.40; $p = 0.005$) and survival to hospital discharge with Cerebral Performance Categories score of 1 or 2 (13.9% [18/130] vs 5.1% [7/138]; OR, 3.28; 95% CI, 1.17–9.20; $p = 0.02$). Moreover, patients assigned to the VSE group with post-resuscitation shock had higher probability of survival to hospital discharge with CPC scores of 1 or 2 (21.1% [16/76] vs 8.2% [6/73]; OR, 3.74; 95% CI, 1.20–11.62; $p = 0.02$). Despite the promising results of the above-mentioned trials, it is difficult to evaluate the contribution of steroids because of the mixed intervention.

7.3.5   Other Drugs

The second most common intracellular cation after potassium is magnesium. Magnesium provides systemic and coronary vasodilation [42] and its use include the treatment of polymorphic VT associated with a prolonged QT interval [43]. In a few small RCTs, magnesium (2–5 g) was administered to patients as an adjunct to standard ACLS treatment when defibrillation had failed [44–48]. These trials failed to show any association between magnesium administration and survival to hospital discharge or either ROSC. However, the small sample size of these studies cannot rule out a type II error.

During cardiac arrest and CPR maneuvers, respiratory and metabolic acidosis arises from the retention of carbon dioxide and from the anaerobic metabolism with lactic acidosis. Severe acidosis both reduces the responsiveness to catecholamines and impairs the myocardial contractility. Before 1986, sodium bicarbonate was routinely used during CPR, regardless the patient's acid-base status. The administration of sodium bicarbonate in cardiac arrest changed due to the potential adverse effects of buffer therapy and due to the studies that failed to demonstrate any clinical benefits of its use [49]. A RCT by Dybvik et al. investigated the effect of sodium bicarbonate in 502 patients with OHCA. These patients were randomized to receive 250 mL sodium bicarbonate or normal saline. No difference was found in survival to hospital admission or discharge [50].

In an animal study on resuscitation from 2003, the administration of hypertonic solutions was found to improve myocardial blood flow, cerebral perfusion, and the incidence of ROSC after cardiac arrest [51]. The same group of researchers in 2012, randomized 203 patients with OHCA in order to compare the infusion of either 2 mL/kg of hypertonic saline (7.2% normal saline with 6% hydroxyethyl starch 200,000/0.5) versus hydroxyethyl starch alone [52]. However, the authors found no significant difference between groups in survival and hospital admission or discharge.

7.4   Discussion and Conclusions

High-quality RCTs of OHCA and IHCA are difficult to conduct and are rare. The use of vasopressors in CA has been a major component of resuscitation for decades, despite limited data supporting its efficacy. The differences between OHCA and IHCA are many, especially regarding patient characteristics and significantly faster drug administration during CPR. The impact on the outcome of epinephrine after IHCA could be very different when compared to OHCA and should be explored in further research. In summary, initial high iv dose epinephrine in CA may increase CPP and improve ROSC, but it may lead to post-arrest myocardial dysfunction. Current recommendations on epinephrine use state that: it can be given to patients in CA (Class 1; Level of Evidence B-R); on the basis of the protocols applied in clinical trials, it is reasonable to administer 1 mg every 3–5 min (Class 2a; Level of Evidence C-LD) [53]. The administration of high doses of epinephrine did not improve long-term survival and neurological outcome when used as initial therapy. Accordingly, higher doses of epinephrine are not recommended for routine use (Class 3: No Benefit; Level of Evidence B-R) [53].

Several gaps remain in the assessment of the optimal timing for vasopressor administration in CA due to non-shockable rhythms and also in the timing of vasopressor administration with respect to defibrillation shockable CA. These questions needs to be further addressed in well-designed randomized controlled studies. Updated 2019 recommendations state that, with respect to timing, for non-shockable CA, epinephrine should be administered as soon as possible (Class 2a; Level of Evidence C-LD) and for shockable CA, it may be reasonable to administer epinephrine after the failure of initial defibrillation attempts (Class 2b; Level of Evidence C-LD) [53].

Available data from current literature presents considerable controversy concerning the first-line antiarrhythmic agent for ventricular arrhythmia. Data on long-term survival and neurologic sequelae remain inconclusive, largely due to underpowered sample sizes of the RCTs. Existing randomized trials did not investigate the timing or the sequence of the administration of amiodarone versus epinephrine. No randomized trials were identified which addressed the use of amiodarone during IHCA. The 2018 recommendations for the use of antiarrhythmic drugs in adults during resuscitation from VF/pVT CA state that amiodarone or lidocaine may be considered for VF/pVT non-responding to shock. These medications may be useful especially in patients with witnessed arrest, for whom the time to drug administration may be shorter (Class IIb; Level of Evidence B-R) [54].

So far, no antiarrhythmic agent has shown to improve long-term survival or together with good neurological outcome. All the current treatment guidelines rely on potential benefits that were found in short-term outcomes (such as ROSC or survival to hospital admission). CPR and defibrillation are the only therapeutic strategies associated with improved survival in patients with VF/pVT [55]. The optimal sequence of interventions during ACLS maneuvers for VF/pVT CA, including the administration of a vasopressor or antiarrhythmic agents and the timing of drug administration in relation to shock delivery is still unclear and should represent a field of future randomized trials.

References

1. Benjamin EJ, Virani SS, Callaway CW, et al. Heart disease and stroke statistics-2018 update: a report from the American Heart Association. Circulation. 2018;137:e67–e492.
2. Hawkes C, Booth S, Ji C, et al. Epidemiology and outcomes from out-of-hospital cardiac arrests in England. Resuscitation. 2017;110:133–40.
3. Bigham BL, Koprowicz K, Aufderheide TP, et al. Delayed prehospital implementation of the 2005 American Heart Association guidelines for cardio-pulmonary resuscitation and emergency cardiac care. Prehosp Emerg Care. 2010;14(3):355–60.
4. Benjamin EJ, Blaha MJ, Chiuve SE, et al. Heart disease and stroke statistics-2017 update: a report from the American Heart Association. Circulation. 2017;135:e146–603.
5. Holmberg M, Ross C, Chan P, et al. Incidence of adult in-hospital cardiac arrest in the United States. In: Abstract presented at: American Heart Association resuscitation science symposium, Chicago, IL, 10–11 November 2018.
6. Nichol G, Thomas E, Callaway CW, et al. Regional variation in out-of-hospital cardiac arrest incidence and outcome. JAMA. 2008;300:1423–31.
7. Keller SP, Halperin HR. Cardiac arrest: the changing incidence of ventricular fibrillation. Curr Treat Options Cardiovasc Med. 2015;17:392.
8. Hasselqvist-Ax I, Riva G, Herlitz J, et al. Early cardiopulmonary resuscitation in out-of-hospital cardiac arrest. N Engl J Med. 2015;372(24):2307–15.
9. Andersen LW, Holmberg MJ, Berg KM, Donnino MW, Granfeldt A. In-hospital cardiac arrest: a review. JAMA. 2019;321(12):1200–10.

10. Neumar RW, Shuster M, Callaway CW, et al. Part 1: executive summary: 2015 American Heart Association guidelines update for cardiopulmonary resuscitation and emergency cardiovascular care. Circulation. 2015;132:S315–67.

11. Weisfeldt ML, Becker LB. Resuscitation after cardiac arrest: a 3-phase time- sensitive model. JAMA. 2002;288:3035–8.

12. De Maio VJ, Stiell IG, Wells GA, Spaite DW. Optimal defibrillation response intervals for maximum out-of-hospital cardiac arrest survival rates. Ann Emerg Med. 2003;42:242–50.

13. Kowey PR. Pharmacological effects of antiarrhythmic drugs. Review and update. Arch Intern Med. 1998;158:325–32.

14. Paradis NA, Martin GB, Rivers EP, Goetting MG, Appleton TJ, Feingold M, Nowak RM. Coronary perfusion pressure and the return of spontaneous circulation in human cardiopulmonary resuscitation. JAMA. 1990;263:1106–13.

15. Gordon E. Special report cardiocerebral resuscitation.The new cardiopulmonary resuscitation. Circulation. 2005;111:2134–42.

16. Olasveengen TM, Sunde K, Brunborg C, Thowsen J, Steen PA, Wik L. Intravenous drug administration during out-of-hospital cardiac arrest: a randomized trial. JAMA. 2009;302:2222–9.

17. Kudenchuk PJ, Cobb LA, Copass MK, Cummins RO, Doherty AM, Fahrenbruch CE, et al. Amiodarone for resuscitation after out-of-hospital cardiac arrest due to ventricular fibrillation. N Engl J Med. 1999;341:871–8.

18. Dorian P, Cass D, Schwartz B, Cooper R, Gelaznikas R, Barr A. Amiodarone as compared with lidocaine for shock- resistant ventricular fibrillation. N Engl J Med. 2002;346(12):884–90.

19. Somberg JC, Bailin SJ, Haffajee CI, Paladino WP, Kerin NZ, Bridges D, et al. Intravenous lidocaine versus intravenous amiodarone (in a new aqueous formulation) for incessant ventricular tachycardia. Am J Cardiol. 2002;90(8):853–9.

20. Kudenchuk PJ, Leroux BG, Daya M, et al. Antiarrhythmic drugs for nonshockable- turned-shockable out-of-hospital cardiac arrest: the ALPS study (amiodarone, lidocaine, or placebo). Circulation. 2017;136(22):2119–31.

21. Tiku PE, Nowell PT. Selective inhibition of K+-stimulation of Na,K-ATPase by bretylium. Br J Pharmacol. December 1991;104(4):895–900.

22. Nowak RM, Bodnar TJ, Dronen S, Gentzkow G, Tomlanovich MC. Bretylium tosylate as initial treatment for cardiopulmonary arrest: randomized comparison with placebo. Ann Emerg Med. 1981;10(8):404–7.

23. Haynes RE, Chinn TL, Copass MK, et al. Comparison of bretylium tosylate and lidocaine in management of out of hospital ventricular fibrillation: a randomized clinical trial. Am J Cardiol. 1981;48(2):353–6.

24. Olson DW, Thompson BM, Darin JC, et al. A randomized comparison study of bretylium tosylate and lidocaine in resuscitation of patients from out-of-hospital ventricular fibrillation in a paramedic system. Ann Emerg Med. 1984;13(9 Pt 2):807–10.

25. Ahlquist RP. A study of the adrenotropic receptors. Am J Phys. 1948;153:586–600.

26. Yakaitis RW, Otto CW, Blitt CD. Relative importance of alpha and beta adrenergic receptors during resuscitation. Crit Care Med. 1979;7:293–6.

27. Tang W, Weil MH, Sun S, Noc M, Yang L, Gazmuri RJ. Epinephrine increases the severity of postresuscitation myocardial dysfunction. Circulation. 1995;92:3089–93.

28. Jacobs IG, Finn JC, Jelinek GA, Oxer HF, Thompson PL. Effect of adrenaline on survival in out-of-hospital cardiac arrest: a randomised double-blind placebo- controlled trial. Resuscitation. 2011;82:1138–43.

29. Perkins GD, Ji C, Deakin CD, Quinn T, Nolan JP, Scomparin C, Regan S, Long J, Slowther A, Pocock H, JJM B, Moore F, Fothergill RT, Rees N, O'Shea L, Docherty M, Gunson I, Han K, Charlton K, Finn J, Petrou S, Stallard N, Gates S, Lall R, PARAMEDIC2 Collaborators. A randomized trial of epinephrine in out-of-hospital cardiac arrest. N Engl J Med. 2018;379(8):711–21. https://doi.org/10.1056/NEJMoa1806842.

30. Gueugniaud PY, Mols P, Goldstein P, et al. A comparison of repeated high doses and repeated standard doses of epinephrine for cardiac arrest outside the hospital. European epinephrine study group. N Engl J Med. 1998;339(22):1595–601.

31. Neumar RW, Otto CW, Link MS, et al. Part 8: adult advanced cardiovascular life support: 2010 American Heart Association guidelines for cardiopulmonary resuscitation and emergency cardiovascular care. Circulation. 2010;122(18 Suppl 3):S729–67.
32. Wenzel V, Lindner KH, Krismer AC, et al. Survival with full neurologic recovery and no cerebral pathology after prolonged cardiopulmonary resuscitation with vasopressin in pigs. J Am Coll Cardiol. 2000;35(2):527–33.
33. Lindner KH, Strohmenger HU, Endinger H. Stress hormone response during and after cardiopulmonary resuscitation. Anesthesiology. 1992;77:662–8.
34. Lindner KH, Dirks B, Strohmenger HU. Randomized comparison of epinephrine and vasopressin in patients with out-of-hospital ventricular fibrillation. Lancet. 1997;349:535–7.
35. Wenzel V, Krismer AC, Arntz HR, Sitter H, Stadlbauer KH, Lindner KH. A comparison of vasopressin and epinephrine for out-of-hospital cardiopulmonary resuscitation. N Engl J Med. 2004;350:105–13.
36. Ong ME, Tiah L, Leong BS, Tan EC, Ong VY, Tan EA, Poh BY, Pek PP, Chen Y. A randomised, double-blind, multi-Centre trial comparing vasopressin and adrenaline in patients with cardiac arrest presenting to or in the emergency department. Resuscitation. 2012;83:953–60.
37. Kim JJ, Lim YS, Shin JH, Yang HJ, Kim JK, Hyun SY, et al. Relative adrenal insufficiency after cardiac arrest: impact on postresuscitation disease outcome. Am J Emerg Med. 2006;24(6):684–8.
38. Chalkias A, Xanthos T. Post-cardiac arrest syndrome: mechanisms and evaluation of adrenal insufficiency. World J Crit Care Med. 2012;1(1):4–9.
39. Peberdy MA, Callaway CW, Neumar RW, Geocadin RG, Zimmerman JL, Donnino M, et al. Part 9: post-cardiac arrest care: 2010 American Heart Association guidelines for cardiopulmonary resuscitation and emergency cardiovascular care. Circulation. 2010;122(18 Suppl 3):S768–86.
40. Mentzelopoulos SD, Zakynthinos SG, Tzoufi M. Vasopressin, epinephrine, and corticosteroids for in-hospital cardiac arrest. Arch Intern Med. 2009;169:15–24.
41. Mentzelopoulos SD, Malachias S, Chamos C. Vasopressin, steroids, and epinephrine and neurologically favorable survival after in-hospital cardiac arrest: a randomized clinical trial. JAMA. 2013;310:270–9.
42. Fawcett WJ, Haxby EJ, Male DA. Magnesium: physiology and pharmacology. Br J Anaesth. 1999;83:302–20.
43. Thomas SH, Behr ER. Pharmacological treatment of acquired QT prolongation and torsades de pointes. Br J Clin Pharmacol. 2015; https://doi.org/10.1111/bcp.12726.
44. Miller B, Craddock L, Hoffenberg S, Heinz S, Lefkowitz D, Callender ML, Battaglia C, Maines C, Masick D. Pilot study of intravenous magnesium sulfate in refractory cardiac arrest: safety data and recommendations for future studies. Resuscitation. 1995;30:3–14.
45. Allegra J, Lavery R, Cody R, Birnbaum G, Brennan J, Hartman A, Horowitz M, Nashed A, Yablonski M. Magnesium sulfate in the treatment of refractory ventricular fibrillation in the prehospital setting. Resuscitation. 2001;49:245–9.
46. Hassan TB, Jagger C, Barnett DB. A randomised trial to investigate the efficacy of magnesium sulphate for refractory ventricular fibrillation. Emerg Med J. 2002;19:57–62.
47. Thel MC, Armstrong AL, McNulty SE, Califf RM, O'Connor CM. Randomised trial of magnesium in in-hospital cardiac arrest. Duke internal medicine housestaff. Lancet. 1997;350:1272–6.
48. Fatovich DM, Prentice DA, Dobb GJ. Magnesium in cardiac arrest (the magic trial). Resuscitation. 1997;35:237–41.
49. Aufderheide TP, Martin DR, Olson DW, et al. Prehospital bicarbonate use in cardiac arrest: a 3-year experience. Am J Emerg Med. 1992;10(1):4–7.
50. Dybvik T, Strand T, Steen PA. Buffer therapy during out-of-hospital cardiopulmonary resuscitation. Resuscitation. 1995;29:89–95.
51. Breil M, Krep H, Sinn D, Hagendorff A, Dahmen A, Eichelkraut W, Hoeft A, Fischer M. Hypertonic saline improves myocardial blood flow during CPR, but is not enhanced further by the addition of hydroxy ethyl starch. Resuscitation. 2003;56:307–17.

52. Breil M, Krep H, Heister U, Bartsch A, Bender R, Schaefers B, Hoeft A, Fischer M. Randomised study of hypertonic saline infusion during resuscitation from out-of-hospital cardiac arrest. Resuscitation. 2012;83:347–52.

53. Soar J, Maconochie I, Wyckoff MH, Olasveengen TM, Singletary EM, Greif R, Aickin R, Bhanji F, Donnino MW, Mancini ME, et al. 2019 international consensus on cardiopulmonary resuscitation and emergency cardiovascular care science with treatment recommendations: summary from the basic life support; advanced life support; pediatric life support; neonatal life support; education, implementation, and teams; and first aid task forces. Circulation. 2019;140:e826–80.

54. Soar J, Donnino MW, Andersen LW, Berg KM, Böttiger BW, Callaway CW, Deakin CD, Drennan I, Neumar RW, Nicholson TC, O'Neil BJ, Paiva EF, Parr MJ, Reynolds JC, Ristagno G, Sandroni C, Wang TL, Welsford M, Nolan JP, Morley PT. Antiarrhythmic drugs for cardiac arrest in adults and children consensus on science and treatment recommendations. Brussels: International Liaison Committee on Resuscitation (ILCOR) Advanced Life Support Task Force. 2018. https://costr.ilcor.org/document/antiarrhythmic-drugs-for-cardiac-arrest-adults. Accessed 30 July 2018.

55. Neumar RW, Otto CW, Link MS, Kronick SL, Shuster M, Callaway CW, Kudenchuk PJ, Ornato JP, McNally B, Silvers SM, Passman RS, White RD, Hess EP, Tang W, Davis D, Sinz E, Morrison LJ. Part 8: adult advanced cardiovascular life support: 2010 American Heart Association guidelines for cardiopulmonary resuscitation and emergency cardiovascular care. Circulation. 2010;122(suppl 3):S729–67.

Non-pharmacological Management of Cardiac Arrest

8

Evgeny Fominskiy, Egor I. Zakharchenko, and Valery A. Nepomniashchikh

Contents

8.1   General Principles

Cardiac arrest is the cessation of cardiac mechanical activity, as confirmed by the absence of signs of circulation [1]. It represents a serious worldwide public health concern [1, 2]. In the United States, the incidence of out-of-hospital cardiac arrest (OHCA) in adults is about 141 per 100,000 people (347,322 per year) while in-hospital cardiac arrest (IHCA) is near 1.99 per 1000 hospitalization days. Millions more occur across the rest of North America, Europe, and Asia [2, 3]. While global survival after OHCA has significantly increased in the past 40 years, it remains unacceptably low at hospital discharge, accounting of 8.8% (95% confidence interval (CI), 8.2–9.4%) [4]. Survival at hospital discharge does not exceed 20% in IHCA according to the actual largest studies [5].

E. Fominskiy (✉)
Department of Anaesthesia and Intensive Care, IRCCS San Raffaele Scientific Institute, Milan, Italy
e-mail: fominskiy.evgeny@hsr.it

E. I. Zakharchenko
Altai State Medical University, Barnaul, Russia

V. A. Nepomniashchikh
Department of Anaesthesia and Intensive Care, Meshalkin National Medical Research Center, Novosibirsk, Russia
e-mail: nepomna57@mail.ru

© Springer Nature Switzerland AG 2021
G. Landoni et al. (eds.), *Reducing Mortality in Critically Ill Patients*,
https://doi.org/10.1007/978-3-030-71917-3_8

The pathophysiology of cardiac arrest and the subsequent post-cardiac arrest syndrome is very complex [6]. Cessation of the circulation determines acute ischemia which, together with ischemia-reperfusion injury triggers a series of events including endothelial activation, systemic inflammatory response, activation of immunological pathways and coagulation, mitochondrial damage, and microvascular dysfunction. Consequently, this leads to the post-cardiac arrest syndrome development, characterized by impaired myocardial function, macrocirculatory failure, global brain injury, and increased susceptibility to infections. The cardiac arrest etiology, duration, underlying precipitating factors and diseases and delay in cardiopulmonary resuscitation (CPR) may further complicate the clinical course [6].

In 2015, both the American Heart Association and the European Resuscitation Council published the update for cardiopulmonary resuscitation and emergency cardiovascular care [7, 8]. These guidelines provide the essential treatment algorithms for resuscitation including, among others, adult basic and advanced life support, use of automated external defibrillation and post-resuscitation care. Finally, both documents underline the necessity for further research in cardiac arrest and peri-arrest management.

8.2 Main Evidence

The current European Resuscitation Council guidelines for resuscitation in adults consider automated external defibrillation (AED) as a part of basic life support, underlining that the prompt use of AED is one of the key components for improving survival from OHCA [9]. Each minute of delay to defibrillation reduces the probability of survival to discharge by 10–12% [10]. Early defibrillation provided by emergency medical technician (EMT) was studied within a multilevel response system [11]. It consisted of the first level by EMT trained to provide cardiopulmonary resuscitation (CPR) and the second level by paramedic that was able to deliver advanced cardiac life support. For the study, 406 EMTs received training in recognition of ventricular fibrillation (VF) and operation of a defibrillator. Along 3 years, researchers compared the effect of rapid defibrillation by EMT combined with paramedic care with that of standard EMT and paramedic care on survival from 540 witnessed patients with OHCA caused by VF. Only for 179 cases, the emergency care was provided randomly between the two types of services. Overall, survival was not significantly different between the two groups. However, when the cases were stratified by time intervals between arrival of EMTs and arrival of paramedics, 19% of cases treated with basic EMT, and paramedic care were discharged compared with 42% of patients treated with EMT defibrillation and paramedic care ($p < 0.05$) in time interval greater than 4 min. Furthermore, when this interval was more than 12 min, there were no discharged patients in basic EMT group, but 60% of patients in the EMT defibrillation survived at hospital discharge ($p < 0.05$).

Another strategy to provide early defibrillation is to deliver it even earlier, before emergency service arrival, by laypersons with the public-access AEDs. This strategy could reduce the time to defibrillation that was about 3.8 min (standard deviation (SD), 1.7) in the previously discussed study [11]. The Public Access Defibrillator Trial examined the effect of AED therapy (1600 AEDs) that was accessible to more than 11,000 trained lay volunteers without aspecific duty to respond [12]. Volunteers were recruited in 622 community units such as shopping malls and apartment complexes during averaged period of 21.5 months; the units were randomly assigned to an emergency-response system involving volunteers trained in CPR or CPR plus the use of AEDs. The use of AEDs increased survival to hospital discharge (30 survivors of 128 definite cardiac arrests vs. 15 of 107, $p = 0.03$) without a decrement in the neurological function of survivors. The PAD trial raised several important organizational and research problems for OHCA management. Out-of-hospital cardiac arrests were uncommon in the public units; the observed numbers of arrests were substantially lower than anticipated. This led to the study extension by 6 months to maintain the specified power level. The finding also emphasizes the difficulty of prospectively identifying locations where OHCA might occur. Another crucial point is that the majority of OHCA happens at home [13]. This category of patients remains unprotected even if such exemplary program would be implemented on a widespread basis.

One of the early attempts to enhance the efficacy of the pre-hospital CPR was a maneuver of the differential application of intrathoracic pressure: during chest compression to provide ventilation at high airway pressure to increase peripheral perfusion, while during chest compression release phase to decrease airway pressure to zero that allowed venous return from extrathoracic veins to occur [14]. This alternating maneuver resulted in a peripheral arteriovenous pressure gradient and hence, forwarded blood flow. Sixteen computer-driven cardiocompressors were built for this purpose. The machines provided 40 chest compressions per minute and synchronized simultaneous ventilation at 80 mmHg. Moreover, abdominal binders to further increase intrathoracic pressure during chest compressions were manufactured. Personnel of 12 rescue stations of fire department was randomly selected on one of the three shifts by study months to perform standard CPR or simultaneous compression and ventilation CPR. During 2 years, 994 patients were enrolled. Survival to hospital admission and to discharge was superior in the conventional CPR group as compared to the experimental group ($p < 0.01$ for both). Unfortunately, authors did not describe how such high airway pressure was provided in the simultaneous compression and ventilation CPR group; there was also no information about respiratory support in the control group. The lack of important methods details makes it difficult to completely explain the observed differences between groups. However, modern data in a large patient population show higher survival rate among patients who received chest compressions at a rate of 100–120 per minute, as compared to more or less frequencies [15]. Concerning the optimal respiratory support, ventilation strategy during CPR is still a broad field of research [16]. The current guidelines recommend ventilating the lungs at approximately 10 breaths per minute and avoiding hyperventilation (both excessive respiratory rate and tidal volume) [8].

The limited efficacy of conventional manual CPR contributed to the development of alternative techniques to deliver chest compressions as with the use of mechanical chest compressors. The active compression-decompression (ACD) device provided compressions depth from 2.5 to 5 cm and had a built-in monitoring system to regulate the force of compressions as to maintain similar chest compressions [17]. Active chest decompression was performed by active device withdrawal against the resistance of the patient chest wall until its full expansion. Along a 11-month period, the hospital resuscitation team randomized 53 IHCA patients to either standard manual CPR or to the ACD CPR. Mean duration of CPR was 18 min (SD, 11). Primary endpoints demonstrated that only 24-h survival was higher in the ACD CPR as compared with standard CPR (12 [48%] of 25 vs. 6 [21%] of 28, respectively, $p < 0.05$), whereas survival at hospital discharge was not different between groups. These results should be interpreted with caution because of the composite character of the primary outcome. Moreover, the compression rate might have been slightly different between the groups, and the resuscitation team was unblinded.

To further increase efficacy of ACD CPR, an inspiratory impedance threshold device (ITD) was proposed. It is a small device that fits on a face mask or an endotracheal tube. Pressure-sensitive valves within the ITD impede the influx of inspiratory gas during chest decompression in ACD CPR, thereby augmenting the amplitude and duration of the vacuum within the thorax and, consequently, increasing venous return. Patients with OHCA were sequentially randomized to ACD + ITD CPR ($n = 103$) or standard CPR ($n = 107$) by the advanced life support team [18]. The primary endpoint of 1-h survival after a witnessed arrest as well as 24-h survival rates were significantly higher with ACD + ITD CPR (55% and 41%, respectively) versus standard CPR (33% and 23%, respectively; $p < 0.05$ for both). Patients randomized ≥ 10 min after the call for help to the ACD + ITD CPR had a three times higher 1-h survival rate than control subjects ($p < 0.05$). As the study could not be blinded, there were greater numbers of unwitnessed cardiac arrest and patients not in VF in the standard CPR group, these categories of patients have less favorable outcomes after OHCA.

Besides ACD devices, there are other devices that provide active chest compression but passive chest decompression. One of these was studied in the context of IHCA that happened only in the intensive care units of four teaching hospitals [19]. The device had the audible feedback that provided the ICU staff the information to shift between the compression and decompression phases. A higher return of spontaneous circulation rate in the experimental group as compared to the control group (29 [72%] of 40 vs. 14 [35%] of 40, respectively; $p = 0.001$) was observed. It should be noted that the study groups were not well balanced: CPR guidelines adherence was significantly higher in the intervention group as well as the dosage of administered antiarrhythmics.

Another potential device that could improve CPR outcomes is integrated load-distributing band device that squeezes the patient's entire chest during CPR. The Circulation Improving Resuscitation Care (CIRC) Trial found equivalent survival in adult OHCA patients who received integrated load-distributing band CPR (iA-CPR) as compared to standard CPR [20]. However, the authors performed a pre-planned secondary analysis where they hypothesized that chest compression duration that was increased in the iA-CPR group would lead to a survival benefit when compared to standard CPR [21]. Chest compressions duration was defined as the total minutes spent on compressions during resuscitation and identified from transthoracic impedance and accelerometer data recorded by the emergency care defibrillator. When adjusting for chest compression duration, there was a survival benefit to hospital discharge with iA-CPR in patients with OHCA requiring more than 16.5 min of chest compressions (odds ratio 1.86 [95% CI, 1.16–3.00]; $p < 0.001$). Of note, 1360/2012 (68%) iA-CPR cases and 1260/2002 (63%) M-CPR cases had more than 16.5 min of chest compressions. Nevertheless, results should be considered as the secondary analysis data. Moreover, the researchers were only able to analyze compressions that were provided after the defibrillator was turned-on and the defibrillator pads attached on the patient chest. Thus, it is unknown how long patients were resuscitated prior to application of the defibrillation pads.

The smaller trial investigating the same device of iA-CPR versus standard CPR in OHCA patients found that 24-h survival rate was significantly higher in the iA-CPR group than in the standard CPR group (27 [39.1%] of 69 vs. 14 [21.9%] of 64, respectively; $p = 0.03$) [22]. The hospital discharge rate was also higher in the iA-CPR CPR group than in the standard CPR group (13 [18.8%] of 69 vs. 4 [6.3%] of 64, respectively; $p = 0.03$). Both outcomes represented the secondary study endpoints.

The analysis of the above-presented randomized controlled trials (RCTs) revealed that research in cardiac arrest clinical context is very challenging, partially due to the difficulty to predict cardiac arrest (especially OHCA), variety of environments where it can happen (home vs. public place, witnessed vs. unwitnessed, etc.), heterogeneity of its causes, lack of widespread community systems to deal with OHCA. On June 24, 2019 65 published manuscripts assessing the interventions in the intra- and post-cardiac arrest period were identified [23]. Almost the same number of trials was published from 2015 to 2019 as compared to all trials published prior to 2015, most of which were small with a median sample size of 90 participants and few trials with more than 500 participants. Only 6% of the included trials studied IHCA clinical context [23]. Almost all the above-discussed trials were also small studies in OHCA and, therefore, were underpowered to investigated clinically significant outcomes. Six of the eight studies investigated different devices aimed to increase the external heart massage quality during CPR compared with standard manual chest compression. However, despite the fact that these devices had technical feasibility and some experimental and clinical data of successful usage during CPR, recent findings demonstrated, in both swine model and OHCA patients, that lung edema is more prominent after mechanical chest compression as compared to manual chest compression [24] because mechanical chest compression was characterized by higher intrathoracic pressure swings which led to increased lung weight, reduced oxygenation, and respiratory system compliance. Thus, the concept of Cardiopulmonary resuscitation-associated lung edema underlines that we are only in the active search of the optimal CPR technologies and further RCTs are needed to make any definitive conclusions.

In conclusion, owing to the low quality of available evidence, it is impossible to determine conclusively whether early defibrillation and manual/mechanical chest compression devices can increase survival after cardiac arrest as compared with standard CPR. There is a need for further rigorous research through additional high-quality RCTs, including larger sample sizes and proper subgroup analysis.

References

1. Jacobs I, Nadkarni V, Bahr J, et al. Cardiac arrest and cardiopulmonary resuscitation outcome reports: update and simplification of the Utstein templates for resuscitation registries: a statement for healthcare professionals from a task force of the International Liaison Committee on Resuscitation (American Heart Association, European Resuscitation Council, Australian Resuscitation Council, New Zealand Resuscitation Council, Heart and Stroke Foundation of Canada, InterAmerican Heart Foundation, Resuscitation Councils of Southern Africa). Circulation. 2004;23:3385–97.
2. Virani SS, Alonso A, Benjamin EJ, et al. Heart disease and stroke statistics-2020 update: a report from the American Heart Association. Circulation. 2020;141:e139–596.
3. Berdowski J, Berg RA, Tijssen JGP, Koster RW. Global incidences of out-of-hospital cardiac arrest and survival rates: systematic review of 67 prospective studies. Resuscitation. 2010;81:1479–87.
4. Yan S, Gan Y, Jiang N, et al. The global survival rate among adult out-of-hospital cardiac arrest patients who received cardiopulmonary resuscitation: a systematic review and meta-analysis. Crit Care. 2020;24:61.
5. Sandroni C, Nolan J, Cavallaro F, Antonelli M. In-hospital cardiac arrest: incidence, prognosis and possible measures to improve survival. Intensive Care Med. 2007;33:237–45.
6. Nolan JP, Neumar RW, Adrie C, et al. Post-cardiac arrest syndrome: epidemiology, pathophysiology, treatment, and prognostication. A Scientific Statement from the International Liaison Committee on Resuscitation; the American Heart Association Emergency Cardiovascular Care Committee; the Council on Cardiovascular Surgery and Anesthesia; the Council on Cardiopulmonary, Perioperative, and Critical Care; the Council on Clinical Cardiology; the Council on Stroke. Resuscitation. 2008;79:350–79.
7. Neumar RW, Shuster M, Callaway CW, et al. Part 1: executive summary: 2015 American Heart Association guidelines update for cardiopulmonary resuscitation and emergency cardiovascular care. Circulation. 2015;132(18 Suppl 2):S315–67.
8. Monsieurs KG, Nolan JP, Bossaert LL, et al. European resuscitation council guidelines for resuscitation 2015: section 1. Executive summary. Resuscitation. 2015;95:1–80.
9. Perkins GD, Handley AJ, Koster RW, et al. European resuscitation council guidelines for resuscitation 2015: section 2. Adult basic life support and automated external defibrillation. Resuscitation. 2015;95:81–99.
10. Blom MT, Beesems SG, Homma PCM, et al. Improved survival after out-of-hospital cardiac arrest and use of automated external defibrillators. Circulation. 2014;18:1868–75.
11. Eisenberg MS, Hallstrom AP, Copass MK, et al. Treatment of ventricular fibrillation. Emergency medical technician defibrillation and paramedic services. JAMA. 1984;251:1723–6.
12. Hallstrom AP, Ornato JP, Weisfeldt M, et al. Public-access defibrillation and survival after out-of-hospital cardiac arrest. N Engl J Med. 2004;351:637–46.
13. Becker L, Eisenberg M, Fahrenbruch C, Cobb L. Public locations of cardiac arrest. Implications for public access defibrillation. Circulation. 1998;97:2106–9.
14. Krischer JP, Fine EG, Weisfeldt ML, et al. Comparison of prehospital conventional and simultaneous compression-ventilation cardiopulmonary resuscitation. Crit Care Med. 1989;17:1263–9.

15. Idris AH, Guffey D, Pepe PE, et al. Chest compression rates and survival following out-of-hospital cardiac arrest. Crit Care Med. 2015;43:840–8.
16. Charbonney E, Grieco DL, Cordioli RL, et al. Ventilation during cardiopulmonary resuscitation: what have we learned from models? Respir Care. 2019;64:1132–8.
17. Tucker KJ, Galli F, Savitt MA, et al. Active compression-decompression resuscitation: effect on resuscitation success after in-hospital cardiac arrest. J Am Coll Cardiol. 1994;24:201–9.
18. Wolcke BB, Mauer DK, Schoefmann MF, et al. Comparison of standard cardiopulmonary resuscitation versus the combination of active compression-decompression cardiopulmonary resuscitation and an inspiratory impedance threshold device for out-of-hospital cardiac arrest. Circulation. 2003;108:2201–5.
19. Amir Vahedian-Azimi A, Mohammadreza Hajiesmaeili M, Ali Amirsavadkouhi A, et al. Effect of the cardio first angel™ device on CPR indices: a randomized controlled clinical trial. Crit Care. 2016;20:147.
20. Wik L, Olsen J, Persse D, et al. Manual vs. integrated automatic load-distributing band CPR with equal survival after out of hospital cardiac arrest. The randomized CIRC trial. Resuscitation. 2014;85:741–8.
21. Olsen J, Lerner EB, Persse D, et al. Chest compression duration influences outcome between integrated load-distributing band and manual CPR during cardiac arrest. Acta Anaesthesiol Scand. 2016;60:222–9.
22. Gao C, Chen Y, Peng H, et al. Clinical evaluation of the AutoPulse automated chest compression device for out-of-hospital cardiac arrest in the northern district of Shanghai, China. Arch Med Sci. 2016;12:563–70.
23. Andersen LW, Lind PC, Vammen L, et al. Adult post-cardiac arrest interventions: an overview of randomized clinical trials. Resuscitation. 2020;147:1–11.
24. Magliocca A, Rezoagli E, Zani D, et al. Cardiopulmonary resuscitation-associated lung edema (CRALE) - a translational study. Am J Respir Crit Care Med. 2021;203:447–57.

Avoidance of Deep Sedation

9

Pasquale Nardelli, Stefano Fresilli, and Marta Mucchetti

Contents

9.1 General Principles

In spite of advances in support of all organ functions over the last decades, cognitive aspects of intensive care unit admission rarely take the central light. It is a common belief that patients admitted to the ICU are completely asleep at all times, but that does not correspond to truth. In fact, a large and growing body of evidence has shown that sedation is harmful, increasing the risk of infection, delirium, and death, and prolonging the time on mechanical ventilation in the ICU and hospital [1–3]. Modern approach to intensive care aims to a comprehensive approach to the patient well-being, including aspects related to pain, agitation/sedation, delirium, immobility, and sleep disruption [4].

A prompt understanding and a correct treating of the underlying cause of distress should be the cornerstone of today practice in intensive care unit sedation. The use

P. Nardelli (✉) · S. Fresilli · M. Mucchetti
Department of Anesthesia and Intensive Care, IRCCS San Raffaele Scientific Institute, Milan, Italy
e-mail: nardelli.pasquale@hsr.it; mucchetti.marta@hsr.it

© Springer Nature Switzerland AG 2021
G. Landoni et al. (eds.), *Reducing Mortality in Critically Ill Patients*,
https://doi.org/10.1007/978-3-030-71917-3_9

of nonpharmacological strategies should also be considered and implemented prior to the use of sedative drugs [5].

Distress in patients admitted to ICU may be caused by a mix of conditions, including anxiety, pain, delirium, dyspnea, and neuromuscular blockade.

- *Anxiety* may be due to fear of death, fear of suffering, and inability to communicate.
- *Pain* during ICU routine care or due to position, immobility, devices, and tubes is reported by a significant proportion of patients after discharge.
- *Delirium* may occur in up to 80% of patients admitted to ICU [6] although often underrecognized and may be caused by medications, infections, environment, electrolyte imbalances, malnutrition, or end organ dysfunction. Understanding and treating delirium using dedicated assessment tools may have an impact over ICU length of stay, duration of mechanical ventilation, and long-term cognitive function.
- *Dyspnea* may occur in spite of acceptable blood gas parameters. Adjusting ventilator settings to find the optimal adaptation should be tried before resuming to medications.
- *Neuromuscular blockade* requires sedation, as paralysis without sedation and pain control may be unpleasant and scary.

Screening and correcting the abovementioned conditions is the cornerstone of treating agitation in the ICU. Nonpharmacological strategies, including frequent communication, family visits, reestablishment of normal circadian cycles (including sleep and meals), but also relaxation therapy, guided imagery, and music therapy should be considered before resorting to pharmacological sedation [7]. Sedation is indicated if the agitation cannot be adequately controlled after correcting all causes of distress and after nonpharmacological interventions were proven to be insufficient.

9.2   Light Versus Deep Sedation

Current Society of Critical Care Medicine (SCCM) Guidelines suggest using light sedation in critically ill, mechanically ventilated adults, although the low overall quality of literature evidence only allowed to issue a conditional recommendation [4]. The scarcity of scientific evidence about light sedation is also worsened by the lack of a universally accepted definition of light sedation. Richmond Agitation-Sedation Scale (RASS, Table 9.1) [8] is frequently used to define the level of sedation in the ICU. The SCCM Guidelines suggest that a RASS score of −2 to +1 is generally considered a light sedation although they admit that this level of sedation is probably deeper than required for the average ICU patient. The ideal sedation goal is for the patient to be awake and comfortable with minimal to no distress (RASS score 0) [9]. Nevertheless, some patients may require higher sedation levels. The correct sedation level should be patient-tailored, evaluated at the bedside on a daily basis. In fact, sedation should be based on observed distress rather than

Table 9.1 Richmond agitation-sedation scale (RASS)

Score	Term	Description
+4	Combative	Overtly combative or violent; immediate danger to staff
+3	Very agitated	Pulls on or removes tube(s) or catheter(s) or has aggressive behavior toward staff
+2	Agitated	Frequent nonpurposeful movement or patient–ventilator dyssynchrony
+1	Restless	Anxious or apprehensive but movements not aggressive or vigorous
0	Alert and calm	Spontaneously pays attention to caregiver
−1	Drowsy	Not fully alert, but has sustained (>10 s) awakening, with eye contact, to voice
−2	Light sedation	Briefly (less than 10 seconds) awakens with eye contact to voice
−3	Moderate sedation	Any movement (but no eye contact) to voice
−4	Deep sedation	No response to voice, but any movement to physical stimulation

Adapted from: Sessler CN, Gosnell MS, Grap MJ, et al. The Richmond Agitation-Sedation Scale: validity and reliability in adult intensive care unit patients. Am J Respir Crit Care Med 2002;166:1338–1344

anticipated to avoid oversedation [10]. A light level of sedation has been associated with a shorter time to extubation and a reduced tracheostomy rate; however, it was not associated with a reduction in the rate of delirium outcomes [11, 12]. A slightly increased risk of self-extubation was described in randomized controlled trials [13] although not statistically significative. While randomized controlled trials failed to demonstrate that sedation depth influences mortality [14, 15], observational studies suggested benefits in reduced risk of death at day 90 [16]. A recent meta-analysis, including both randomized and non-randomized studies, revealed that deep sedation was associated with increased mortality and lengths of stay [17].

9.3   Sedation-Sparing Protocols

Evidences on the harms of excessive sedation are sufficient to justify efforts to minimize use of sedatives in the ICU [1–3]. Uninterrupted sedative-analgesic infusion to sedate critically ill patients should be avoided [18]. Since the groundbreaking Awakening and Breathing Controlled (ABC) Trial was published in 2008 [19], a protocol that paired spontaneous awakening trials (SATs), i.e., daily interruption of sedatives, with spontaneous breathing trials (SBTs)—the so-called *wake up and breathe*, was endorsed by guidelines and become routine in many centers around the world. A two-step process focuses on creating a synergy between SAT and SBT protocols. These protocols typically incorporate safety screens and failure criteria (Fig. 9.1). Many different strategies aiming at this target have been proposed, including protocol-driven intermittent infusions, daily interruption of sedation, nursing-protocolized sedation, or a combination of the above mentioned.

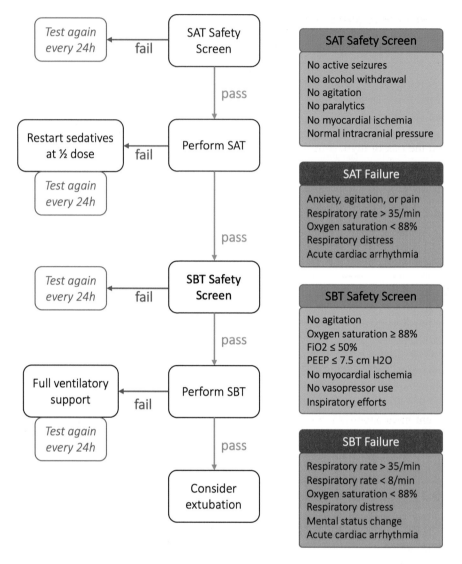

Fig. 9.1 "Wake up and breathe" protocol: spontaneous awakening trials (SATs) + spontaneous breathing trials (SBTs). Adapted from: Vanderbilt University "Wake up and breathe protocol"—https://uploads-ssl.webflow.com/5b0849daec50243a0a1e5e0c/5babf80c5116b561c618063c_ABCDEF-Wake-Up-And-Breathe.pdf

Daily Interruption of Sedation Daily interruption of sedation consists in discontinuing the continuous infusion of sedatives until the patient is awake and obeying to orders, or until agitation or discomfort occurs. This method allows a better neurological evaluation, avoiding unnecessary transportation for imaging, and also allows a constant reevaluation of patient's sedation needs [20].

Nursing-Protocolized Sedation Nursing-protocolized sedation consists in an established sedation protocol implemented by nurses at the bedside, who are allowed to titrate medications to reach the prescribed sedation level [21].

Light sedation can be properly achieved by using either method or a combination of the two. Benefits arising from these strategies have been proven by randomized controlled trials and meta-analyses in terms of reduction of length of ICU stay and mechanical ventilation [22, 23]. Concerns about long-term psychological sequelae and the risk of myocardial ischemia and their relation to light sedations have been disproven by multiple observational trials [24, 25]. However, some important pitfalls need to be addressed: if on the one side it is important to remember that these protocols increase nursing workload, on the other side a brief daily interruption of sedation should not justify the use of deep sedation for the rest of the day when it is not indicated. Regardless of the protocol used, ICU staff should attempt to achieve light levels of sedation in the majority of patients the majority of the time.

9.4 Sedative Agents: Old School and New School

Sedative agents commonly used for sedation and analgesia in the ICU include benzodiazepines, opioids, propofol, dexmedetomidine, ketamine, and antipsychotics (haloperidol and quetiapine). Paracetamol, non-steroidal anti-inflammatory, and antiepileptics may be used as adjuvants. Barbiturates must be avoided as they cause cardiovascular and respiratory depression, and they reduce cerebral blood flow [26]. Halogenated-based (e.g., sevoflurane) ICU sedation is a promising strategy, as a recent meta-analysis reported shorter awakening and extubation times, and a possible myocardial protective effect after cardiac surgery [27]. Further clinical trials are needed to confirm these findings.

Evidence in the literature is not sufficient to support the use of one agent over others in all clinical situations [28, 29]. However, 2018 SCCM Guidelines recommend to avoid benzodiazepines due to improved short-term outcomes such as ICU length of stay, duration of mechanical ventilation, and delirium [4].

Propofol is considered the agent of choice for sedation after cardiac surgery, [30] while propofol or dexmedetomidine should be considered in all other surgical or medical patients [31, 32]. Choosing a sedative agent should take into consideration the etiology of the distress: opioids should be used in case of pain or dyspnea. Paracetamol, low-dose ketamine, or neuropathic pain medication (in neuropathic pain management) can be considered in adjunction to reduce opioid dosage. Antipsychotics or dexmedetomidine may be considered in cases of significative distress induced by delirium. It is important to remember, however, that no agent to date is proven to prevent delirium. Combination therapies are rather common in the ICU since many patients experience a multifactorial distress. Drug interaction, age, body weight, and organ function should always be carefully taken into account when selecting a sedative agent and its dosage [33].

Propofol Versus Dexmedetomidine A few randomized controlled trials were conducted [34–36], but failed to show differences in terms of time to extubation, bradycardia, or hypotension between patients sedated with propofol and dexmedetomidine. Associated harm or benefit with these two drugs was minimal and not clinically significant. Both propofol and dexmedetomidine can be used for ICU sedation, in accordance to local practice and drug availability. Dexmedetomidine should not be used when deep sedation is required, with or without neuromuscular paralysis [37].

Benzodiazepines: Do They Still Have a Role? Benzodiazepines are still widely used in low-income areas and might play a fundamental role in selected clinical scenarios—including hemodynamically unstable patients, patients in need of deep sedation, at risk for delirium, or with signs of alcohol withdrawal [38, 39]. Also, the role of intermittent administration of benzodiazepines in the context of an analgesia-based approach is an interesting topic, which requires further investigation.

Enteral Sedation The possibility to administer sedation enterally rather than intravenously also deserves some consideration, as this route is cheaper and may result in lighter sedations. A recent study conducted in 12 Italian ICUs compared the enteral administration of hydroxyzine, lorazepam, and melatonin to intravenous sedation with midazolam or propofol in critically ill patients [40]. Although less self-extubations were observed in the intravenous group, the target RASS was achieved similarly in both groups, postulating a cultural change in regard to the enteral route when it comes to "gentle patient sedation" in the ICU.

9.5   Monitoring of Sedation: Analogic and Digital

Sedated patients need frequent reassessments to determine if the distress and/or agitation that required sedation at first are being properly managed. Several scales have been proposed to assess patients' levels of pain, sedation, and delirium. These scales are fundamental tools to determine the right amount of medications required to correctly manage ICU patients.

Sedation The Richmond Agitation-Sedation Scale (RASS, Table 9.1) [8] and the Riker Sedation-Agitation Scale (SAS, Table 9.2) [41] are the most commonly used to assess sedation in the ICU. RASS score ranges between −5 (unarousable) and +4 (combative). SAS score ranges between 1 (unarousable) and 7 (dangerous agitation).

Pain Unidimensional scales (e.g., visual analog scale, numeric rating scale) are quicker and easy to apply in the ICU environment. The Behavioral Pain Scale (BPS, Table 9.3) [42] and the Critical-Care Pain Observation Tool (CPOT, Table 9.4) [43] represent the golden standard to assess pain in the ICU.

Delirium The Confusion Assessment Method for the ICU (CAM-ICU, Table 9.5) [44] is the delirium assessment tool recommended by SCCM Guidelines. Results of CAM-ICU can be presence or absence of delirium, but cannot help in quantifying it.

Table 9.2 Riker sedation-agitation scale (SAS)

Score	Term	Description
7	Dangerous	Pulling at ET tube, trying to remove catheters, climbing over bedrail, striking at staff, thrashing side-to-side
6	Very agitated	Requiring restraint and frequent verbal reminding of limits, biting ETT
5	Agitated	Anxious or physically agitated, calms to verbal instructions
4	Calm and cooperative	Calm, easily arousable, follows commands
3	Sedated	Difficult to arouse but awakens to verbal stimuli or gentle shaking, follows simple commands but drifts off again
2	Very sedated	Arouses to physical stimuli but does not communicate or follow commands, may move spontaneously
1	Unarousable	Minimal or no response to noxious stimuli, does notcommunicate or follow commands

Adapted from: Riker RR, Picard JT, Fraser GL. Prospective evaluation of the Sedation-Agitation Scale for adult critically ill patients. Crit Care Med 1999;27:1325–1329

Table 9.3 Behavioral pain scale

Item	Description	Score
Facial expression	Relaxed	1
	Partially tightened (e.g., brow lowering)	2
	Fully tightened (e.g., eyelid closing)	3
	Grimacing	4
Upper limbs	No movement	1
	Partially bent	2
	Fully bent with finger flexion	3
	Permanently retracted	4
Compliance with ventilation	Tolerating movement	1
	Coughing but tolerating ventilation for most of the time	2
	Fighting ventilator	3
	Unable to control ventilation	4

Adapted from: Payen JF, Bru O, Bosson JL, et al. Assessing pain in critically ill sedated patients by using a behavioral pain scale. Crit Care Med 2001;29:2258–2263

Bispectral Index (BIS) Patients under neuromuscular blockers cannot be assessed with any of the above-mentioned scales. Historically, vital signs have been assessed as indicators of distress, but this method is neither sensible nor specific. Objective monitoring should be used in these patients to assess if the proper level of sedation is being obtained. BIS monitoring translates electroencephalographic data into a number ranging between 0 and 100, estimating the level of sedation. BIS is routinely used in the operative room but not in the ICU, due to possibility that artifacts may alter the reliability of data. According to 2018 SCCM Guidelines, [4] BIS monitoring appears best suited for sedative titration during deep sedation or neuromuscular blockade though observational data suggest potential benefit with lighter sedation as well.

Table 9.4 Critical-care pain observation tool (CPOT)

Item	Description	Description	Score
Facial expression	Relaxed, neutral	No muscle tension observed	0
	Tense	Presence of frowning, orbit tightening, levator contraction, or any other change (e.g., opening eyes or tearing during nociceptive procedures)	1
	Grimacing	All previous facial movements plus eyelid tightly closed	2
Upper limbs	Absence of movements or normal position	Does not move at all or normal position (movements not aimed toward the pain site)	0
	Protection	Slow, cautious movements, touching, or rubbing the pain site, seeking attention through movements	1
	Restlessness	Pulling tube, attempting to sit up, moving limbs, not following commands, trying to climb out of bed	2
Compliance with ventilation (intubated patient)	Tolerating ventilator or movement	Alarms not activated, easy ventilation	0
	Coughing but tolerating	Coughing, alarms may be activated	1
	Fighting ventilator	Asynchrony: blocking ventilation, alarms frequently activated	2
Vocalization (*non-intubated patient*)	Talking in normal tone or no sound	Talking in normal tone or no sound	0
	Sighing, moaning	Sighing, moaning	1
	Crying out, sobbing	Crying out, sobbing	2
Muscle tension *Evaluation by passive flexion and extension of upper limbs (in rest or when patient is being turned)*	Relaxed	No resistance to passive movements	0
	Tense, rigid	Resistance to passive movements	1
	Very tense or rigid	Strong resistance to passive movements, inability to complete them	2

Adapted from: Gélinas C, Johnston C. Pain assessment in the critically ill ventilated adult: validation of the Critical-Care Pain Observation Tool and physiologic indicators. Clin J Pain 2007;23:497–505

9.6   Limiting Physical Restraints

Use of effect physical restraints in modern-era ICU remains controversial. The frequency of use of physical restraints widely varies in the world. While most ICU personnel claims that their use is needed to reduce self-extubation and falls, prevent device removal, and protect staff from combative patients, no randomized

Table 9.5 Confusion assessment method for the ICU (CAM-ICU)

	Criteria	Present
Feature 1: Alteration/fluctuation in mental status		
Is the patient's mental status different than his/her baseline? **OR**	If **yes** for either question >	☐
Has the patient had any fluctuation in mental status in the past 24 h as evidenced by fluctuation on a sedation scale (e.g., RASS, Glasgow coma scale [GCS]), or previous delirium assessment?		
Feature 2: Inattention 1: Alteration/fluctuation in mental status		
Letters attention test: Tell the patient "I am going to read to you a series of ten letters. Whenever you hear the letter 'A,' squeeze my hand" **SAVEAHAART** *Count errors (each time patient fails to squeeze on the letter "A" and squeezes on a letter other than "A")*	If more than two errors >	☐
Feature 3: Altered level of consciousness (LOC)		
Present if the RASS score is anything other than alert and calm (zero) **OR**	If RASS≠0 or SAS ≠ 4 >	☐
If SAS is anything other than calm (4)		
Feature 4: Disorganized thinking		
Yes/no questions: ask the patient to respond: 1. Will a stone float on water? 2. Are there fish in the sea? 3. Does 1 pound weigh more than 2 pounds? 4. Can you use a hammer to pound a nail? *Count errors (each time patient answers incorrectly)* Commands: ask the patient to follow your instructions: (a) "Hold up this many fingers" (hold 2 fingers in front of the patient) (b) "Now do the same thing with the other hand" (do not demonstrate the number of fingers this time) – If unable to move both arms, for part "b" of command ask patient to "hold up one more finger" *Count errors if patient is unable to complete the entire command*	If combined number of errors >1 >	☐

If features 1 and 2 are both present and either features 3 or 4 are present:
CAM-ICU is positive, delirium is present

Adapted from: Ely EW, Margolin R, Francis J, et al. Evaluation of delirium in critically ill patients: validation of the Confusion Assessment Method for the Intensive Care Unit (CAM-ICU). Crit Care Med2001;29:1370–1379

controlled trials exist demonstrating the safety and efficacy of physical restraint in critically ill patients [14, 15]. On the contrary, a few studies report a paradox increase in unplanned extubations, unintentional device removal, longer ICU stays, and higher needs of sedatives in physically restraint patients [45]. While physical restraints have been eliminated from daily routine in a few countries [46], this required a high nurse-to-patient ratio and possibly higher levels of sedation. Therefore, risks and benefits of physical restraints should be carefully considered before applying them.

9.7 Conclusions

As intensive care approaches to modern era and the quality of care improves worldwide, the focus on cognitive and psychological aspects of ICU stay are growing worldwide. As lighter levels of sedation closely affect the outcome, all efforts must be taken to avoid deep sedation and to increase the use of nonpharmacological strategies to relieve stress, anxiety, and ICU-related pain. Bridging the patient toward normality, aiming to normalize circadian rhythms, physiological sleep, enteral route of drug administration, and avoidance of physical constrictions should constitute the cornerstone of medical treatment of the next generation of intensive care units.

References

1. Kollef MH, Levy NT, Ahrens TS, et al. The use of continuous i.v. sedation is associated with prolongation of mechanical ventilation. Chest. 1998;114:541–8.
2. Pandharipande P, Shintani A, Peterson J, et al. Lorazepam is an independent risk factor for transitioning to delirium in intensive care unit patients. Anesthesiology. 2006;104:21–6.
3. Shehabi Y, Bellomo R, Kadiman S, Sedation Practice in Intensive Care Evaluation (SPICE) Study Investigators, The Australian and New Zealand Intensive Care Society Clinical Trials Group, et al. Sedation intensity in the first 48 hours of mechanical ventilation and 180-day mortality: a multinational prospective longitudinal cohort study. Crit Care Med. 2018;46:850–9.
4. Devlin JW, Skrobik Y, Gélinas C, et al. Clinical practice guidelines for the prevention and management of pain, agitation/sedation, delirium, immobility, and sleep disruption in adult patients in the ICU. Crit Care Med. 2018;46:e825–73.
5. Fontaine DK. Nonpharmacologic management of patient distress during mechanical ventilation. Crit Care Clin. 1994;10:695–708.
6. Milbrandt EB, Deppen S, Harrison PL, et al. Costs associated with delirium in mechanically ventilated patients. Crit Care Med. 2004;32:955–62.
7. Bradt J, Dileo C. Music interventions for mechanically ventilated patients. Cochrane Database Syst Rev. 2014;2014:CD006902.
8. Sessler CN, Gosnell MS, Grap MJ, et al. The Richmond agitation-sedation scale: validity and reliability in adult intensive care unit patients. Am J Respir Crit Care Med. 2002;166:1338–44.
9. Hughes CG, McGrane S, Pandharipande PP. Sedation in the intensive care setting. Clin Pharmacol. 2012;4:53–63.
10. SRLF Trial Group. Impact of oversedation prevention in ventilated critically ill patients: a randomized trial-the AWARE study. Ann Intensive Care. 2018;8:93.
11. Treggiari M. Randomized trial of light versus deep sedation on mental health after critical illness. Crit Care Med. 2010;38:349–50.
12. Tanaka LM, Azevedo LC, Park M, et al. ERICC study investigators early sedation and clinical outcomes of mechanically ventilated patients: a prospective multicenter cohort study. Crit Care. 2014;18:R156.
13. Muller L, Chanques G, Bourgaux C, et al. Impact of the use of propofol remifentanil goal-directed sedation adapted by nurses on the time to extubation in mechanically ventilated ICU patients: the experience of a French ICU. Ann Fr Anesth Reanim. 2008;27:481.e1–8.
14. Shehabi Y, Bellomo R, Reade MC, Sedation Practice in Intensive Care Evaluation Study Investigators, Australian and New Zealand Intensive Care Society Clinical Trials Group, et al. Early goal-directed sedation versus standard sedation in mechanically ventilated critically ill patients: a pilot study. Crit Care Med. 2013;41:1983–91.

15. Bugedo G, Tobar E, Aguirre M, et al. The implementation of an analgesia-based sedation protocol reduced deep sedation and proved to be safe and feasible in patients on mechanical ventilation. Rev Bras Ter Intensiva. 2013;25:188–96.
16. Shehabi Y, Chan L, Kadiman S, Sedation Practice in Intensive Care Evaluation (SPICE) Study Group Investigators, et al. Sedation depth and long-term mortality in mechanically ventilated critically ill adults: a prospective longitudinal multicentre cohort study. Intensive Care Med. 2013;39:910–8.
17. Stephens RJ, Dettmer MR, Roberts BW, et al. Practice patterns and outcomes associated with early sedation depth in mechanically ventilated patients: a systematic review and meta-analysis. Crit Care Med. 2018;46:471–9.
18. Roberts DJ, Haroon B, Hall RI. Sedation for critically ill or injured adults in the intensive care unit: a shifting paradigm. Drugs. 2012;72:1881–916.
19. Girard TD, Kress JP, Fuchs BD, et al. Efficacy and safety of a paired sedation and ventilator weaning protocol for mechanically ventilated patients in intensive care (awakening and breathing controlled trial): a randomised controlled trial. Lancet. 2008;371:126–34.
20. Mehta S, Burry L, Cook D, et al. Daily sedation interruption in mechanically ventilated critically ill patients cared for with a sedation protocol: a randomized controlled trial. JAMA. 2012;308:1985–92.
21. de Wit M, Gennings C, Jenvey WI, Epstein SK. Randomized trial comparing daily interruption of sedation and nursing-implemented sedation algorithm in medical intensive care unit patients. Crit Care. 2008;12:R70.
22. Burry L, Rose L, McCullagh IJ, Fergusson DA, Ferguson ND, Mehta S. Daily sedation interruption versus no daily sedation interruption for critically ill adult patients requiring invasive mechanical ventilation. Cochrane Database Syst Rev. 2014;2014:CD009176.
23. Minhas MA, Velasquez AG, Kaul A, Salinas PD, Celi LA. Effect of protocolized sedation on clinical outcomes in mechanically ventilated intensive care unit patients: a systematic review and meta-analysis of randomized controlled trials. Mayo Clin Proc. 2015;90:613–23.
24. Devlin JW, Tanios MA, Epstein SK. Intensive care unit sedation: waking up clinicians to the gap between research and practice. Crit Care Med. 2006;34:556–7.
25. Mehta S, Burry L, Fischer S, et al. Canadian survey of the use of sedatives, analgesics, and neuromuscular blocking agents in critically ill patients. Crit Care Med. 2006;34:374–80.
26. Evers A, Crowder C. General anesthetics. In: Hardman JG, Limbird LE, Gilman AG, editors. Goodman and Gilman's the pharmacological basis of therapeutics. 10th ed. New York: McGraw-Hill; 2001. p. 337–65.
27. Kim HY, Lee JE, Kim HY, Kim J. Volatile sedation in the intensive care unit: a systematic review and meta-analysis. Medicine. 2017;96:e8976.
28. Jakob SM, Ruokonen E, Grounds RM, et al. Dexmedetomidine vs midazolam or propofol for sedation during prolonged mechanical ventilation: two randomized controlled trials. JAMA. 2012;307:1151–60.
29. Paliwal B, Rai P, Kamal M, et al. Comparison between dexmedetomidine and propofol with validation of bispectral index for sedation in mechanically ventilated intensive care patients. J Clin Diagn Res. 2015;9:UC01–UC5.
30. Snellen F, Lauwers P, Demeyere R, et al. The use of midazolam versus propofol for short-term sedation following coronary artery bypass grafting. Intensive Care Med. 1990;16:312–6.
31. Fraser GL, Devlin JW, Worby CP, et al. Benzodiazepine versus non benzodiazepine-based sedation for mechanically ventilated, critically ill adults: a systematic review and meta-analysis of randomized trials. Crit Care Med. 2013;41:S30–8.
32. Venn RM, Grounds RM. Comparison between dexmedetomidine and propofol for sedation in the intensive care unit: patient and clinician perceptions. Br J Anaesth. 2001;87:684–90.
33. Kollef MH, Levy NT, Ahrens TS, Schaiff R, Prentice D, Sherman G. The use of continuous i.v. sedation is associated with prolongation of mechanical ventilation. Chest. 1998;114:541–8.
34. Srivastava VK, Agrawal S, Kumar S, et al. Comparison of dexmedetomidine, propofol and midazolam for short-term sedation in post-operatively mechanically ventilated neurosurgical patients. J Clin Diagn Res. 2014;8:GC04–7.

35. Jakob SM, Ruokonen E, Grounds RM, Dexmedetomidine for Long-Term Sedation Investigators, et al. Dexmedetomidine vs midazolam or propofol for sedation during prolonged mechanical ventilation: two randomized controlled trials. JAMA. 2012;307:1151–60.
36. Herr DL, Sum-Ping ST, England M. ICU sedation after coronary artery bypass graft surgery: Dexmedetomidine-based versus propofol-based sedation regimens. J Cardiothorac Vasc Anesth. 2003;17:576–84.
37. Ruokonen E, Parviainen I, Jakob SM, et al. Dexmedetomidine versus propofol/midazolam for long-term sedation during mechanical ventilation. Intensive Care Med. 2009;35:282–90.
38. Hui D. Benzodiazepines for agitation in patients with delirium: selecting the right patient, right time, and right indication. Curr Opin Support Palliat Care. 2018;12(4):489–94.
39. Skrobik Y. Counterpoint: should benzodiazepines be avoided in mechanically ventilated patients? No Chest. 2012;142:285.
40. Mistraletti G, Umbrello M, Salini S, et al. Enteral versus intravenous approach for the sedation of critically ill patients: a randomized and controlled trial. Crit Care. 2019;23:3.
41. Riker RR, Picard JT, Fraser GL. Prospective evaluation of the sedation-agitation scale for adult critically ill patients. Crit Care Med. 1999;27:1325–9.
42. Payen JF, Bru O, Bosson JL, et al. Assessing pain in critically ill sedated patients by using a behavioral pain scale. Crit Care Med. 2001;29:2258–63.
43. Gélinas C, Johnston C. Pain assessment in the critically ill ventilated adult: validation of the critical-care pain observation tool and physiologic indicators. Clin J Pain. 2007;23:497–505.
44. Ely EW, Margolin R, Francis J, et al. Evaluation of delirium in critically ill patients: validation of the confusion assessment method for the intensive care unit (CAM-ICU). Crit Care Med. 2001;29:1370–9.
45. Minnick A, Leipzig RM, Johnson ME. Elderly patients' reports of physical restraint experiences in intensive care units. Am J Crit Care. 2001;10:168–71.
46. Martin B, Mathisen L. Use of physical restraints in adult critical care: a bicultural study. Am J Crit Care. 2005;14:133–42.

Hydrocortisone in Sepsis

10

Federico Longhini, Eugenio Garofalo, and Andrea Bruni

Contents

10.1 General Principles

Sepsis is a life-threatening organ dysfunction caused by a dysregulated host response to infection. Sepsis may worsen in septic shock, which is characterized by underlying circulatory, cellular, and metabolic abnormalities, associated with an increased risk of mortality [1]. Each year, millions of people around the world are affected by sepsis or septic shock with a mortality close to 25% [2].

Septic shock is characterized by a hypotension defined by a mean arterial pressure <65 mmHg, despite fluid resuscitation, and requiring the administration of vasopressors [1].

F. Longhini (✉)
Anesthesia and Intensive Care Unit, "Mater Domini" University Hospital, "Magna Graecia" University, Catanzaro, Italy

Department of Medical and Surgical Sciences, Magna Graecia University, Catanzaro, Italy
e-mail: flonghini@unicz.it

E. Garofalo · A. Bruni
Anesthesia and Intensive Care Unit, "Mater Domini" University Hospital, "Magna Graecia" University, Catanzaro, Italy
e-mail: eugenio.garofalo@unicz.it; andreabruni@unicz.it

© Springer Nature Switzerland AG 2021
G. Landoni et al. (eds.), *Reducing Mortality in Critically Ill Patients*,
https://doi.org/10.1007/978-3-030-71917-3_10

However, some patients affected by septic shock are unresponsive to vaso-pressors. Indeed, cytokines produced during septic shock may suppress the cortisol response to the adrenocorticotropic hormone (ACTH), with a prevalence of adrenal insufficiency of 50% of patients. Adrenal insufficiency is defined as a maximal post-ACTH cortisol increase ≤9 μg/dL. These patients may potentially benefit of steroid therapy, which may reverse the shock and may also improve survival [3].

Several trials have been conducted to assess the potential benefit on survival of intravenous hydrocortisone to treat septic shock patients.

10.2   Physiological Basis

Steroids have been a topic of particular focus because of their influence on the immune response. Several molecular mechanisms of action of corticosteroids have been considered beneficial to counteracting the uncontrolled inflammation that may characterize sepsis. Steroids modulate the inflammatory response through the regulation of white blood cells, cytokines, and nitric oxide. However, up to 50% of septic patients may be affected by adrenal insufficiency [4]. In addition, steroids receptors may be under-expressed during septic shock and their affinity may be low, inducing a state of body tissues resistance. Since the hypothalamic-pituitary-adrenal axis is a major determinant of the host response to stress, researchers have hypothesized that the administration of exogenous corticosteroids would improve the survival of patients with septic shock.

In an early study conducted in animal model of sepsis, pharmacologic doses of steroid increased the survival rate. In rodents, lower doses of corticosteroids were then demonstrated to improve hemodynamic and organ function, to favorably modulate the inflammatory response, and prolonged survival [5–7].

Low dose of steroids was also tested in healthy volunteers who had received intravenous injection of *Escherichia coli* lipopolysaccharide 12 h before. Steroids reduced the release of pro-inflammatory cytokines, prevented endothelial cell and neutrophil activation, and inhibited the acute phase response without altering coagulation and fibrinolysis balance [8].

In a prospective observational study, a short course (2 days) of hydrocortisone attenuated the inflammatory response in 57 surgical septic patients [9]. Furthermore, in another trial enrolling 40 patients with septic shock, low doses of hydrocortisone were shown also to increase mean arterial pressure, systemic vascular resistance, and to reduce heart rate, cardiac index, and norepinephrine requirement [10]. According to these findings, the administration of corticosteroids or hydrocortisone may potentially improve the survival rate of patients affected by septic shock. For these reasons, several trials have been conducted in the attempt to assess whether or not these physiological benefits would translate into outcome improvements.

10.3   Main Evidences on Mortality

In 1999, Briegel et al. reported the result of a controlled trial randomizing 40 septic shock patients to receive or not hydrocortisone. In particular, hydrocortisone was started with a loading dose of 100 mg in 30 min, followed by a continuous infusion of 0.18 mg/kg/h. At septic shock reversal, hydrocortisone was reduced to 0.08 mg/kg/h. Although hydrocortisone produced some physiological advantage, such as the reduction of the time on vasopressor support and hemodynamic status, no difference on survival was observed [11]. A multicenter placebo-controlled, randomized trial of 300 septic shock patients to receive either hydrocortisone (50-mg intravenous bolus every 6 h) and fludrocortisone (50-μg tablet once daily) or placebo for 7 days [12]. Vasopressor therapy was terminated within 28 days in 57% of patients in the corticosteroid group, while in 40% in the placebo group ($p = 0.001$). Overall, steroid therapy reduced time to shock reversal with no difference in the rate of adverse events (including gastrointestinal bleed, infection, psychiatric disorder, dysrhythmia, myocardial infarction, and ischemia). However, in the overall population, the 28-day, ICU, hospital and 1-year mortalities were similar between treatments. When stratifying patients in responders and non-responders to a short corticotropin test, no differences were also found in responders' cohort, while in non-responders steroids reduced the 28-day, ICU, and hospital mortalities [12].

Following these results, steroids were widespread accepted as adjunctive treatment for septic shock, until 2008, when the Corticosteroid Therapy of Septic Shock (CORTICUS) study was published [13]. In this multicenter trial, 499 patients were randomized to receive 50 mg of intravenous hydrocortisone or placebo every 6 h for 5 days; the dose was then tapered during a 6-day period. The trial failed to demonstrate any survival improvement operated by the hydrocortisone in patients with septic shock, either overall or in patients who did not have a response to corticotropin [13].

In 2016, Tongyoo et al. reported that, compared to placebo, hydrocortisone improved the pulmonary function and gas exchange, in 197 patients with septic shock; however, no survival improvement was observed [14]. In keeping with these trials, other studies reported different benefits of physiological outcomes, without any survival improvements [15].

More recently, a randomized controlled trial (ADRENAL trial) compared a continuous infusion of hydrocortisone (200 mg per day) with placebo for 1 week, in 3800 patients with septic shock [16]. Although hydrocortisone fastened the resolution of the shock and reduced the time spent under mechanical ventilation, no significant differences in 28-day or 90-day mortalities were observed between treatments [16].

On the opposite, some studies reported outcome improvement in patients with septic shock receiving low doses of hydrocortisone [17–19]. However, these trials are of limited quality of evidence, due to a retrospective design or small sample.

Given the contradictory results from the literature, several systematic reviews have been conducted in the attempt to clarify the role of hydrocortisone in septic shock. However, a large part of these reviews lacks of some studies to be included and has several limitations. Very recently, a Cochrane systematic review, with pooled data analysis, has been conducted in the attempt to clarify the literature evidence [20]. From the results of 50 trials, that accounted for a total of 1233 participants, the authors reported that the risk ratio (RR) of dying at 28 days was 0.91 (95% confidence interval (CI) 0.84 to 0.99; $p = 0.04$). However, heterogeneity was evident in the results, limiting the strength of these findings for inconsistency [20]. Furthermore, a subgroup analysis of 1079 patients with adrenal insufficiency from 12 studies also did not show any survival improvement (47.8% versus 52.5% in steroids and control groups, respectively; RR of dying 0.92 [95% CI 0.82 to 1.03; $p = 0.16$]) [20].

Indeed, the recent Surviving Sepsis Campaign guidelines suggest against the use of intravenous hydrocortisone to treat septic shock patients, if adequate fluid resuscitation and vasopressor therapy are able to restore hemodynamic stability. However, when patients are hemodynamically unstable, despite fluid resuscitation and administration of vasopressors, a low dose (200 mg daily) of intravenous hydrocortisone may be used [2]. It must be mentioned, however, that the use of low-dose hydrocortisone in septic shock patients may produce an increase of hyperglycemia and hypernatremia, which physicians should consider as potential side effects [2].

10.4 Conclusions

Considering the contradictory evidences from the literature and trials, the use of hydrocortisone seems to not add any benefit on survival in septic shock patients. Indeed, the current guidelines on septic shock suggest against using intravenous hydrocortisone in all septic shock patients. However, in case of persistence of unstable hemodynamic despite fluid resuscitation and administration of vasopressors, a low dose of hydrocortisone may be used.

References

1. Shankar-Hari M, Phillips GS, Levy ML, Seymour CW, Liu VX, Deutschman CS, Angus DC, Rubenfeld GD, Singer M. Developing a new definition and assessing new clinical criteria for septic shock: for the third international consensus definitions for sepsis and septic shock (Sepsis-3). JAMA. 2016;315:775–87.
2. Rhodes A, Evans LE, Alhazzani W, Levy MM, Antonelli M, Ferrer R, Kumar A, Sevransky JE, Sprung CL, Nunnally ME, Rochwerg B, Rubenfeld GD, Angus DC, Annane D, Beale RJ, Bellinghan GJ, Bernard GR, Chiche JD, Coopersmith C, De Backer DP, French CJ, Fujishima S, Gerlach H, Hidalgo JL, Hollenberg SM, Jones AE, Karnad DR, Kleinpell RM, Koh Y, Lisboa TC, Machado FR, Marini JJ, Marshall JC, Mazuski JE, McIntyre LA, McLean AS, Mehta S, Moreno RP, Myburgh J, Navalesi P, Nishida O, Osborn TM, Perner A, Plunkett CM, Ranieri M, Schorr CA, Seckel MA, Seymour CW, Shieh L, Shukri KA, Simpson SQ, Singer M,

Thompson BT, Townsend SR, Van der Poll T, Vincent JL, Wiersinga WJ, Zimmerman JL, Dellinger RP. Surviving sepsis campaign: international guidelines for management of sepsis and septic shock: 2016. Crit Care Med. 2017;45:486–552.

3. Annane D, Bellissant E, Bollaert PE, Briegel J, Confalonieri M, De Gaudio R, Keh D, Kupfer Y, Oppert M, Meduri GU. Corticosteroids in the treatment of severe sepsis and septic shock in adults: a systematic review. JAMA. 2009;301:2362–75.

4. Annane D, Sebille V, Troche G, Raphael JC, Gajdos P, Bellissant E. A 3-level prognostic classification in septic shock based on cortisol levels and cortisol response to corticotropin. JAMA. 2000;283:1038–45.

5. Vachharajani V, Vital S, Russell J, Scott LK, Granger DN. Glucocorticoids inhibit the cerebral microvascular dysfunction associated with sepsis in obese mice. Microcirculation. 2006;13:477–87.

6. Tsao CM, Ho ST, Chen A, Wang JJ, Li CY, Tsai SK, Wu CC. Low-dose dexamethasone ameliorates circulatory failure and renal dysfunction in conscious rats with endotoxemia. Shock. 2004;21:484–91.

7. Heller AR, Heller SC, Borkenstein A, Stehr SN, Koch T. Modulation of host defense by hydrocortisone in stress doses during endotoxemia. Intensive Care Med. 2003;29:1456–63.

8. de Kruif MD, Lemaire LC, Giebelen IA, Struck J, Morgenthaler NG, Papassotiriou J, Elliott PJ, van der Poll T. The influence of corticosteroids on the release of novel biomarkers in human endotoxemia. Intensive Care Med. 2008;34:518–22.

9. Briegel J, Kellermann W, Forst H, Haller M, Bittl M, Hoffmann GE, Buchler M, Peter K, Uhl W, Schild A, Hanisch E, Waydhas C, Muller K, Entholzner E, Zugel M, Busch EW. Low-dose hydrocortisone infusion attenuates the systemic inflammatory response syndrome. Clin Investig. 1994;72:782–7.

10. Keh D, Boehnke T, Weber-Cartens S, Schulz C, Ahlers O, Bercker S, Volk HD, Doecke WD, Falke KJ, Gerlach H. Immunologic and hemodynamic effects of "low-dose" hydrocortisone in septic shock - a double-blind, randomized, placebo-controlled, crossover study. Am J Respir Crit Care. 2003;167:512–20.

11. Briegel J, Forst H, Haller M, Schelling G, Kilger E, Kuprat G, Hemmer B, Hummel T, Lenhart A, Heyduck M, Stoll C, Peter K. Stress doses of hydrocortisone reverse hyperdynamic septic shock: a prospective, randomized, double-blind, single-center study. Crit Care Med. 1999;27:723–32.

12. Annane D, Sebille V, Charpentier C, Bollaert PE, Francois B, Korach JM, Capellier G, Cohen Y, Azoulay E, Troche G, Chaumet-Riffaut P, Bellissant E. Effect of treatment with low doses of hydrocortisone and fludrocortisone on mortality in patients with septic shock. JAMA. 2002;288:862–71.

13. Sprung CL, Annane D, Keh D, Moreno R, Singer M, Freivogel K, Weiss YG, Benbenishty J, Kalenka A, Forst H, Laterre PF, Reinhart K, Cuthbertson BH, Payen D, Briegel J, Grp CS. Hydrocortisone therapy for patients with septic shock. N Engl J Med. 2008;358:111–24.

14. Tongyoo S, Permpikul C, Mongkolpun W, Vattanavanit V, Udompanturak S, Kocak M, Meduri GU. Hydrocortisone treatment in early sepsis-associated acute respiratory distress syndrome: results of a randomized controlled trial. Crit Care. 2016;20:329.

15. Gordon AC, Mason AJ, Perkins GD, Stotz M, Terblanche M, Ashby D, Brett SJ. The interaction of vasopressin and corticosteroids in septic shock: a pilot randomized controlled trial. Crit Care Med. 2014;42:1325–33.

16. Venkatesh B, Finfer S, Cohen J, Rajbhandari D, Arabi Y, Bellomo R, Billot L, Correa M, Glass P, Harward M, Joyce C, Li Q, McArthur C, Perner A, Rhodes A, Thompson K, Webb S, Myburgh J, Investigators AT, A-NZI C. Adjunctive glucocorticoid therapy in patients with septic shock. N Engl J Med. 2018;378:797–808.

17. Torgersen C, Luckner G, Schroder DCH, Schmittinger CA, Rex C, Ulmer H, Dunser MW. Concomitant arginine-vasopressin and hydrocortisone therapy in severe septic shock: association with mortality. Intensive Care Med. 2011;37:1432–7.

18. Katsenos CS, Antonopoulou AN, Apostolidou EN, Ioakeimidou A, Kalpakou GT, Papanikolaou MN, Pistiki AC, Mpalla MC, Paraschos MD, Patrani MA, Pratikaki ME, Retsas TA, Savva AA, Vassiliagkou SD, Lekkou AA, Dimopoulou I, Routsi C, Mandragos KE, Grp HSS. Early administration of hydrocortisone replacement after the advent of septic shock: impact on survival and immune response. Crit Care Med. 2014;42:1651–7.
19. Cicarelli DD, Vieira JE, Bensenor FEM. Early dexamethasone treatment for septic shock patients: a prospective randomized clinical trial. Sao Paulo Med J. 2007;125:237–41.
20. Annane D, Bellissant E, Bollaert PE, Briegel J, Keh D, Kupfer Y, Pirracchio R, Rochwerg B. Corticosteroids for treating sepsis in children and adults. Cochrane Database Syst Rev. 2019;12:CD002243.

Goal-Directed Therapy

11

Pasquale Nardelli, Giacomo Senarighi,
and Carmine D. Votta

Contents

11.1 General Principles

Since the publication of the landmark paper by Dr. Emanuel Rivers in The New England Journal of Medicine in 2001, the world of critical care massively adopted his protocol for the resuscitation of severe sepsis and/or septic shock—which was named "early goal-directed therapy" [1]. The concept of goal-directed therapy rapidly arose from sepsis and was applied to shock in general in the intensive care unit. Goal-directed therapy is a bundle of care that embraces the use of fluids, blood transfusion, and inotropes aiming to precise hemodynamic targets [2]. In case of hypotension or lactate raise, a fluid challenge of 30 ml/kg of crystalloid solution is administered to the patient. Fluid responsiveness is assessed in terms of low central venous pressure (CVP) and decreases in heart rate. In the following hours, hemodynamic targets include: a CVP of 8–12 mmHg, a superior vena cava oxygen saturation ($ScvO_2$) >70% or a mixed venous oxygen saturation (SvO_2) >65%, a mean arterial pressure (MAP) $\geq$65 mmHg, and a urine output $\geq$0.5 mL/kg/h. Strategies to

P. Nardelli (✉) · G. Senarighi · C. D. Votta
Department of Anesthesia and Intensive Care, IRCCS San Raffaele Scientific Institute,
Milan, Italy
e-mail: nardelli.pasquale@hsr.it; votta.carmine@hsr.it

© Springer Nature Switzerland AG 2021   99
G. Landoni et al. (eds.), *Reducing Mortality in Critically Ill Patients*,
https://doi.org/10.1007/978-3-030-71917-3_11

achieve these target involve additional fluids, transfusion of packed red blood cells or inotrope infusion. In the original study, the application of this protocol reduced mortality by more of one third and halved that of patients with severe sepsis [1].

In spite of being a medical dogma for over a decade, three recent multicenter trials (ProCESS [3], ARISE [4], and ProMISe [5]) published in the New England Journal of Medicine failed to show any benefit from early goal-directed therapy. Consequently, the PRISM patient-level meta-analysis was also performed and published on the same Journal [6] and to confirm that early goal-directed therapy did not result in better outcomes than usual care and was associated with higher hospitalization costs. However, taking a closer look at the results of these trials, it appears evident that the usual care groups didn't differ much than the early goal-directed therapy group in the Rivers' trial [7]. The increased awareness of sepsis and efforts related to the Surviving Sepsis Campaign caused an evolution of usual care, which now includes early volume resuscitation. In modern-era intensive care, the approach should always be patient-tailored and invasive care, including blood transfusions and use of pulmonary artery catheter, should be carefully considered in each case, rather than routinely applied.

11.2 Intravenous Fluids

Pathogenesis of sepsis usually implies intravascular hypovolemia due not only to peripheral vasodilation, but also to endothelial injury with altered vascular permeability [8]. Severe intravascular hypovolemia in sepsis must be promptly treated. The rapid infusion of 30 ml/kg of fluids is indicated as initial therapy for septic shock, unless a significant pulmonary edema is concurrently present. While in the earlier days the goal-directed therapy included the administration of up to 5 l of fluids, modern studies demonstrated that 2–3 l are sufficient for most patients. Administration of extra fluids should be tailored on clinical or hemodynamic indicators of fluid responsiveness. Predefined (e.g., 500 ml) boluses of fluids should be rapidly infused. After each bolus, the clinical and hemodynamic response and the presence of pulmonary edema must be assessed. Fluid boluses can be repeated until blood pressure and tissue perfusion are acceptable in the absence of complications.

Randomized trials and meta-analyses failed to show a significant difference between albumin and crystalloid solutions in this setting, but they identified potential harm of synthetic colloids.

Albumin vs Crystalloids Many randomized controlled trials comparing albumin with crystalloids in sepsis failed to assess a difference in hard clinical outcomes [9–11]. Consequently, most meta-analysis could not report any difference although one suggests a trend toward reduced 90-day mortality in severe sepsis patients resuscitated with albumin [12]. In the absence of hard evidence in favor of albumin, due to the limited availability and the higher costs, crystalloids are the standard of care in clinical practice. No guidelines suggest which crystalloid to use in resuscitation from septic shock.

Colloids vs Crystalloids The "6S" Scandinavian Starch for Severe Sepsis and Septic Shock trial, [13] and the Efficacy of Volume Substitution and Insulin Therapy in Severe Sepsis (VISEP) trial [14] compared hydroxyethyl starch and pentastarch to crystalloids, respectively. Use of colloids resulted in increased mortality and renal replacement therapy.

11.3 Monitoring Fluid Response

Goal-directed therapy requires a strict assessment of clinical, hemodynamic, and laboratory parameters. Most patients respond to fluid administration within the first 6–24 h. However, some patients require intensive monitoring for days or weeks. Fluid responsiveness, entailing an increase by 10–20% in cardiac output and in tissue perfusion after the administration of intravenous fluid, should be carefully monitored during fluid resuscitation.

Clinical Parameters Clinical monitoring is the cornerstone of tailoring an adequate goal-directed therapy. Main targets of goal-directed therapy are a mean arterial pressure (MAP) ≥ 65 mmHg and urine output ≥ 0.5 mL/kg/h. Many trials were performed to assess the appropriate MAP during goal-directed therapy, and concluded that target should be individualized within a range between 60 and 70 mmHg, as higher MAPs are potentially harmful [15, 16].

Hemodynamic Parameters Current guidelines suggest that dynamic hemodynamic indexes are more accurate than static measures at predicting fluid responsiveness. Static measures include central venous pressure (usual target 8–12 mmHg) and (central) venous mixed O_2 saturation (ScvO$_2$, usual target $\geq 70\%$; SvO$_2$, usual target $\geq 65\%$).

Dynamic parameters include pulse pressure variation (PPV), stroke volume variation (SVV), oximetric waveform variation, respiratory changes in the vena cava diameter, femoral vein diameter and Doppler of portal, hepatic, or renal veins.

Pulse Pressure Variation (PPV) The difference between systolic and diastolic pressure (defined pulse pressure) varies during positive pressure ventilation. Variation in pulse pressure depends on the individual response to preload, according to the Frank-Starling Curve. A low variation in the pulse pressure indicates a lack of fluid responsiveness, while a variation in pulse pressure over 15% denotes fluid responsiveness [17]. PPV is usually averaged over three or more breaths, and calculated as:

$$\frac{\text{maximum pulse pressure } (\text{PPmax}) - \text{minimum pulse pressure } (\text{PPmin})}{\text{mean pulse pressure } (\text{PPmean})}$$

Stroke Volume Variation (SVV) Stroke volume has a linear correlation with pulse pressure; therefore, SVV relies on the same physiologic principle as PPV. Studies consistently found that SVV >10% is associated with fluid responsiveness [18]. Analogous to PPV, SVV is averaged over several respiratory cycles and calculated as:

$$\frac{\text{maximum stroke volume } (SVmax) - \text{minimum stroke volume } (SVmin)}{\text{mean stroke volume } (SVmean)}$$

The stroke volume can be calculated from the arterial pressure waveform with special arterial catheter capable of measuring vascular resistance and arterial compliance. SVV has the same limitations as PPV although it may also be applied to spontaneously breathing patients [19].

Oximetric Waveform Variation Variation in the pulse oximeter waveform has been proposed as a predictor of fluid responsiveness; however, it showed a modest prediction of fluid responsiveness in the ICU in recent trials [20].

Vena Cava Assessment A change in inferior vena cava diameter of more than 12% with respiration has been associated with fluid responsiveness [21]. Due to the lack of clear evidence and the operator-dependent nature of this technique, vena cava assessment should not be used as a sole indicator of volume responsiveness.

Femoral Vein Diameter Measuring the diameter of femoral vein in mechanically ventilated patients has been proposed to estimate central venous pressure. Further studies are warranted to validate these findings [22].

Doppler of Portal, Hepatic, or Renal Veins Doppler flow in the portal, hepatic, or renal veins has been proposed to assess fluid responsiveness. Pulsatile flows in these vessels imply venous congestion and can be early markers of end-organ injury [23].

Pulmonary Artery Catheterization Routine use of a pulmonary artery catheter (PAC) does not improve outcome in septic patients, as wedge pressure is a poor predictor of fluid responsiveness, cardiac output can be measured with less invasive tests and the ability to measure SvO_2 does not justify its use—as $ScvO_2$ can be easily obtained from a CVC [24]. PAC use must be considered when a concomitant cardiac dysfunction is present, as it may guide the administration of the correct inotropic therapy [25].

Laboratory Parameters Include measures which are usually obtained from point-of-care arterial blood gases (including lactate levels) and laboratory measures.

Arterial Blood Gases Acidosis severity and type must be closely monitored during goal-directed therapy, as hyperchloremic acidosis may occur after resolution of metabolic acidosis. Moreover, a drop in the arterial partial pressure of oxygen: fraction of inspired oxygen ratio may be caused by pulmonary edema from excessive fluid resuscitation.

Lactate Clearance Lactate clearance is defined as [(initial lactate—lactate >2 h later)/initial lactate] × 100. Lactate-guided resuscitation resulted in a reduction in mortality [26]. However, lactate level poorly relates to tissue perfusion after the restoration of perfusion [27].

Laboratory Measures A strict monitoring of laboratory values, with special focus on platelet count, serum chemistries, and liver function tests should be performed. Hyperchloremia should be avoided or treated using low chloride solutions.

11.4 Non-responders to Goal-Directed Therapy

If hypoperfusion persists after fluid resuscitation, a complete reassessment including fluid responsiveness, control of any septic focus, proper antimicrobial treatment, identification, and correction of unexpected complications or coexisting problems must be performed. Vasopressors, inotropes, steroids, and blood transfusion should be considered after fluid status has been restored to correct hypoperfusion.

Vasopressors Noradrenaline should be considered as first-line agent in patients who remain hypotensive despite adequate fluid resuscitation [28, 29]. Guidelines suggest additional agents including vasopressin (as noradrenaline-sparing) or adrenaline, nevertheless current practice is not homogeneous [30]. The addition of vasopressin may reduce the incidence of atrial fibrillation although no impact on hard clinical outcomes was reported in a recent meta-analysis. In patients with refractory shock associated with a low cardiac output, dobutamine was associated with improved survival [31].

Therefore, initial choice of vasopressor must be patient-tailored and should take into consideration the presence of conditions including heart failure, arrhythmias, or end-organ dysfunction. In patients with significant tachycardia, vasopressin should be considered as it does not have any ß-adrenergic effects, while dopamine may be used in those with significant bradycardia.

Steroids While routine use of glucocorticoids is not recommended by current guidelines, it must be considered if shock is refractory to adequate fluid resuscitation and vasopressors.

Red Blood Cell Transfusions Current guidelines only endorse red blood cell transfusions for patients with a ≤7 g/dl of hemoglobin or if concurrent hemorrhagic shock or myocardial ischemia are suspected. These guidelines are derived from large randomized clinical trials [32] and expert consensus [33, 34], reporting no benefit to more liberal transfusion strategies.

11.5 Responders to Goal-Directed Therapy

If patients respond to fluid resuscitation, a proper de-escalation of fluid administration must be performed to avoid overload and development of pulmonary edema. The rate of fluid should be carefully reduced or stopped, vasopressor support weaned, and, if necessary, diuretics administered. Fluids may be harmful when the patient is no longer fluid responsive, as circulatory overload may rapidly cause respiratory insufficiency. A restrictive approach to fluids has been associated with shorter mechanical ventilation and ICU stay [35]. Also, fluid overload has been reported as common in patients with sepsis [36]. As cardiac function may be already partly impaired by sepsis, avoidance of fluid overload once fluid status has been restored is fundamental in treating shock in critically ill patients.

References

1. Rivers E, Nguyen B, Havstad S, et al. Early goal-directed therapy in the treatment of severe sepsis and septic shock. N Engl J Med. 2001;345(19):1368–77. https://doi.org/10.1056/NEJMoa010307.
2. Gordon AC, Russell JA. Goal directed therapy: how long can we wait? Crit Care. 2005;9(6):647–8. https://doi.org/10.1186/cc3951.
3. Investigators PCESS, Yean DM, Kellum JA, et al. A randomized trial of protocol-based care for early septic shock. N Engl J Med. 2014;370(18):1683–93. https://doi.org/10.1056/NEJMoa1401602.
4. Investigators ARISE, ANZICS Clinical Trials Group, Peake SL, et al. Goal-directed resuscitation for patients with early septic shock. N Engl J Med. 2014;371(16):1496–506. https://doi.org/10.1056/NEJMoa1404380.
5. Mouncey PR, Osborn TM, Power GS, et al. Trial of early, goal-directed resuscitation for septic shock. N Engl J Med. 2015;372(14):1301–11. https://doi.org/10.1056/NEJMoa1500896.
6. Investigators PRISM, Rowan KM, Angus DC, et al. Early, goal-directed therapy for septic shock - a patient-level meta-analysis. N Engl J Med. 2017;376(23):2223–34. https://doi.org/10.1056/NEJMoa1701380.
7. Edriss H. What comes after the early goal directed therapy for sepsis era? J Thorac Dis. 2017;9(10):3514–7. https://doi.org/10.21037/jtd.2017.09.27.
8. Russell JA, Rush B, Boyd J. Pathophysiology of septic shock. Crit Care Clin. 2018;34(1):43–61. https://doi.org/10.1016/j.ccc.2017.08.005.
9. Finfer S, Bellomo R, Boyce N, et al. A comparison of albumin and saline for fluid resuscitation in the intensive care unit. N Engl J Med. 2004;350(22):2247–56. https://doi.org/10.1056/NEJMoa040232.
10. Caironi P, Tognoni G, Masson S, et al. Albumin replacement in patients with severe sepsis or septic shock. N Engl J Med. 2014;370(15):1412–21. https://doi.org/10.1056/NEJMoa1305727.
11. Park CHL, de Almeida JP, de Oliveira GQ, et al. Lactated Ringer's versus 4% albumin on lactated Ringer's in early sepsis therapy in cancer patients: a pilot single-center randomized trial. Crit Care Med. 2019;47(10):e798–805. https://doi.org/10.1097/CCM.0000000000003900.
12. Xu JY, Chen QH, Xie JF, et al. Comparison of the effects of albumin and crystalloid on mortality in adult patients with severe sepsis and septic shock: a meta-analysis of randomized clinical trials. Crit Care. 2014;18(6):702. https://doi.org/10.1186/s13054-014-0702-y.
13. Perner A, Haase N, Guttormsen AB, et al. Hydroxyethyl starch 130/0.42 versus Ringer's acetate in severe sepsis. N Engl J Med. 2012;367(2):124–34. https://doi.org/10.1056/NEJMoa1204242.

14. Brunkhorst FM, Engel C, Bloos F, et al. Intensive insulin therapy and pentastarch resuscitation in severe sepsis. N Engl J Med. 2008;358(2):125–39. https://doi.org/10.1056/NEJMoa070716.
15. Asfar P, Meziani F, Hamel JF, et al. High versus low blood-pressure target in patients with septic shock. N Engl J Med. 2014;370(17):1583–93. https://doi.org/10.1056/NEJMoa1312173.
16. Lamontagne F, Meade MO, Hébert PC, et al. Higher versus lower blood pressure targets for vasopressor therapy in shock: a multicentre pilot randomized controlled trial. Intensive Care Med. 2016;42(4):542–50. https://doi.org/10.1007/s00134-016-4237-3.
17. Marik PE, Cavallazzi R, Vasu T, Hirani A. Dynamic changes in arterial waveform derived variables and fluid responsiveness in mechanically ventilated patients: a systematic review of the literature. Crit Care Med. 2009;37(9):2642–7. https://doi.org/10.1097/CCM.0b013e3181a590da.
18. Biais M, Nouette-Gaulain K, Cottenceau V, Revel P, Sztark F. Uncalibrated pulse contour-derived stroke volume variation predicts fluid responsiveness in mechanically ventilated patients undergoing liver transplantation. Br J Anaesth. 2008;101(6):761–8. https://doi.org/10.1093/bja/aen277.
19. Lanspa MJ, Grissom CK, Hirshberg EL, Jones JP, Brown SM. Applying dynamic parameters to predict hemodynamic response to volume expansion in spontaneously breathing patients with septic shock. Shock. 2013;39(2):155–60. https://doi.org/10.1097/SHK.0b013e31827f1c6a.
20. Maughan BC, Seigel TA, Napoli AM. Pleth variability index and fluid responsiveness of hemodynamically stable patients after cardiothoracic surgery. Am J Crit Care. 2015;24(2):172–5. https://doi.org/10.4037/ajcc2015864.
21. Orso D, Paoli I, Piani T, Cilenti FL, Cristiani L, Guglielmo N. Accuracy of ultrasonographic measurements of inferior vena cava to determine fluid responsiveness: a systematic review and meta-analysis. J Intensive Care Med. 2020;35(4):354–63. https://doi.org/10.1177/0885066617752308.
22. Cho RJ, Williams DR, Leatherman JW. Measurement of femoral vein diameter by ultrasound to estimate central venous pressure. Ann Am Thorac Soc. 2016;13(1):81–5. https://doi.org/10.1513/AnnalsATS.201506-337BC.
23. Beaubien-Souligny W, Benkreira A, Robillard P, et al. Alterations in portal vein flow and intrarenal venous flow are associated with acute kidney injury after cardiac surgery: a prospective observational cohort study. J Am Heart Assoc. 2018;7(19):e009961. https://doi.org/10.1161/JAHA.118.009961.
24. Richard C, Warszawski J, Anguel N, et al. Early use of the pulmonary artery catheter and outcomes in patients with shock and acute respiratory distress syndrome: a randomized controlled trial. JAMA. 2003;290(20):2713–20. https://doi.org/10.1001/jama.290.20.2713.
25. Parker MM, Peruzzi W. Pulmonary artery catheters in sepsis/septic shock. New Horiz. 1997;5(3):228–32.
26. Hernández G, Ospina-Tascón GA, Damiani LP, et al. Effect of a resuscitation strategy targeting peripheral perfusion status vs serum lactate levels on 28-day mortality among patients with septic shock: the ANDROMEDA-SHOCK randomized clinical trial. JAMA. 2019;321(7):654–64. https://doi.org/10.1001/jama.2019.0071.
27. Forsythe SM, Schmidt GA. Sodium bicarbonate for the treatment of lactic acidosis. Chest. 2000;117(1):260–7. https://doi.org/10.1378/chest.117.1.260.
28. De Backer D, Aldecoa C, Njimi H, Vincent JL. Dopamine versus norepinephrine in the treatment of septic shock: a meta-analysis*. Crit Care Med. 2012;40(3):725–30. https://doi.org/10.1097/CCM.0b013e31823778ee.
29. Vasu TS, Cavallazzi R, Hirani A, Kaplan G, Leiby B, Marik PE. Norepinephrine or dopamine for septic shock: systematic review of randomized clinical trials. J Intensive Care Med. 2012;27(3):172–8. https://doi.org/10.1177/0885066610396312.
30. McIntyre WF, Um KJ, Alhazzani W, et al. Association of vasopressin plus catecholamine vasopressors vs catecholamines alone with atrial fibrillation in patients with distributive shock: a systematic review and meta-analysis. JAMA. 2018;319(18):1889–900. https://doi.org/10.1001/jama.2018.4528.

31. Nguyen HB, Lu S, Possagnoli I, Stokes P. Comparative effectiveness of second vasoactive agents in septic shock refractory to norepinephrine. J Intensive Care Med. 2017;32(7):451–9. https://doi.org/10.1177/0885066616647941.
32. Holst LB, Haase N, Wetterslev J, et al. Lower versus higher hemoglobin threshold for transfusion in septic shock. N Engl J Med. 2014;371(15):1381–91. https://doi.org/10.1056/NEJMoa1406617.
33. Hébert PC, Wells G, Blajchman MA, et al. A multicenter, randomized, controlled clinical trial of transfusion requirements in critical care. Transfusion requirements in critical care investigators, Canadian critical care trials group. N Engl J Med. 1999;340(6):409–17. https://doi.org/10.1056/NEJM199902113400601.
34. Retter A, Wyncoll D, Pearse R, et al. Guidelines on the management of anaemia and red cell transfusion in adult critically ill patients. Br J Haematol. 2013;160(4):445–64. https://doi.org/10.1111/bjh.12143.
35. National Heart, Lung, and Blood Institute Acute Respiratory Distress Syndrome (ARDS) Clinical Trials Network, Wiedemann HP, Wheeler AP, et al. Comparison of two fluid-management strategies in acute lung injury. N Engl J Med. 2006;354(24):2564–75. https://doi.org/10.1056/NEJMoa062200.
36. Silversides JA, Major E, Ferguson AJ, et al. Conservative fluid management or deresuscitation for patients with sepsis or acute respiratory distress syndrome following the resuscitation phase of critical illness: a systematic review and meta-analysis. Intensive Care Med. 2017;43(2):155–70. https://doi.org/10.1007/s00134-016-4573-3.

Levosimendan in Cardiogenic Shock and Low Cardiac Output Syndrome

12

Vladimir Lomivorotov, Martina Baiardo Redaelli, and Vladimir Boboshko

Contents

12.1 General Principles

Low cardiac output syndrome (LCOS) is the most common and the most serious complication after cardiac surgery and is associated with increased rates of morbidity and mortality [1]. This syndrome is characterized by impaired heart function, causing a reduced oxygen delivery with further hypoxia [2]. The universally

V. Lomivorotov (✉)
Department of Anesthesiology and Intensive Care, E. Meshalkin National Medical Research Center, Novosibirsk, Russia

Department of Anaesthesiology and Intensive Care, Novosibirsk State University, Novosibirsk, Russia
e-mail: vvlom@mail.ru

M. Baiardo Redaelli
Department of Anesthesia and Intensive Care, IRCCS San Raffaele Scientific Institute, Milan, Italy
e-mail: baiardoredaelli.martina@hsr.it

V. Boboshko
Department of Anesthesiology and Intensive Care, E. Meshalkin National Medical Research Center, Novosibirsk, Russia

© Springer Nature Switzerland AG 2021
G. Landoni et al. (eds.), *Reducing Mortality in Critically Ill Patients*,
https://doi.org/10.1007/978-3-030-71917-3_12

definition of LCOS includes decreases in the cardiac index (CI) to less than 2.0 L/min/m^2 and a systolic blood pressure below 90 mmHg, associated with tissue hypoperfusion (clammy skin, cold periphery, oliguria, elevated lactate level, confusion) in the absence of hypovolemia.

Cardiogenic shock (CS) is caused by severe reduction of myocardial pump function that results in decreased cardiac output, organ hypoperfusion, and hypoxia. Usually, this presents as hypotension state refractory to volume infusion with signs of end-organ hypoperfusion often requiring pharmacological or mechanical support [3]. Left ventricular (LV) dysfunction due to acute myocardial infarction (MI) remains the most frequent cause of CS. Despite an early revascularization strategy and advancing patients care, CS is still the leading cause of death in this population with high hospital mortality rate, approaching 50% [4, 5]. Treatment of patients with LCOS and CS is challenging, as many will require a combination of inotropic/vasoactive medications and mechanical support.

Levosimendan is a novel calcium sensitizer with inotropic/vasodilatory action and other specific pharmacologic properties which, unlike traditional inotropes such as catecholamines, improves myocardial contractility without influence on myocardial oxygen consumption and impairing diastolic function, and with no pro-arrhythmic effects [6]. Due to these favorable features, levosimendan may represent an ideal agent to be administered in patients with LCOS and CS. In the last few years, there was a very high interest in using this drug for the treatment of cardiac complications after surgery and in critically ill patients [7]. In the recently updated web-based consensus conference on mortality reduction in critically ill patients, levosimendan was confirmed as one of the drugs/techniques/strategies, which have been proven by high-quality randomized evidence to reduce mortality in the perioperative period [8].

12.2   Pharmacologic Properties

Unlike classic inotropic drugs, levosimendan uniquely increases troponin C affinity to calcium without increasing intracellular calcium concentration. Cardiac contractility thus improves without an increase in myocardial oxygen consumption [9]. The binding of levosimendan to troponin C is dependent on cytosolic calcium content, which is consistently reduced during diastole; this avoids the side effects of traditional inotropes such as lusitropy reduction and arrhythmias [6]. Levosimendan also induces vasodilation by acting on potassium channels in the peripheral smooth musculature.

Moreover, levosimendan has been recently shown to have anti-apoptotic and anti-inflammatory properties, which may contribute to a cardioprotective action and further improve long-term outcomes in the failing heart [10].

12.3   Main Evidences

The use of levosimendan has been widely studied in different clinical settings such as cardiac surgery, intensive care, and heart failure.

12.3.1 Perioperative Levosimendan in Cardiac Surgery

Several meta-analyses and randomized trials suggested that levosimendan might prevent LCOS and reduce morbidity and mortality after cardiac surgery. In 2008, a randomized controlled trial (RCT) by Levin et al. found that levosimendan was superior to dobutamine to treat postoperative LCOS [11]. The study enrolled 137 patients: 69 were treated with levosimendan, while 68 received dobutamine. Although hemodynamic parameters improved in both groups, the effect of levosimendan was more obvious and emerged earlier than that of dobutamine. Also, levosimendan treatment resulted in less need for an additional inotropic (8.7% vs 36.8%; $p < 0.05$), a vasopressor drugs (11.6% vs 30.9%; $p < 0.05$), an intra-aortic balloon pump (IABP) counterpulsation (2.9% vs 14.7%; $p < 0.05$), lower incidence of major postoperative complications andlower postoperative mortality (8.7% vs 25%; $p < 0.05$).

In a further trial by Levin et al., preoperative levosimendan treatment was found to be superior to placebo in patients with severe LV dysfunction (left ventricle ejection fraction (LVEF) <25%) undergoing coronary artery bypass surgery (CABG). Patients treated with levosimendan had a lower incidence of complicated weaning from cardiopulmonary bypass (2.4% versus 9.6%; $p < 0.05$), a decreased mortality (3.9% versus 12.8%; $p < 0.05$), and a lower incidence of LCOS (7.1% versus 20.8%; $p < 0.05$) compared with placebo. The study group also had a lower requirement for inotropes (7.9% versus 58.4%; $p < 0.05$), vasopressors (14.2% versus 45.6%; $p < 0.05$), and IABP (6.3% versus 30.4%; $p < 0.05$) [12]. Recently, three large multicenter RCTs investigated the perioperative use of levosimendan: the LICORN (Levosimendan on Low Cardiac Output Syndrome in Patients With Low Ejection Fraction Undergoing Coronary Artery Bypass Grafting With Cardiopulmonary Bypass) trial [13], the CHEETAH (Levosimendan to Reduce Mortality in High Risk Cardiac Surgery Patients) trial [14], and the LEVO-CTS (Levosimendan in Patients with Left Ventricular Systolic Dysfunction Undergoing Cardiac Surgery Requiring Cardiopulmonary Bypass) trial [15]. Contrary to the results of many previous smaller investigations which yielded promising results with the use of levosimendan in the perioperative setting, these three studies were either neutral or inconclusive.

In the LEVO-CTS trial, patients with a reduced LVEF undergoing cardiac surgery with the use of CPB were assigned to receive either a levosimendan or placebo infusion starting before surgery and continued after surgery. The study population included 882 patients with LVEF <35% undergoing scheduled or urgent cardiac surgery. All patients were considered at risk of developing postoperative LCOS. Levosimendan (0.2 μg/kg/min for 60 min, followed by 0.1 μg/kg/min for 23 h) or placebo were started at the induction of anesthesia. The study did not find a statistically significant difference between the two groups in a composite primary endpoint of death, perioperative MI, and need for renal replacement therapy (RRT) or a mechanical ventricular assist device. Nevertheless, there were fewer deaths in the levosimendan group: 20/428 (4.7%) versus 30/421 (7.1%), odds ratio 0.64, 95% confidence interval [CI] 0.37–1.13 ($p = 0.12$). In addition, patients who received levosimendan experienced significantly fewer LCOS events (78 vs 108; $p = 0.007$) and needed less inotropic support 24 h after initiation of infusion (235 vs. 264; $p = 0.02$).

In a subanalysis of the LEVO-CTS trial, the authors demonstrated a beneficial effect of levosimendan in terms of both 30-day (1.8% vs 5.4%; hazard ratio [HR] 0.32; 95% CI 0.11–0.88) and 90-day all-cause mortality (2.1% vs 7.9%; HR, 0.26; 95% CI, 0.11–0.64) in patients with reduced LVEF undergoing isolated (CABG). Levosimendan was also associated with a lower incidence of LCOS (interaction P 1/4 0.118) and secondary inotropes use beyond 24 h (interaction P 1/4 0.423), and with a greater CI than placebo (interaction P 1/4 0.051). However, these data were not confirmed in patients undergoing isolated valve surgery, as well as in patients undergoing combined procedures [16].

In the LICORN trial, 336 patients with LVEF ≤40% undergoing CABG were recruited from 13 hospitals. The study drug was started after induction of anesthesia and infused at a rate of 0.1 μg/kg/min for 24 h. Postoperative LCOS was determined using a composite criteria including need for inotropic drugs beyond 48 h following discontinuation of levosimendan; need for postoperative assist devices or failure to wean from these devices; need for RRT. The primary endpoint occurred in 87/167 patients (52%) in the levosimendan group compared with 101/168 (61%) in the control group (absolute risk reduction −7%, 95% CI: −17% to +3%, $p = 0.15$). There were no statistically significant inter-group differences in mortality or length of intensive care unit stay.

Unlike the two trials discussed above, the CHEETAH trial investigated the effects of levosimendan used for the treatment rather than for prophylaxis of post-operative LCOS in patients undergoing cardiac surgery [14]. Either levosimendan or placebo was administered to cardiac surgery patients who, according to pre-defined criteria, developed postoperative LCOS. The median preoperative LVEF was 50% in both groups, with 11% of patients having a LVEF <25%. A total of 248 patients received levosimendan and 258 received placebo. The mean dose and duration of levosimendan infusion were 0.07 μg/kg/min and 33 h, respectively. There was no significant difference in 30-day mortality between the levosimendan and placebo groups: 32 patients (12.9%) versus 33 (12.8%); absolute risk difference 0.1 percentage points; 95% CI −5.7 to +5.9 percentage points; $p = 0.97$).

12.3.2 Levosimendan in Cardiogenic Shock and in Takotsubo Syndrome

The standard of care in cardiogenic shock consists of primary percutaneous coronary intervention for AMI, inotropes, vasopressors, fluid therapy, and mechanical assist devices [17]. Levosimendan has been evaluated in large RCTs against dobutamine or placebo in patients with decompensated heart failure [18], septic shock [19], and LCOS after cardiac surgery [14], but not thoroughly in cardiogenic shock. Fuhrman and colleagues studied 32 patients with refractory CS. Patients meeting the inclusion criteria were randomly allocated to receive either levosimendan or enoximone. The survival rate at 30 days was significantly higher in the levosimendan group compared with the enoximone group (69% vs 37%, $p = 0.023$). Levosimendan induced a trend toward higher CI, stroke volume, and mixed venous oxygen saturation (SvO2). Also, lower cumulative values for catecholamines infusion at 72 h and for clinical signs of inflammation were seen in the levosimendan group. Multiple organ failure with subsequent death occurred only in the enoximone group (4 out of 16 patients) [20].

LCOS caused by Takotsubo syndrome (TS), also known as broken-heart syndrome or stress cardiomyopathy, is an increasingly diagnosed form of transient LV dysfunction that is often completely reversible [21]. It is recognized in ≈1–2% of patients initially presenting with symptoms suggestive of acute coronary syndrome [22]. In a prospective, randomized, double-blinded study by Guo et al., 200 consecutive patients (>65 years) with TS were randomly assigned to either a levosimendan ($n = 100$) or a control group ($n = 100$). On the days 30 and 180 after treatment, LVEF was significantly higher, and NYHA class and N-terminal pro-brain natriuretic peptide levels were significantly lower, in the levosimendan group as compared with the control group ($p < 0.05$ for all). The main finding of this study was mortality reduction in the levosimendan group compared with the control group (1% vs 8%, $p = 0.041$).

12.4 Therapeutic Use

In a current clinical practice levosimendan is administered with or without an initial bolus with further intravenous continuous infusion. It has approximately 1-h half-life. The steady-state concentration can be achieved within 4 h (without loading dose) and active metabolite plasma concentration peaking at 2 days after infusion. The drug has total clearance 175–250 ml/h/k, primarily through liver metabolism and with a smaller part metabolized through the intestine. Its prolonged action (up to 7–9 days) is not due to the drug itself but mainly due to its active metabolite OR-1896 (approximately 80 h half-life). The unique inotropic and cardioprotective properties of levosimendan can provide persistent effects for several days with subsequent reducing the rate of postoperative complications.

According to expert opinion, the agreed-upon recommended dose of levosimendan to be administered preoperatively or perioperatively in patients undergoing cardiac surgery was 0.1 µg/kg/min for 24 h, or to the end of the vial. The day prior to planned surgery was proposed as the optimal time frame for starting a preoperative levosimendan therapy. When levosimendan infusion is started during or after induction of anesthesia, the addition of a bolus is considered to be a feasible option. Experts advised against a bolus dose when used outside the operation room. Levosimendan can be administered in any hospital setting with adequate hemodynamic monitoring [23]. Several previously published trials have used infusion rates of 0.2 µg/kg/min with variable bolus doses. Another way to exert a preconditioning effect of levosimendan is administration for up to 24 h before surgery [24]. Higher doses could produce more potent hemodynamic effects, but at the expense of a greater vasodilatation and hypotension. In case of vasodilation, the experts suggest to combine levosimendan with vasopressors (norepinephrine, vasopressin). Dobutamine should be the preferred drug if additional inotropic support becomes necessary in a levosimendan-treated patient.

12.5   Discussion and Conclusion

According to available literature, levosimendan has been studied in more than 40 clinical trials in cardiac surgery. Earlier studies showed that it could prevent the development of LCOS and be useful in treating postoperative LCOS. Considering all the existing data, including the results of the three most recent large studies, we can conclude that levosimendan is a safe and effective drug for the treatment of patients undergoing cardiac surgery and requiring inotropic support. Nevertheless, available data showed that despite its unique mechanism of action, levosimendan has no evident advantage over classic inotropic drugs for the treatment of perioperative LCOS in patients undergoing cardiac surgery. For this reason, levosimendan currently cannot be recommended for routine use in all cardiac surgery patients with the aim of reducing mortality. A possible area of levosimendan use might be its application in patients during extracorporeal life support withdrawal, based on the rationale of the ongoing "Weanilevo" trial (NCT04158674).

There are currently no high-quality studies assessing the use of levosimendan in CS. When analyzing the existing data, it becomes clear that, levosimendan has no effect on short-term and long-term mortality, ischemic events, acute kidney injury, arrhythmias, or hospital length of stay when compared with dobutamine [25]. On the other hand, levosimendan can be well tolerated in combination with increased vasopressor support. The main drug-specific changes during levosimendan treatment include an increase in CI, cardiac power index, SvO2 and decrease in left ventricular pressure [26]. Additionally based on a low-quality study, levosimendan appears to be more useful in refractory cardiogenic shock secondary to MI when compared with enoximone [20]. Altogether, despite very promising aforementioned properties and based on existing evidence, levosimendan should be considered as a second-line therapy in well-selected patients with CS. Well-designed RCTs are warranted to address the gap between the potential use of levosimendan in CS and evident proof. The role of levosimendan in this setting will be evaluated in the LevoHeartShock study, which will include 634 patients in France (NCT04020263).

The therapeutic management of TS is still under debate and remains empirical with no evidence from RCTs available to date. Moreover, the use of catecholamine infusion is controversial and should be rather avoided in compromised TS patients since it may likely induce or worsen ventricle dysfunction. The potential role of levosimendan in this setting deserves further research.

References

1. Maganti M, Badiwala M, Sheikh A, et al. Predictors of low cardiac output syndrome after isolated mitral valve surgery. J Thorac Cardiovasc Surg. 2010;140:790–6.
2. Vincent J-L, De Backer D. Circulatory shock. N Engl J Med. 2013;369:1726–34.
3. van Diepen S, Katz JN, Albert NM, Henry TD, Jacobs AK, Kapur NK, Kilic A, Menon V, Ohman EM, Sweitzer NK, Thiele H, Washam JB, Cohen MG. Contemporary management of cardiogenic shock: a scientific statement from the American Heart Association. Circulation. 2017;136:e232–68.
4. Fox KAA, Steg PG, Eagle KA, Goodman SG, Anderson FA Jr, Granger CB, et al. Decline in rates of death and heart failure in acute coronary syndromes, 1999–2006. JAMA. 2007;297:1892–900.
5. Thiele H, Zeymer U, Neumann FJ, Ferenc M, Olbrich HG, Hausleiter J, et al. IABP-SHOCK II trial investigators: Levosimendan in patients with cardiogenic shock. Intraaortic balloon support for myocardial infarction with cardiogenicshock. N Engl J Med. 2012;367:1287–96.
6. Toller WG, Stranz C. Levosimendan, a new inotropic and vasodilator agent. Anesthesiology. 2006;104:556–69.
7. Landoni G, Biondi-Zoccai G, Greco M, et al. Effects of levosimendan on mortality and hospitalization. A meta-analysis of randomized controlled studies. Crit Care Med. 2012;40:634–46.
8. Landoni G, Pisano A, Lomivorotov V, et al. Randomized evidence for reduction of periop- erative mortality: an updated consensus process. J Cardiothorac Vasc Anesth. 2017;31(2):719–30.
9. Papp Z, Édes I, Fruhwald S, et al. Levosimendan: molecular mechanisms and clinical implications: consensus of experts on the mechanisms of action of levosimendan. Int J Cardiol. 2012;159:82–7.
10. Trikas A, Antoniades C, Latsios G, et al. Long-term effects of levosimendan infusion on inflammatory processes and sFas in patients with severe heart failure. Eur J Heart Fail. 2006;8:804–9.
11. Levin RL, Degrange MA, Porcile R, Salvagio F, Blanco N, Botbol AL, Tanus E, del Mazo CD. The calcium sensitizer levosimendan gives superior results to dobutamine in postoperative low cardiac output syndrome. Rev Esp Cardiol. 2008;61(5):471–9.
12. Levin R, Degrange M, Del Mazo C, et al. Preoperative levosimendan decreases mortality and the development of low cardiac output in high-risk patients with severe left ventricular dysfunction undergoing coronary artery bypass grafting with cardiopulmonary bypass. Exp Clin Cardiol. 2012;17:125–30.
13. Cholley B, Caruba T, Grosjean S, et al. Effect of Levosimendan on low cardiac output syndrome in patients with low ejection fraction undergoing coronary artery bypass grafting with cardiopulmonary bypass: the LICORN randomized clinical trial. JAMA. 2017;318:548–56.
14. Landoni G, Lomivorotov VV, Alvaro G, et al. CHEETAH study group. Levosimendan for hemodynamic support after cardiac surgery. N Engl J Med. 2017;376(21):2021–31.
15. Mehta RH, Leimberger JD, van Diepen S, et al. LEVO-CTS investigators. Levosimendan in patients with left ventricular dysfunction undergoing cardiac surgery. N Engl J Med. 2017;376(21):2032–42.
16. van Diepen S, Mehta RH, Leimberger JD, Goodman SG, Fremes S, Jankowich R, et al. Levosimendan in patients with reduced left ventricular function undergoing isolated coronary or valve surgery. J Thorac Cardiovasc Surg. 2020;159:2302–9.
17. Steg PG, James SK, Atar D, et al. Task force on the management of ST-segment elevation acute myocardial infarction of the European Society of Cardiology (ESC): ESC guidelines for the management of acute myocardial infarction in patients presenting with ST-segment elevation. Eur Heart J. 2012;33:2569–619.
18. Mebazaa A, Nieminen MS, Packer M, et al. SURVIVE investigators. Levosimendan vs dobutamine for patients with acute decompensated heart failure: the SURVIVE randomized trial. JAMA. 2007;297:1883–91.
19. Gordon AC, Perkins GD, Singer M, et al. Levosimendan for the prevention of acute organ dysfunction in sepsis. N Engl J Med. 2016;375:1638–48.

20. Fuhrmann JT, Schmeisser A, Schulze MR, Wunderlich C, Schoen SP, Rauwolf T, Weinbrenner C, Strasser RH. Levosimendan is superior to enoximone in refractory cardiogenic shock complicating acute myocardial infarction. Crit Care Med. 2008;36(8):2257–66. https://doi.org/10.1097/CCM.0b013e3181809846.
21. Akashi YJ, Goldstein DS, Barbaro G, Ueyama T. Takotsubo cardiomyopathy. Circulation. 2008;118:2754–62.
22. Kurowski V, Kaiser A, von Hof K, Killermann DP, Mayer B, Hartmann F, Schunkert H, Radke PW. Apical and midventricular transient left ventricular dysfunction syndrome (tako-tsubo cardiomyopathy) frequency, mechanisms, and prognosis. Chest. 2007;132:809–16.
23. Toller W, Heringlake M, Guarracino F, et al. Preoperative and perioperative use of levosimendan in cardiac surgery: European expert opinion. Int J Cardiol. 2015;184:323–36.
24. Levin R, Degrange M, Del Mazo C, et al. Preoperative levosimendan decreases mortality and the development of low cardiac output in high-risk patients with severe left ventricular dysfunction undergoing coronary artery bypass grafting with cardiopulmonary bypass. Exp Clin Cardiol. 2012;17(3):125–30.
25. Schumann J, Henrich EC, Strobl H, et al. Inotropic agents and vasodilator & strategies for the treatment of cardiogenic shock or low cardiac output syndrome. Cochrane Database Syst Rev. 2018;1:CD009669.
26. Fang M, Cao H, Wang Z. Levosimendan in patients with cardiogenic shock complicating myocardial infarction: a meta-analysis. Med Intensiva. 2017;42:409–15.

Drugs in Myocardial Infarction

13

Margherita Tozzi, Martina Di Piazza, and Paolo Meani

Contents

M. Tozzi · M. Di Piazza
Department of Anesthesia and Intensive Care, IRCCS San Raffaele Scientific Institute,
Milan, Italy
e-mail: tozzi.margherita@hsr.it

P. Meani (✉)
ECLS Centrum, Cardio-Thoracic Surgery Department, Heart & Vascular Centre, Maastricht
University Medical Centre (MUMC), Maastricht, The Netherlands
e-mail: paolo.meani@mumc.nl

© Springer Nature Switzerland AG 2021
G. Landoni et al. (eds.), *Reducing Mortality in Critically Ill Patients*,
https://doi.org/10.1007/978-3-030-71917-3_13

13.1 General Principles

According to the "Fourth universal definition of myocardial infarction," Acute Myocardial Infarction (AMI) is a "myocardial injury detected by abnormal cardiac biomarkers with clinical evidence of acute myocardial ischemia" [1]. The criteria include abnormal cardiac troponin (cTn) values with at least one value above the 99th percentile upper reference limit (URL), and at least one of the following:

- symptoms of myocardial ischemia,
- new ischemic electrocardiogram (ECG) changes,
- development of pathological Q waves,
- new loss of myocardium/new regional wall motion abnormality (imaging evidence),
- coronary thrombus (identification at angiography or autopsy).

These criteria were developed to differentiate type 1 MI (due to atherothrombotic coronary artery disease), type 2 MI (oxygen supply and demand mismatch), and type 3 MI (patient dies before obtaining blood for cTn but presentation was typical for MI). Type 4A, 4B, and 5 are coronary procedure-related MIs and the previous criteria are not to be used in order to make a diagnosis.

In the United States, the overall prevalence for AMI is 3.0% in people ≥20 years of age, and the estimated annual incidence is 605,000 new attacks and 200,000 recurrent attacks [2].

The patient may present with typical symptoms such as chest discomfort, nausea and/or vomiting, dyspnea and weakness, or have no symptoms at all; 12-lead ECG should be performed and evaluated for ischemic changes whenever AMI is suspected, and serial biomarker testing (i.e., cTn) should be done to confirm diagnosis [3].

ST-segment elevation MI (STEMI) is diagnosed if ST-segment elevation is found in at least two contiguous leads and symptoms indicating ischemia are present [4]. Non-ST-segment elevation MI (NSTEMI) is diagnosed in patients who do not have ST-segment elevation [5]. Serial biomarker testing is also used to subclassify an acute coronary syndrome without ST-segment elevation as NSTEMI or unstable angina (described as myocardial ischemia at rest or minimal exertion in the absence of cardiomyocyte necrosis) [3, 6].

13.2 Pathophysiological Principles

The most diagnosed type of MI is type 1 [4], caused by the erosion or rupture of an atherosclerotic coronary plaque that leads to the exposure of circulating blood to highly thrombogenic materials [7]. STEMI is usually the result of a totally occluding thrombus, with transmural ischemia, while NSTEMI or unstable angina are the result of partial occlusion or occlusion in the presence of collateral circulation [4, 5]. An evidence of coronary artery disease (CAD), diagnosed with angiography, is not mandatory for MI diagnosis [8]: in the absence of CAD, MI is called "Myocardial Infarction with Non-Obstructive Coronary Arteries" (MINOCA).

13.3 Treatment

13.3.1 Primary Percutaneous Coronary Intervention (STEMI and NSTEMI)

Primary percutaneous coronary intervention (PCI) is the ideal reperfusion strategy if patient presents within 12 h of symptoms onset, but it should be performed within 120 min from a diagnosis of STEMI [4]. For NSTEMI patients, an early invasive strategy (coronary angiography performed within 24 h of hospital admission) is recommended in high-risk patients [5, 9]. With similar delay to treatment, primary PCI is shown superior to intravenous fibrinolytic therapy in reducing mortality or other complications in STEMI patients [10, 11]. PCI is the most common intervention, but depending on clinical and anatomical features, coronary artery bypass graft (CABG) surgery could be performed instead of PCI.

Dual anti-platelet therapy (DAPT: aspirin and a $P2Y_{12}$ inhibitor) should be administered to patients undergoing primary PCI, plus a parenteral anticoagulant. The $P2Y_{12}$ inhibitor of choice should be prasugrel or ticagrelor, but they should be avoided in patients who take oral anticoagulants, with previous hemorrhagic complications or moderate-to-severe liver disease [4]. When both medications are contraindicated, clopidogrel is another possibility [12]. Unfractionated heparin (UFH), bivalirudin, and enoxaparin are the anticoagulants of choice for primary PCI, while fondaparinux is not recommended [13].

About 6–8% of patients undergoing PCI have an indication for long-term oral anticoagulation (OAC) with vitamin K antagonists (VKA) or direct oral anticoagulants (DOACs), due to various conditions such as atrial fibrillation, venous thromboembolism, or mechanical heart valves [5]. Interruption of OAC and bridging with parenteral anticoagulants to perform PCI may lead to an increase in both thromboembolic episodes and bleeds [14]. The safety of PCI on DOACs without additional parenteral anticoagulation is unknown, while no parenteral anticoagulation is needed if the international normalized ratio (INR) is >2.5 in VKA-treated patients [15].

13.3.2 Fibrinolytic Therapy (STEMI)

Fibrinolysis could be the most indicated option when primary PCI is neither feasible nor immediate. The STrategic Reperfusion Early After Myocardial infarction (STREAM) trial [16] randomized early STEMI patients to immediate fibrinolysis, followed by routine early angiography, or transfer to primary PCI (immediate PCI was not possible): the two groups reported similar outcomes. The median delay to PCI was 78 min, while 9 min was the median time from randomization to fibrinolytic therapy. In the 2017 ESC Guidelines for the management of STEMI [4], 10 min became the time-limit from STEMI diagnosis for the bolus of fibrinolytic therapy.

A fibrin-specific agent (i.e., tenecteplase, alteplase, or reteplase) should be favored for fibrinolysis [17]. Streptokinase is an option as well, but being a bacterial product, it can cause an immune response and lead to allergic reactions if used for a second time. Anti-platelet and anticoagulation agents can be considered in addition, and the benefits of aspirin and fibrinolytics seem to sum up [18]. Clopidogrel as well should be added to aspirin in case of fibrinolysis: the risk of cardiovascular events and overall mortality was reduced in previous trials [19, 20]. The Assessment of the Safety and Efficacy of a New Thrombolytic 3 (ASSENT-3) Trial showed that enoxaparin was better than UFH when administered in combination with tenecteplase [21]. In the OASIS-6 Trial [13], Fondaparinux reduced death and reinfarction when compared to UFH or placebo. In the Hirulog and Early Reperfusion or Occlusion (HERO)-2 Trial, compared to UFH, bivalirudin reduced reinfarctions when given with streptokinase (fibrin-specific agents were not studied) [22].

13.3.3 Different Perspectives (NSTEMI)

Another approach has to be considered for NSTEMI, where the clot is platelet-enriched, and the coronary artery is only partially occluded by the clot's fibrin cap. STEMI is caused instead by a fibrin-rich clot. Therefore, in NSTEMI platelets could be released into circulation by thrombolysis or fibrinolysis, possibly leading to the development of further thrombosis. Hence, the risk of thrombolysis outweighs the benefits in NSTEMI patients [23].

NSTEMI can be managed with an invasive approach and treated with PCI/CABG [5, 9]. Conversely, various trials explore a noninvasive management of NSTEMI [24, 25].

The management strategy of NSTEMI has no effect on the need for initiation of $P2Y_{12}$ inhibitors after the diagnosis [26, 27]. Aspirin administration is suggested as well [28]. Ischemic events in NSTEMI are reduced by parenteral anticoagulation, with a further reduction if anticoagulation is combined with platelet inhibitors [29].

13.3.4 Other Medications

- Oxygen: it should be administered only with arterial oxygen saturation (SaO2) <90% since hyperoxia could have detrimental effects in non-complicated MI [30].
- Betablockers: acute malignant ventricular arrhythmias in patients undergoing fibrinolysis are reduced by intravenous beta-blocker treatment, but effects on long-term clinical outcomes are unknown [31]. Hemodynamically stable patients undergoing primary PCI could benefit from early administration of beta-blockers [32, 33].

- Statins: they are a keystone of secondary prevention [34], and also patients with acute coronary syndrome may benefit from their early administration, according to literature [35, 36].
- Nitrates: their routine use in STEMI is not recommended because it was not beneficial in a randomized controlled trial against placebo [37]. In chronic situations, they can be used to control angina symptoms.
- Angiotensin-converting enzyme inhibitors (ACE-I) and angiotensin II receptor blockers (ARBs): an impaired left ventricle ejection fraction (<40%) is an indication for ACE-I, and their administration is also recommended in patients who initially suffered from heart failure [38]. ARBs should be given to patients intolerant to ACE-I. Valsartan was found to be non-inferior to captopril in the VALsartan In Acute myocardial iNfarcTion (VALIANT) trial [39].

13.4 Main Evidences

13.4.1 Dual Anti-Platelet Therapy

The Dual Anti-Platelet Therapy dramatically changed the acute coronary syndrome (ACS) treatment. Compared with aspirin alone, results of randomized trials have shown that clopidogrel plus aspirin reduces the risk of ischemic events in patients undergoing PCI, and in those with non-ST-elevation ACS [40, 41].

ST-elevation acute coronary syndromes were deeply investigated by COMMIT-CCS2 (ClOpidogrel and Metoprolol in Myocardial Infarction Trial—Second Chinese Cardiac Study), one of the largest randomized placebo-controlled trials of the emergency treatment of patients with suspected AMI [19]: 45,852 patients were included among 1250 hospitals, those scheduled for primary PCI were excluded. ST-segment elevation or bundle branch block was found in 93% patient at the admission. Patients were randomized to clopidogrel 75 mg daily or matching placebo in addition to aspirin 162 mg daily. The main results showed how the allocation to clopidogrel led to a consistent 9% proportional death, reinfarction, or stroke reduction. This was independent of other treatments being used and no significant excess major bleeding risk was recorded. These findings clearly demonstrated the reduction of mortality and major vascular events in hospital when clopidogrel was daily added to aspirin and other standard treatments in a large population with AMI. The authors underlined that aspirin might have a substantial role at preventing recurrent clinical events, rather than at maintaining coronary artery patency [42]. On the contrary, clopidogrel might be more effective in acute setting by preventing re-occlusion or by limiting the microvascular effects of platelet activation.

13.4.2 Novel Anti-Platelet Medication

The PLATO, a multicenter, double-blind, randomized trial showed a significant reduction of deaths from vascular causes, myocardial infarction, or stroke in patients who have an acute coronary syndrome with or without ST-segment elevation. Ticagrelor (180 mg loading dose, 90 mg twice daily thereafter) was compared with clopidogrel (300–600 mg loading dose, 75 mg daily thereafter) for the prevention of cardiovascular events in 18,624 acute coronary syndromes. The occurrence of death from vascular causes, myocardial infarction or stroke, evaluated at 12 months, was 9.8% in patients treated with ticagrelor as compared with 11.7% in those receiving clopidogrel. Myocardial infarction alone occurred in 5.8% in the ticagrelor group, whereas in 6.9% of patients receiving clopidogrel. However, ticagrelor was associated with a higher rate of major procedure-related bleeding (4.5% vs. 3.8%, $p = 0.03$) [43].

The TRITON-TIMI is another crucial trial, which compared prasugrel (a 60 mg loading dose and a 10 mg daily maintenance dose) with clopidogrel (a 300 mg loading dose and a 75 mg daily maintenance dose) in 13,608 patients with moderate-to-high-risk acute coronary syndromes scheduled to percutaneous coronary intervention. Prasugrel was associated with significantly reduced rates of ischemic events (hazard ratio for prasugrel vs. clopidogrel, 0.81; 95% confidence interval [CI], 0.73 to 0.90; $p < 0.001$), including stent thrombosis (2.4% vs. 1.1%; $p < 0.001$), but with an increased risk of major bleeding, including fatal bleeding (0.4% vs. 0.1%; $p = 0.002$). However, the overall mortality did not differ significantly between treatment groups [44].

13.4.3 Thrombolysis

The thrombolytic therapy was a milestone in the AMI treatment, being a crucial step before the ongoing percutaneous revascularization therapy.

The Grampian Region Early Anistreplase Trial (GREAT) was one of the largest trials investigating the effects of thrombolysis. First, this trial demonstrated the high benefit of earlier thrombolysis in AMI. In fact, Rawles et al. [45] showed delaying thrombolytic treatment by 1 h increases the hazard ratio of death by 20%, equivalent to the loss of 43/1000 lives within the next 5 years. Furthermore, delaying thrombolytic treatment by 30 min reduces the average expectation of life by 1 year. They compared two groups undergoing intravenous administration of anistreplase either before hospital admission or in the hospital, at a median time of 105 and 240 min, respectively, after onset of symptoms. By 5 years, 25% of patients included in the pre-hospital group had died compared with 36% of those treated in the hospital group. Pre-hospital and hospital Kaplan–Meier survival curves were clearly separated throughout the 5-year follow-up period. Furthermore, if compared to in-hospital thrombolysis, administrating anistreplase at home resulted in a reduction in mortality, fewer cardiac arrests, fewer Q-wave infarcts, and better left ventricular function.

For instance, a substudy of GREAT trial [46] found a 50% relative reduction in cardiac mortality when anistreplase was given at home [11/163 cases (6.7%) vs 20/148 (13.5%), difference −6.8%, $p = 0.05$]. Again, fewer deaths or resuscitation from cardiac arrest occurred in patients treated at home compared with patients treated in hospital [13/163 (8.0%) vs 24/148 (16.2%), difference −8.2%, $p = 0.02$]. The benefits of home thrombolysis also led to a better myocardial performance. Since the reduction in Q-wave infarction with home thrombolysis was greater in the group who received the home injection (in particular those treated within 2 h of the onset of symptoms), the survivors in the early branch showed a better left ventricular function in the short term which may explain the middle-long-term survival benefit.

Secondly, The GREAT Trial group confirmed the feasibility and safety of domiciliary thrombolysis by general practitioners. The study included 311 patients with suspected AMI visited at home within four h of onset of symptoms. Patients with contraindications to thrombolytic therapy were excluded. Anistreplase was administered by general practitioners at home 101 min after onset of symptoms. Adverse events after thrombolysis were infrequent and, apart from cardiac arrest, not a serious one occurred before admission to hospital. However, no obvious association between the thrombolytic therapy and cardiac arrest was found. Moreover, its occurrence was less common in the anistreplase group compared with placebo, indicating the coronary occlusion might be the primary cause leading to fatal arrhythmias. Yet, few patients suffered from hematemesis, but only one required a transfusion and none had significant blood loss before arrival to hospital.

Although the results from GREAT trial were positive, the thrombolysis may fail. Sarullo et al. [47] demonstrated that an additional thrombolytic administration in patients with unsuccessful thrombolysis is feasible and provides significant infarct extension reduction. Ninety patients hospitalized for suspected AMI who underwent thrombolytic therapy within 4 h of the symptom onset, experienced pain, and showed persistent ST-segment elevation 120 min after starting thrombolysis, were randomized into two groups. The first group included patients who received an additional 50 mg recombinant Tissue Plasminogen Activator (rt-PA), whereas only conventional therapy was administrated in the second one. Among patients who received the additional dose, 77.7% showed reperfusion compared to 26.6% in the control group. Furthermore, markers of myocardial injury such as CK (creatine kinase) and CK-MB (CK myocardial band) showed lower peaks, as well as pre-discharge echocardiogram ejection fraction which was higher. This led to a lower mortality in patients treated with additional thrombolytic dose (6.6% vs 28.8%), and the bleeding risk increase was acceptable. In fact, only one major bleeding was recorded (non-fatal stroke), and 44.4% patients suffered from minor bleeding. However, the rescue thrombolysis does not guarantee a stable coronary reperfusion since 55.5% of patient who received a rescue thrombolysis had a recurrent ischemia event (reinfarction or angina).

References

1. Thygesen K, Alpert JS, Jaffe AS, et al. Fourth universal definition of myocardial infarction. Circulation. 2018;138:e618–51.
2. Benjamin EJ, Muntner P, Alonso A, et al. Heart disease and stroke statistics-2019 update: a report from the American Heart Association. Circulation. 2019 Mar 5;139(10):e56–e528.

3. Anderson JL, Morrow DA. Acute myocardial infarction. N Engl J Med. 2017;376:2053–64.
4. Ibanez B, James S, Agewall S, et al. 2017 ESC guidelines for the management of acute myocardial infarction in patients presenting with ST-segment elevation. Eur Heart J. 2018;39:119–77.
5. Collet JP, Thiele H, Barbato E, et al. 2020 ESC guidelines for the management of acute coronary syndromes in patients presenting without persistent ST-segment elevation. Eur Heart J. 2020:ehaa575. https://doi.org/10.1093/eurheartj/ehaa575.
6. Braunwald E, Morrow DA. Unstable angina: Is it time for a requiem? Circulation. 2013;127:2452–7.
7. Libby P. Mechanisms of acute coronary syndromes and their implications for therapy. N Engl J Med. 2013;368:2004–13.
8. Agewall S, Beltrame JF, Reynolds HR, et al. ESC working group position paper on myocardial infarction with non-obstructive coronary arteries. Eur Heart J. 2017;38(3):143–53.
9. Fox KAA, Dabbous OH, Goldberg RJ, et al. Prediction of risk of death and myocardial infarction in the six months after presentation with acute coronary syndrome: prospective multinational observational study (GRACE). BMJ. 2006;333(7578):1091.
10. Zijlstra F, Hoorntje JC, de Boer MJ, et al. Long-term benefit of primary angioplasty as compared with thrombolytic therapy for acute myocardial infarction. N Engl J Med. 1999;341(19):1413–9.
11. Keeley EC, Boura JA, Grines CL. Primary angioplasty versus intravenous thrombolytic therapy for acute myocardial infarction: a quantitative review of 23 randomised trials. Lancet. 2003;361(9351):13–20.
12. Mehta SR, Tanguay JF, Eikelboom JW, et al. Double-dose versus standard-dose clopidogrel and high-dose versus low-dose aspirin in individuals undergoing percutaneous coronary intervention for acute coronary syndromes (CURRENT-OASIS 7): a randomized factorial trial. Lancet. 2010;376(9748):1233–43.
13. Yusuf S, Mehta SR, Chrolavicius S, et al. Effects of fondaparinux on mortality and reinfarction in patients with acute ST-segment elevation myocardial infarction: the OASIS-6 randomized trial. JAMA. 2006;295(13):1519–30.
14. Gilard M, Blanchard D, Helft G, et al. Antiplatelet therapy in patients with anticoagulants undergoing percutaneous coronary stenting (from STENTing and oral antiCOagulants [STENTICO]). Am J Cardiol. 2009;104:338–42.
15. Dewilde WJM, Janssen PW, Kelder JC, et al. Uninterrupted oral anticoagulation versus bridging in patients with long-term oral anticoagulation during percutaneous coronary intervention: subgroup analysis from the WOEST trial. Euro Intervention. 2015;11(4):381–90.
16. Armstrong PW, Gershlick AH, Goldstein P, et al. Fibrinolysis or primary PCI in ST-segment elevation myocardial infarction. N Engl J Med. 2013;368(15):1379–87.
17. The GUSTO Investigators. An international randomized trial comparing four thrombolytic strategies for acute myocardial infarction. N Engl J Med. 1993;329(10):673–82.
18. ISIS-2 (Second International Study of Infarct Survival) Collaborative Group. Randomised trial of intravenous streptokinase, oral aspirin, both, or neither among 17,187 cases of suspected acute myocardial infarction: ISIS-2. Lancet. 1988;2(8607):349–60.
19. Chen ZM, Jiang LX, Chen YP, et al. & COMMIT (ClOpidogrel and metoprolol in myocardial infarction trial) collaborative group. Addition of clopidogrel to aspirin in 45,852 patients with acute myocardial infarction: randomised placebo-controlled trial. Lancet. 2005;366(9497):1607–21.
20. Sabatine MS, Cannon CP, Gibson CM, et al. Addition of clopidogrel to aspirin and fibrinolytic therapy for myocardial infarction with ST-segment elevation. N Engl J Med. 2005;352(12):1179–89.
21. Assessment of the Safety and Efficacy of a New Thrombolytic Regimen (ASSENT)-3 Investigators. Efficacy and safety of tenecteplase in combination with enoxaparin, abciximab, or unfractionated heparin: the ASSENT-3 randomised trial in acute myocardial infarction. Lancet. 2001;358(9282):605–13.
22. White H. Hirulog and early reperfusion or occlusion (HERO)-2 trial investigators. Thrombin-specific anticoagulation with bivalirudin versus heparin in patients receiving

fibrinolytic therapy for acute myocardial infarction: the HERO-2 randomised trial. Lancet. 2001;358(9296):1855–63.

23. Anderson HV, Cannon CP, Stone PH, et al. One-year results of the thrombolysis in myocardial infarction (TIMI) IIIb clinical trial. J Am Coll Cardiol. 1995;26(7):1643–50.

24. Roe MT, Armstrong PW, Fox KAA, et al. Prasugrel versus clopidogrel for acute coronary syndromes without revascularization. N Engl J Med. 2012;367:1297–309.

25. James SK, Roe MT, Cannon CP, et al. Ticagrelor versus clopidogrel in patients with acute coronary syndromes intended for non-invasive management: substudy from prospective randomised PLATelet inhibition and patient outcomes (PLATO) trial. BMJ. 2011;342:d3527.

26. Hamm CW, Bassand JP, Agewall S, et al. ESC guidelines for the management of acute coronary syndromes inpatients presenting without persistent ST-segment elevation: the task force for the management of acute coronary syndromes (ACS) in patients presenting without persistent ST-segment elevation of the European Society of Cardiology (ESC). Eur Heart J. 2011;32:2999–3054.

27. Bellemain-Appaix A, Brieger D, Beygui F, et al. New P2Y12 inhibitors versus clopidogrel in percutaneous coronary intervention: a meta-analysis. J Am Coll Cardiol. 2010;56:1542–51.

28. Antithrombotic Trialists' Collaboration. Collaborative meta-analysis of randomized trials of antiplatelet therapy for prevention of death, myocardial infarction, and stroke in high risk patients. BMJ. 2002;324:71–86.

29. Eikelboom JW, Anand SS, Malmberg K, et al. Unfractionated heparin and low-molecular-weight heparin in acute coronary syndrome without ST elevation: a meta-analysis. Lancet. 2000;355:1936–42.

30. Stub D, Smith K, Bernard S, et al. Air versus oxygen in ST-segment-elevation myocardial infarction. Circulation. 2015;131(24):2143–50.

31. Chen ZM, Pan HC, Chen YP, et al. Early intravenous then oral metoprolol in 45,852 patients with acute myocardial infarction: randomised placebo-controlled trial. Lancet. 2005;366(9497):1622–32.

32. Ibanez B, Macaya C, Sánchez-Brunete V, et al. Effect of early metoprolol on infarct size in ST-segment-elevation myocardial infarction patients undergoing primary percutaneous coronary intervention: the effect of metoprolol in Cardioprotection during an acute myocardial infarction (METOCARD-CNIC) trial. Circulation. 2013;128(14):1495–503.

33. Roolvink V, Ibáñez B, Ottervanger JP, et al. Early intravenous beta-blockers inpatients with ST-segment elevation myocardial infarction before primary percutaneous coronary intervention. J Am Coll Cardiol. 2016;67(23):2705–15.

34. Baigent C, Keech A, Kearney PM, et al. Efficacy and safety of cholesterol-lowering treatment: prospective meta-analysis of data from 90,056 participants in 14 randomised trials of statins. Lancet. 2005;366(9493):1267–78.

35. Cannon CP, Braunwald E, McCabe CH, et al. Intensive versus moderate lipid lowering with statins after acute coronary syndromes. N Engl J Med. 2004;350(15):1495–504.

36. Schwartz GG, Olsson AG, Ezekowitz MD, et al. Effects of atorvastatin on early recurrent ischemic events in acute coronary syndromes: the MIRACL study: a randomized controlled trial. JAMA. 2001;285(13):1711–8.

37. Holmes DR Jr, Berger PB, Hochman JS, et al. Cardiogenic shock in patients with acute ischemic syndromes with and without ST-segment elevation. Circulation. 1999;100:2067–73.

38. Pfeffer MA, Greaves SC, Arnold JM, et al. Early versus delayed angiotensin-converting enzyme inhibition therapy in acute myocardial infarction. The healing and early afterload reducing therapy trial. Circulation. 1997;95(12):2643–51.

39. Pfeffer MA, McMurray JJV, Velazquez EJ, et al. Valsartan, captopril, or both in myocardial infarction complicated by heart failure, left ventricular dysfunction, or both. N Engl J Med. 2003;349(20):1893–906.

40. Steinhubl SR, Berger PB, Mann JT III, et al. Early and sustained dual oral antiplatelet therapy following percutaneous coronary intervention: a randomized controlled trial. JAMA. 2002;288:2411–20.

41. CURE investigators. Effects of clopidogrel in addition to aspirin in patients with acute coronary syndromes without ST-segment elevation. NEJM. 2001;345:494–502.
42. Roux S, Christeller S, Ludin E. Effects of aspirin on coronary reocclusion and recurrent ischemia after thrombolysis: a meta- analysis. JACC. 1992;19:671–7.
43. Wallentin L, Becker RC, Budaj A, et al. Ticagrelor versus clopidogrel in patients with acute coronary syndromes. N Engl J Med. 2009;361(11):1045–57.
44. Wiviott SD, Braunwald E, McCabe CH, et al. Prasugrel versus clopidogrel in patients with acute coronary syndromes. N Engl J Med. 2007;357(20):2001–15.
45. Rawles JM. Quantification of the benefit of earlier thrombolytic therapy: five-year results of the Grampian region early Anistreplase trial (GREAT). J Am Coll Cardiol. 1997;30(5):1181–6.
46. GREAT Group. Feasibility, safety, and efficacy of domiciliary thrombolysis by general practitioners: Grampian region early anistreplase trial. BMJ. 1992;305(6853):548–53.
47. Sarullo FM, Schicchi R, Schirò M, et al. Sicurezza ed efficacia della trombolisi di salvataggio per via sistemica nell'infarto miocardico acuto [the safety and efficacy of systemic salvage thrombolysis in acute myocardial infarct]. Ital Heart J Suppl. 2000;1(1):81–7.

Tranexamic Acid in Trauma Patients

14

Annalisa Volpi, Silvia Grossi, and Roberta Mazzani

Contents

14.1 General Principles

Traumatic injuries are a considerable public health burden with significant personal and social costs. Hemorrhage is responsible for a third of in-hospital trauma deaths and contributes to deaths due to multiorgan failure [1].

The hemostatic system helps to maintain circulation after severe vascular injury, whether traumatic or surgical in origin. Major surgery and trauma trigger similar hemostatic responses and, in both situations, severe blood loss presents an extreme challenge to the coagulation system, resulting in a stimulation of clot breakdown (fibrinolysis) that might become pathological. Hyperfibrinolysis is demonstrated in severely injured trauma patients contributing to an early coagulopathy associated with increased mortality [2].

A. Volpi (✉) · S. Grossi · R. Mazzani
1st Anaesthesia and Intensive Care Unit, University Hospital of Parma, Parma, Italy
e-mail: avolpi@ao.pr.it; sigrossi@ao.pr.it; rmazzani@ao.pr.it

© Springer Nature Switzerland AG 2021
G. Landoni et al. (eds.), *Reducing Mortality in Critically Ill Patients*,
https://doi.org/10.1007/978-3-030-71917-3_14

Antifibrinolytic agents reduce blood loss in patients with both normal and exaggerated fibrinolytic responses to surgery, without apparently increasing the risk of postoperative complications [3]. In a large multicenter placebo-controlled trial (CRASH-2), early administration of a short course of tranexamic acid (TXA), an inhibitor of fibrinolysis, was proved to have positive effect on survival, leading to validation of its use in trauma patients [4, 5].

14.2   Main Evidences

Reliable evidence that TXA reduces blood transfusion in surgical patients has been available for many years. Several systematic reviews of randomized trials in patients undergoing elective or emergency/urgent surgery treated with TXA identified a reduction in blood transfusion by 30% without serious adverse effects but with no significant reduction in mortality. Although the effect on thromboembolic events remains uncertain, the use of TXA in cardiac surgery did not increase the risk of myocardial infarction (MI), stroke, deep venous thrombosis, pulmonary embolus or renal dysfunction [3, 6, 7] (Table 14.1).

Since the hemostatic responses to surgery and trauma are similar, the effects of TXA on death, vascular occlusive events, and the receipt of blood transfusion on adult trauma patients with significant hemorrhage or at risk of significant hemorrhage, were evaluated by a large multicenter, placebo-controlled trial, the CRASH-2 (Clinical Randomization of an Antifibrinolytic in Significant Hemorrhage 2). Tranexamic acid was administrated within 8 h from injury, with a loading dose of 1 g over 10 min followed by infusion of 1 g over 8 h. The trial included 20,211 patients and treatment with TXA was associated with a reduction in all-cause mortality with no apparent increase in vascular occlusive events, in number of patients receiving blood products and in amount of blood transfused within the two groups (respectively 1.7% vs. 2.0%, 50.4% vs. 51.3%, 6.06 vs. 6.29). The relative risk (RR) of death with TXA was 0.91 (95% Confidence Interval [95%CI] 0.85–0.97, $p = 0.0035$) [4].

Although the reduction of fibrinolysis is a plausible mechanism, no measure on fibrinolytic activity has been performed in the trial. Alternative plausible hypotheses that may explain the effects take into account the reduction of the pro-inflammatory effects of plasmin, hemostasis improvement, or other mechanisms [5].

A further analysis of the CRASH-2 results showed that TXA treatment within 3 h of injury reduced the risk of death due to bleeding by nearly 30% ($p < 0.0001$), and the effect was even greater if the time of administration was less than 1 h from injury (5.3% vs. 7.7%; RR 0.68, 95% CI 0.57–0.82; $p < 0.0001$). Moreover, there were fewer vascular occlusive deaths with TXA and a significant reduction in fatal and non-fatal MI. Treatment given more than 3 h after injury, on the other hand, significantly increased the risk of death due to bleeding (4.4% vs 3.1%). The hypothesized mechanisms leading to reduced risk of death are anti-thrombotic or

Table 14.1 Results of the main meta-analysis comparing tranexamic acid to placebo or no intervention in surgical and trauma patients

Meta-analyses	Size		Mortality		Blood transfusion		Myocardial infarction		Stroke		Pulmonary embolism	
	RCT	pts	RR	95% CI	RR	95% CI	RR	95% CI	RR	95% CI	RR	95% CI
Henry DA [3][a]	252	25,000	0.60	0.33–1.10	0.61	0.53–0.70	0.79	0.41–1.52	1.23	0.49–3.07	0.67	0.23–1.99
Ker K [8][a]	129	10,488	0.61	0.32–1.12	0.63	0.58–0.68	0.68	0.43–1.09	1.14	0.65–2	0.61	0.25–1.47
Ker K [6][a]	104	NR	NR	NR	0.66	0.65–0.67	NR	NR	NR	NR	NR	[b]
Perel P [7][a]	5	372	1.01	0.14–7.3	0.7	0.52–0.24	[b]	[b]	2.79	0.12–67.10	[b]	[b]
Roberts I [9][c]	4	20,548	0.9	0.85–0.97	0.98[d]	0.96–1.03	0.64[d]	0.42–0.97	0.86[d]	0.61–1.23	1.01[d]	0.73–1.41

RCT randomize-controlled trial, *pts* patients, *RR* relative risk, *CI* confidence interval, *NR* not reported

[a]Surgical setting
[b]No cases of myocardial infarction or pulmonary embolism reported in this meta-analysis
[c]Traumatic injury setting
[d]Only the CRASH-2 trial reported

anti-inflammatory effects together with the effect on myocardial oxygen demand and oxygen supply, secondary to the reduction of bleeding [5, 9–11].

A new randomized placebo-controlled trial that evaluates the effects of tranexamic acid on death, disability, vascular occlusive events in patients with traumatic brain injury (CRASH-3) was published in October 2019. Patients with a GCS of 12 or lower or with any intracranial bleeding on CT scan without no major extracranial bleeding were enrolled for this study. The primary study outcome was head injury-related in-hospital death within 28 days of injury. The results show that among patients treated within 3 h of injury, the risk of head injury-related death was 18.5% in the tranexamic acid group versus 19.8% in the placebo group (855 vs 892 events, RR 0.94%). Excluding patients with GCS score of 3 or bilateral unreactive pupils at baseline, the results were 12.5% in the tranexamic acid group vs 14.0% in the placebo group (RR 0.89). The risk of vascular occlusive events and other complications was similar in the two groups. The CRASH-3 trial provides evidence that tranexamic acid is safe in patients with TBI and that treatment within 3 h of injury reduces head injury-related deaths because early administration of tranexamic acid in patients with TBI might prevent or reduce intracranial hemorrhage expansion, brain herniation, and death [12].

14.3 Pharmacologic Properties and Physiopathological Principles

Tranexamic acid is trans-4-aminomethylcyclohexane-carboxylic acid, a lysine-like drug. It is a competitive inhibitor of plasminogen activation and, at higher concentrations, a non-competitive inhibitor of plasmin that prevents dissolution of the fibrin clot. With reduction in plasmin activity, TXA also has an anti-inflammatory effect reducing activation of complement and consumption of C1 esterase inhibitor. Since fibrinolysis normally acts in hours or days, while there is a quick clinical effect of TXA, other mechanism should be involved.

Tranexamic acid activates thrombin generation by contact phase and acts on factor XII and prekallikrein. It also shows some modulatory effect on thrombin: it inhibits competitively the activation of trypsinogen by enterokinase, it inhibits noncompetitively the trypsin and weakly the thrombin, it activates thrombin generation by contact phase, and it acts on factor XII and prekallikrein. Tranexamic acid at usual doses has no effect on blood coagulation parameters (coagulation time or various coagulation factors in whole blood or citrated blood from normal subjects), platelets count, and in vitro aggregation [13, 14].

Although further studies are needed to understand the way TXA reduces the risk of death in bleeding trauma patients, on the basis of evidence, different mechanism should be involved:

- reduction in perioperative bleeding, transfusion requirements, and risk of postoperative complications. In the CRASH-2 trial, the lack of transfusion reduction could be related to the difficulty to estimate blood loss in the emergency

evaluation together with the greater opportunity to receive a blood transfusion by the patients who survived (competing risks)
- activity on hyperfibrinolysis which is associated with increased mortality [2, 15]
- reduction in inflammatory response (17% vs. 42%; $p < 0.05$) and in incidence of vasoplegic shock (0 vs. 27%; $p < 0.01$) [6]

14.4 Therapeutic Use

14.4.1 Pharmacokinetics

After i.v. administration of TXA the plasma concentration showed three mono-exponential decays: the first very rapid, the second with half-life of 1.3–2 h, and the third with half-life of 9–18 h. About half of the dose was recovered unchanged in the urine during the first 3–4 h, 90–95% within 24 h, and 95–99% within 72 h. The half-life of elimination was about one-fourth of the half-life related to availability of the compound (3 h). Tranexamic acid is eliminated by glomerular filtration and neither tubular excretion nor absorption takes place. Impairment of renal function prolongs the biological half-life of the compound with consequent increased plasma concentrations. Tranexamic acid is delivered in the cell compartment and the cerebrospinal fluid with delay. The distribution volume is about 33% of the body mass.

Moreover, TXA is minimally bound to plasma proteins ($\approx$3%) at therapeutic plasma concentrations (5–10 mg/L) [16].

14.4.2 Practical Application: Dosage and Timing

Tranexamic acid use is unlabeled in most fields (hemorrhage associated to trauma, surgery, and fibrinolysis) but large reliable evidence demonstrated its benefit in these circumstances.

In trauma-associated hemorrhage, clinical trials included patients with significant hemorrhage (systolic blood pressure < 90 mmHg, heart rate > 110 bpm, or both) or those at risk of significant hemorrhage. According to studies in surgical patients that showed no significant difference between high and low doses, an i.v. loading dose of 1000 mg over 10 min was recommended for administration, followed by a continuous i.v. infusion of 1000 mg over the next 8 h. In children, the Royal College of Paediatrics and Child Health and the National and Paediatric Pharmacists Group Joint Committee recommended an initial loading dose of 15 mg/kg (maximum 1 g) over 10 min followed by 2 mg/kg/h [17]. In elderly patients, no reduction in dosage is necessary unless there is evidence of renal failure.

Every effort should be made to treat patients as soon as possible. In the CRASH-2 Trial, treatment began within 8 h of injury [4], but further analysis demonstrated a higher benefit with an administration within 3 h of injury, and preferably within 1 h.

Moreover, there is the possibility that late treatment might increase the risk of death due to bleeding although there was no evidence of any increase in all-cause mortality in patients treated after 3 h [5, 10, 18].

14.4.3 Indications and Contraindications

The recommendation in the European guideline on management of bleeding and coagulopathy following major trauma include the early administration of TXA (Grade 1A), preferably within 3 h after injury (Grade 1B), considering the administration of the first dose en route to the hospital (Grade 2C) [19].

The Clinical Guideline of the National Institute for health and Care Excellence (NICE) on major trauma (Major trauma: assessment and initial management NICE guideline [NG39] Published date: 17 February 2016), recommend the use of intravenous tranexamic acid as soon as possible in patients with major trauma and active or suspected active bleeding and advise against its use more than 3 h after injury in patients with major trauma unless there is evidence of hyperfibrinolysis [20].

Moreover, the 18th Expert Committee on the Selection and Use of Essential Medicines was successful to get TXA included in the World Health Organization list of essential medicines for use in adult trauma patients with hemorrhage within 8 h of injury [21].

In the evidence statement "Major Trauma and the Use of Tranexamic Acid in Children," the Royal College of Paediatrics and Child Health and the National and Paediatric Pharmacists Group Joint Committee recommended a pragmatic dosage schedule, but further prospective trials are needed to better define the best dose scheme and the safety profile of these drugs. Administration of TXA or epsilon-aminocaproic acid could potentially be helpful in other settings, such as transplantation, trauma, or massively bleeding children [17].

Contraindications are hypersensitivity to TXA or any of the other ingredients, history of venous or arterial thrombosis, or history of convulsions.

14.5 Conclusion

The evidence collected strongly endorses the importance of early administration of TXA in bleeding trauma patients and suggests that trauma systems should be configured to facilitate this recommendation. In patients presenting late (>3 h after injury), the use has to be limited to patients with evidence of hyperfibrinolysis since the drug after the 3 h is associate with worst outcome.

Clinical summary

Drug	Indications	Cautions	Side-effects	Dose	Notes
Tranexamic Acid	Trauma patient with evidence or at risk of significant hemorrhage	• Pregnancy and lactation • DIC (only with acute severe bleeding) • Renal impairment: reduction of the dose • Upper urinary tract bleeding • Subarachnoid hemorrhage • Uncorrected cardiovascular or cerebrovascular disease • Concomitant use of procoagulant agents (e.g., anti-inhibitor coagulant complex/factor IX complex concentrates, fibrinogen concentrate, oral tretinoin, hormonal contraceptives) • *Contraindicated in active thromboembolic disease*	• Hypersensitivity reactions • Retinal venous and arterial occlusion • Seizure • Thrombotic events (venous and arterial thrombosis or thromboembolism, including central retinal artery/vein obstruction) • Ureteral obstruction • Gastro-intestinal disorders (nausea, vomiting, and diarrhea)	Loading dose of 1 g infused over 10 min, followed by a continuous intravenous infusion of 1 g over 8 h	Before use of TXA, when possible, risk factors of thromboembolic disease should be investigated

References

1. Sauaia A, Moore FA, Moore EE, et al. Epidemiology of trauma deaths: a reassessment. J Trauma. 1995;38:185–93.
2. Brohi K, Cohen MJ, Ganter MT, et al. Acute coagulopathy of trauma: hypoperfusion induces systemic anticoagulation and hyperfibrinolysis. J Trauma. 2008;64:1211–7.
3. Henry DA, Carless PA, Moxey AJ, O'Connel D, Stokes BJ, Fergusson DA, Ker K. Antifibrinolytic use for minimising perioperative allogeneic blood transfusion. Cochrane Database Syst Rev. 2011;19(1):CD001886.
4. The CRASH-2 Collaborators. Effects of TXA on death, vascular occlusive events, and blood transfusion in trauma patients with significant hemorrhage (CRASH-2): a randomised, placebo-controlled trial. Lancet. 2010;376:23–32.
5. The CRASH-2 Collaborators. The importance of early treatment with TXA in bleeding trauma patients: an exploratory analysis of the CRASH-2 randomised controlled trial. Lancet. 2011;377:1096–101.
6. Ker K, Prieto-Merino D, Roberts I. Systematic review, meta-analysis and meta regression of the effect of tranexamic acid on surgical blood loss. Br J Surg. 2013;100:1271–9.
7. Perel P, Ker K, Morales Uribe CH, Roberts I. Tranexamic acid for reducing mortality in emergency and urgent surgery. Cochrane Database Syst Rev. 2013;31(1):CD010245.
8. Ker K, Edwards P, Perel P, Shakur H, Roberts I. Effect of tranexamic acid on surgical bleeding: systematic review and cumulative meta-analysis. BMJ. 2012;344:e30542.
9. Roberts I, Shakur H, Ker K, Coats T, CRASH-2 Trial Collaborators. Antifibrinolytic drugs for acute traumatic injury. Cochrane Database Syst Rev. 2012;1:CD004896.
10. Roberts I, Perel P, Prieto-Merino D, Shakur H, Coats T, Hunt BJ, Lecky F, Brohi K, Willwt K. Effect of tranexamic acid on mortality in patients with traumatic bleeding: prespecified analysis of data from randomised controlled trial. BMJ. 2012;345:e5839.
11. Godier A, Roberts I, Hunt BJ. Tranexamic acid: less bleeding and less thrombosis? Crit Care. 2012;16(3):135.
12. The CRASH-3 Trial Collaborators. Effects of tranexamic acid on death, disability, vascular occlusive events and other morbidities in patients with acute traumatic brain injury (CRASH-3): a randomized, placebo-controlled trial. Lancet. 2019;394(10210):1713–23.
13. Stief TW. Drug-induced thrombin generation: the breakthrough. Hemost Lab. 2010;3:3–6.
14. Dirkmann D, Gorlinger K, Gisbertz C, et al. Factor XIII and TXA but not recombinant factor VIIa attenuate tissue plasminogen activator-induced hyperfibrinolysis in human whole blood. Anesth Analg. 2012;114(6):1182–8.
15. Sawamura A, Hayakawa M, Gando S, et al. Disseminated intravascular coagulation with a fibrinolytic phenotype at an early phase of trauma predicts mortality. Thromb Res. 2009;1214:608–13.
16. Eriksson O, Kjellman H, Pilbrant A, Schannong M. Pharmacokinetics of TXA after intravenous administration to normal volunteers. Eur J Clin Pharmacol. 1974;7:375–80.
17. Faraoni D, Goobie SM. The efficacy of Antifibrinolytic drugs in children undergoing noncardiac surgery: a systematic review of the literature. Anesth Analg. 2014;118:628–36.
18. Morrison JJ, Dubose JJ, Rasmussen TE, Midwinter MJ. Military application of tranexamic acid in trauma emergency resuscitation (MATTERs) study. Arch Surg. 2012;147(2):113–9.
19. Spahn DR, Bouillon B, Cerny V, Coats TJ, Duranteau J, Fernández-Mondéjar E, Filipescu D, Hunt BJ, Komadina R, Nardi G, Neugebauer E, Ozier Y, Riddez L, Schultz A, Vincent J-L, Rossaint R. Management of bleeding and coagulopathy following major trauma: an updated European Guideline. Spahn et al. Critical Care. 2013;17:R76. http://ccforum.com/content/17/2/R76

20. National Institute for Health and Clinical Excellence. Major trauma: assessment and initial management NICE guideline [NG39]. Published date: 17 February 2016.
21. I Roberts, T Kawahara. Proposal for the inclusion of TXA (antifibrinolytic – lysine analogue) in the WHO model list of essential medicines. In: 18th expert committee on the selection and use of essential medicines. Published on 2 June 2010.

Procalcitonin-Guided Antibiotic Discontinuation

15

Marta Mucchetti, Nicolò Maimeri, and Pasquale Nardelli

Contents

15.1 General Principles

Procalcitonin (PCT) is a blood biomarker used in clinical practice to detect bacterial etiology in patients with sepsis or acute respiratory tract infection, to assess infection severity, and to monitor the effectiveness of antibiotic therapy. In February 2017, the U.S. Food and Drug Administration (FDA) approved the use of the first PCT assay to guide antibiotic use in the context of lower respiratory tract infections (LRTI) and sepsis [1].

Antibiotics are the cornerstone of bacterial infection treatment. Unfortunately, the number of multi-drug resistant (MDR) pathogens is constantly increasing and is directly linked to antibiotic overuse. Therefore, many efforts have been done in order to implement antibiotic stewardship in clinical practice. Procalcitonin,

M. Mucchetti (✉) · N. Maimeri · P. Nardelli
Department of Anesthesia and Intensive Care, IRCCS San Raffaele Scientific Institute, Milan, Italy
e-mail: mucchetti.marta@hsr.it

© Springer Nature Switzerland AG 2021
G. Landoni et al. (eds.), *Reducing Mortality in Critically Ill Patients*,
https://doi.org/10.1007/978-3-030-71917-3_15

together with full clinical evaluation, can help physicians to withhold antibiotics prescription when bacterial infection is unlikely and to stop treatment earlier when infection is defeated [2].

Since 2005, an increasing number of randomized controlled trials (RCTs) compared a PCT-guided intervention arm to a standard-of-care arm, showing a safe and significant reduction in antibiotic use. The safety parameters usually considered in these trials were mortality (with a non-inferiority approach), length of hospital/intensive care unit (ICU) stay, and reinfection rate [3].

Among these RCTs, two showed a statistically significant, but conflicting, effect on mortality [4, 5]. These two RCTs are discussed in details in the first part of this chapter, in which the survival effect reported by these investigations is also analyzed in light of the wide literature available on PCT. The second part of the chapter describes PCT physiology and its possible clinical use.

15.2   Main Evidences

Most of the RCTs on PCT guidance to antibiotic therapy aimed to demonstrate a reduction of antibiotic exposure, with potential benefits in term of toxicity, rise of MDR pathogens, and costs. Mortality was investigated in these trials, as primary or secondary outcome, with a non-inferiority approach, i.e., to demonstrate that antibiotic use reduction does not lead to increased mortality.

As mentioned, only two RCTs reported a significant effect on survival: the Stop Antibiotics on Procalcitonin guidance Study (SAPS) showed a reduction in 28-day mortality rate in the interventional (PCT-guided antibiotic therapy) arm among critically ill patients [4], while the BPCTrea trial failed to prove non-inferiority of PCT-guided antibiotic therapy with respect to 3-month mortality among patients with severe acute exacerbation of chronic obstructive pulmonary disease (AECOPD) [5].

15.2.1 The SAPS Trial and PCT Guidance in Critically Ill/Septic Patients

In 2016, de Jong et al. [4] published the Stop Antibiotics on Procalcitonin guidance Study (SAPS), a prospective, multicenter, open-label RCT of 1546 patients from 15 ICUs in the Netherland. Eligible patients had to be admitted to the ICU and to have initiated antibiotic treatment within 24 h before inclusion in the trial for an assumed or proven infection.

The study protocol included daily measurement of PCT levels until ICU discharge or 3 days after antibiotic discontinuation in the interventional arm. Physicians were invited to stop antibiotic treatment when PCT concentration had decreased by 80% or more of its peak value (relative stopping threshold) or when it reached a value of 0.5 µg/L or lower (absolute stopping threshold). In the standard-of-care arm, PCT levels were not measured and antibiotics were used according to local or national guidelines.

No significant difference in baseline characteristics was noted. Despite adherence to the stopping thresholds was low (44%), both antibiotic consumption (i.e., daily defined doses) and antibiotic treatment duration were lower in the interventional arm, respectively, 7.5 vs 9.3 defined daily doses (absolute difference 2.69, 95% confidence interval (CI) 1.26–4.12, $p < 0.0001$) and 5 vs 7 days (absolute difference 1.22, 95% CI 0.65–1.78, $p < 0.0001$). Both 28-day and 1-year mortality were lower in the PCT-guided group. In the intention-to-treat analysis, 20% of patients had died in the PCT group versus 25% in the control group (absolute difference 5.4%, 95% CI 1.2–9.5, $p = 0.012$). The favorable effect on mortality was maintained 1 year after randomization (35% vs 41%, absolute difference 6.1%, 95% CI 1.2–10.9, $p < 0.0158$). Per-protocol analysis confirmed these results [4]. Fragility index was 9, which shows a good robustness compared to other RCTs involving critically ill patients [6].

As stated by the authors themselves, mortality reduction with PCT guidance was an unexpected result, as the study was aiming for non-inferiority. It can be hypothesized that bias and type I error might have played an essential role in obtaining these results. Other important limitations were the absence of blinding and the low adherence to the study protocol. As a matter of fact, the stopping rule was followed only when patients were clinically stable.

The authors speculated several reasons for the observed mortality reduction: first, low PCT levels may have led to consider alternative diagnoses; second, persistent high values may have highlighted inadequate therapy and induced to optimize infection management. Third, unnecessary antibiotics might have led to adverse effects without benefits. However, none of these hypotheses is supported by any data in the study.

While the antibiotic sparing effect of PCT-guided protocols has been confirmed by numerous meta-analyses published both before and after the SAPS trial, an effect on mortality was only shown in subsequent meta-analyses [7–9], with loss of statistical significance when the results of the SAPS trial are omitted.

As a matter of fact, the SAPS trial is the largest RCT of PCT use in critically ill patients, and it is the only one showing a statistically significant mortality reduction. To date, only two trials were designed to detect a survival benefit of PCT guidance and both failed to show a significant mortality reduction [10, 11]. The Placebo-Controlled Trial of Sodium Selenite and Procalcitonin Guided Antimicrobial Therapy in Severe Sepsis (SISPCT) was the only RCT adequately powered for mortality. It was a two-by-two factorial trial investigating the role of sodium selenite and PCT-guided antibiotic therapy in sepsis, in which 1089 patients were enrolled across 33 German ICUs. Therapy optimization was recommended if PCT levels did not drop by at least 50% at day 4 and discontinuation of antibiotics was recommended when PCT values were less than 1 µg/L. There was no significant difference in 28-day mortality between patients assigned to PCT guidance and those not assigned to PCT guidance (25.6% vs 28.2%, $p = 0.34$); PCT guidance resulted in a 4.5% reduction in antibiotic exposure [10]. The Procalcitonin And Survival Study (PASS) had a completely different design, in which a drug-escalation algorithm and intensified diagnostics based on daily PCT measurements were implemented in the

PCT arm. The trial included 1200 patients from nine Danish ICUs. Death from any cause at day 28 did not differ between the interventional and control arm (31.5% vs 32%, respectively); moreover, the length of ICU stay was lower in the control arm [11].

Two more large multicenter RCTs of PCT in critically ill patients investigated mortality [12, 13]. In 2010, the PROcalcitonin to Reduce Antibiotic Treatments in Acutely ill patients (ProRATA) trail enrolled 621 patients from seven French ICUs. In the interventional arm, PCT values were used to decide whether antibiotic treatment should be started (with the exception of situations requiring immediate antibiotic treatment, such as septic shock or purulent meningitis), continued, and stopped. Procalcitonin threshold was 0.5 µg/L. 28-day mortality in the PCT group met the set non-inferiority margin of 10% (21.2% in PCT group vs 20.4% in control group, absolute difference 0.8%, 95% CI −4.6 to 6.2), also 60-day mortality was not significantly different although it was higher in the experimental group (30% in PCT group vs 26% in control group, absolute difference 3.8%, 95% CI −2.1 to 9.7). Duration of antibiotic treatment was significantly lower in the PCT group (6.1 days vs 9.9 days, $p < 0.0001$), but no difference was detected in the length of both ICU and hospital stay. Moreover, the percentage of emerging MDR bacteria isolated from specimens taken for routine microbiological assessments did not differ between the two groups (17.9% in PCT group vs 16.6% in control group, $p = 0.67$) [12]. The only large trial which did not show any reduction in the duration of antibiotic therapy is the Australian ProGUARD. Compared to other trials, this multicenter RCT of 400 patients used a very restrictive PCT threshold to discontinue antibiotics (<0.1 µg/L). The total number of days on antibiotic therapy by 28-day was not significantly different (9 in the PCT group vs 11 in the control group, $p = 0.58$), and no differences were found in the length of ICU and hospital stay and in the emergence of MDR organisms. Also mortality was not significantly different between PCT and control group (60-day all-cause mortality, 18% vs 16%, $p = 0.6$) [13].

15.2.2 BPCTrea Trial and PCT Guidance in Respiratory Tract Infections

The BPCTrea trial is a prospective, multicenter, parallel-group RCT, involving 302 patients from 11 French ICUs. This study was designed to assess the effect of PCT-guided antibiotic therapy on 3-month mortality (with an expected non-inferiority margin of 12%) in ICU patients with severe AECOPD and suspected LRTI with or without pneumonia. Duration of antibiotic exposure was assessed too.

Procalcitonin levels were measured in all patients at the time of randomization, 6 h after randomization, and on days 1, 3, and 5. In the interventional arm, antibiotic therapy was based on PCT levels as follows: strongly discouraged with PCT < 0.1 µg/L (no bacterial infection); encouraged with PCT 0.1–0.25 µg/L (possible bacterial infection); strongly encouraged with PCT > 0.25 µg/L (bacterial infection). In addition, antibiotic discontinuation was recommended when PCT levels were reduced by at least 90% of the peak concentration or less than 0.1 µg/L. In the control group, clinicians were blinded to PCT values and prescribed antibiotics according to current guidelines.

Mortality at 3 months was not statistically different, but the study failed to demonstrate non-inferiority (mortality was 20% in the PCT group vs 14% in the control group; adjusted difference, 6.6%; 90% CI −0.3 to 13.5%). In the subgroup of patients who were not receiving antibiotics at baseline, mortality was significantly higher in PCT group (31% vs 12%, adjusted difference 19.1%; CI 7.2–31.1%). As for antibiotics usage, significantly less patients received antibiotics in the PCT group, but both in-ICU and in-hospital antibiotic exposure duration were similar (5.2 ± 6.5 days in the PCT group vs 5.4 ± 4.4 days in the control group, $p = 0.85$, and 7.9 ± 8 days in the PCT group vs 7.7 ± 5.7 days in the control group, $p = 0.75$, respectively) [5].

These results challenge the wide literature according to which PCT guidance seems to be safe and effective in reducing antibiotic exposure in patients with acute respiratory infections.

No other RCT nor meta-analysis showed an association between PCT-guided antibiotic therapy and increased mortality [14–16]. In a recent meta-analysis by Li et al. which focused on PCT guidance in AECOPD and included the BPCTrea trial, no effect on all-cause mortality was reported (RR 1.05, $p = 0.79$) [15]. Moreover, in a large, individual patient-level data meta-analysis of RCTs (not including data from the BPCTrea study), Schuetz et al. pooled data of 6708 patients from 26 trials and found that PCT-guided antibiotic therapy was associated with a significant reduction in 30-day mortality (9% in PCT group vs 10% in control group, $p = 0.037$) although this result is not statistically robust (fragility index = 0). This meta-analysis included a very heterogeneous population, regarding both the primary diagnosis (ranging from common cold to ventilator-associated pneumonia) and the clinical setting (i.e., primary care, emergency department, and ICU). However, no significant negative effect was detected in subgroup analyses, when focusing on both ICU patients (19% vs 22%, $p = 0.62$) and AECOPD (3% vs 4%, $p = 0.85$) [14]. These positive results are also validated by large observational studies that confirm the results of RCTs in "real life" [17]. The Pro-REAL study included 1759 patients from Switzerland, France, and the USA. Overall algorithm compliance was 68.2%, with differences between diagnoses, outpatients and inpatients, algorithm-experienced and algorithm-naive centers, and countries. Antibiotic therapy duration was significantly shorter if the PCT algorithm was followed compared with when it was overruled (5.9 versus 7.4 days; difference −1.51 days, 95% CI −2.04 to −0.98; $p < 0.001$) [18].

The PCT algorithm of the BPCTrea study is similar to those applied in other trials focusing on LRTI, where PCT guidance is used to both initiate and stop antibiotics. However, in the vast majority of trials focusing on AECOPD patients, the population investigated is generally less severe than the study population of the BPCTrea study, which consists in severely ill patients, requiring ICU. Conversely, in most trials involving critically ill patients, PCT values are used only to discontinue antibiotic therapy, which is usually started according to other clinical criteria and physician's judgment [14, 15, 19, 20]. In fact, only two out of the ten ICU RCTs included in the meta-analysis by Schuetz et al. provided for a PCT cut-off to start antibiotic therapy in their algorithm [14]. A meta-analysis by Huang et al. comparing different PCT-guided strategies in critically ill patients found that only PCT-guided antibiotic discontinuation (but not PCT-guided antibiotic initiation) was associated with reduced antibiotic use and lower short-term mortality [21]. Consistently, mortality in the BPCTrea trial is not increased when included patients where already receiving antibiotics [5].

The guidelines for the management of adult patients with LRTI recommend that patients with a severe AECOPD who require invasive or noninvasive mechanical ventilation should receive antibiotics [22].

The findings of the BPCTrea study also challenge current literature on PCT efficacy in reducing antibiotic exposure in patients with respiratory infection. Large meta-analyses showed a clinical benefit in terms of antibiotic initiation and exposure [14, 16]. However, the most recent meta-analysis by Li et al., which includes the BPCTrea trial, shows a significant reduction only in antibiotic prescription [15], confirming the results of Daubin et al. Moreover, in the recent ProACT trial, which enrolled 1656 patients presenting at the emergency department with suspected LRTI, PCT guidance did not result in less use of antibiotics compared with usual care [20]. It is possible that the benefits of PCT-guided protocols might be less evident in contests where antibiotic prescription guidelines are highly implemented. As a matter of fact, in the BPCTrea study the control group mean duration of antibiotic therapy was rather low (7.9 ± 8 days in PCT group vs 7.7 ± 5.7 days in control group, $p = 0.75$). This might be due to the fact that almost 80% of the patients were enrolled in three teaching hospitals [5]. In the meta-analysis by Schuertz et al., PCT guidance was associated with a 2.4 day reduction in antibiotic exposure (5.7 days in PCT group vs 8.1 days in control group, $p < 0.0001$) [14]. The same consideration can be done when comparing the two main RCTs of PCT guidance in respiratory infections in the emergency department: the ProHOSP trial and the ProACT trial [19, 20]. The ProHOSP study showed a great reduction in antibiotic treatment duration (5.7 days in the PCT group vs 8.7 in the control group) [19], while no significant difference in antibiotic-days (4.2 vs. 4.3 days, $p = 0.87$) was found between the PCT group and the control group in the ProACT trial, in which clinicians in both arms were provided with national antibiotic guidelines for LRTI [20].

Other characteristics of the BPCTrea trial might have affected the efficacy of PCT guidance for antibiotic therapy in patients with respiratory tract infections. First, the PCT algorithm on antibiotic discontinuation was very restrictive. Most ICU trials recommend to stop antibiotics when PCT is below 0.25 or 0.5 µg/L [14]. Trials focusing on AECOPD are more conservative [15], but they usually deal with less severe patients, with alleged lower PCT concentrations [4, 20, 23]. Second, mean ICU and hospital antibiotic duration was longer than PCT monitoring according to study protocol; therefore in most cases, antibiotic therapy was stopped according to clinical judgment also in the PCT group not for low protocol adherence, but for protocol design [5]. The same issues concerning PCT algorithm and duration of PCT monitoring are also present in the ProGUARD trial, which failed to demonstrate a significant reduction in the median number of days on antibiotic therapy (9 days in the PCT group vs. 11 days in the control group, $p = 0.58$) [13].

15.3 Pathophysiological Principles

Procalcitonin is the precursor of calcitonin, a hormone involved in calcium homeostasis. In physiological conditions, thyroid C cells synthesize preprocalcitonin, a 141 amino acids precursor of calcitonin, which is then rapidly converted into PCT (116 amino acids) by endopeptidases-catalyzed removal of the 25-amino acid signal sequence. Procalcitonin is then converted into the circulation in calcitonin (32 amino acids) and other products. Normal PCT blood concentration is as low as <0.01 µg/L [24].

Severe bacterial infections enhance extra-thyroid production of PCT. Bacterial toxins (e.g., endotoxin) and proinflammatory cytokines (TNFα, IL-1β, IL-6) stimulate PCT secretion in several organs such as liver, lung, pancreas, kidney, and intestine, as well as in leukocytes. Moreover, cleavage of the protein into calcitonin is reduced during bacterial infection [25]. Accordingly, patients with bacterial infections show high blood PCT concentrations. Notably, interferon-γ, that is commonly released in response to viral infection, inhibits PCT synthesis so that its concentration remains low in this type of infections [26].

Procalcitonin levels start to increase within 2–4 h from the onset of sepsis, reaching peak blood values 6–8 h afterward and persisting as long as the inflammatory process continues. Its concentrations correlate with the severity of infection and PCT half-life is usually 20-24 h [27]. Impaired renal function might slow PCT clearance [8]. Peak concentrations also correlate with the pathogen involved and the infection site. Septic patients with proven Gram-negative bacteremia have significantly higher PCT concentrations (median 26 µg/L, IQR 7.7–63.1 µg/L) than patients with Gram-positive bacteremia (median 7.1 µg/L, IQR 2.0–23.3 µg/L) or candidemia (median 4.7 µg/L, IQR 1.9–13.7 µg/L). Moreover, higher PCT values are seen in patients with urogenital infection, followed by abdominal infection, while the lowest values are usually found in patients with respiratory infection [23]. Last, in certain conditions PCT levels may increase significantly even in non-septic patients. In postoperative patients, normal PCT kinetics varies. A physiological rise in PCT concentration is observed due to surgical stress-triggered inflammation. The highest values are measured on the second postoperative day and usually show a sharp decline thereafter [17]. In patients with cardiogenic shock, PCT level might rise up to 10 µg/L within 1–3 days, especially if vasopressor support is required. Severe chronic liver and kidney dysfunctions are associated with a moderate, but constant increase in PCT level (<2 µg/L). In addition, certain types of autoimmune disorders (Kawasaki Syndrome, Good pasture's Syndrome, Anti-neutrophil antibody-positive vasculitis, autoimmune hepatitis, or primary sclerosing cholangitis) may induce significant amounts of PCT level [28].

These features make PCT a useful diagnostic tool to differentiate bacterial infection from inflammatory states with different etiology, mainly in patients with sepsis or acute respiratory tract infection [3]. In a large meta-analysis of 30 observational studies, Wacker et al. evaluated PCT performance in identifying septic patients. Procalcitonin showed a high discriminatory ability (area under the curve (AUC) 0.85); mean sensitivity was 0.77 (95% CI 0.72–0.81) and mean specificity was 0.79 (95% CI 0.74–0.84). The area under the receiver operating characteristic curve was 0.85 (95% CI 0.81–0.88) [29]. In a large observational study, Laukemann compared the ability of several clinical scores and blood biomarkers to predict positive blood cultures. The best biomarker was PCT (AUC 0.803), compared to C-reactive protein (AUC 0.645) and white blood cell counts (AUC 0.544). Combining PCT levels with the Shapiro score further increased the AUC to 0.827 [30].

In addition, several studies proved a good correlation with clinical evolution and prognosis [3].

15.4   Clinical Use

There is no consensus on the use of PCT in clinical practice. Traditionally, this marker is used in situations where differential diagnostic is needed in order to help defining the bacterial origin of an inflammatory status. Tujula et al. performed a systematic search to identify clinical practice guidelines (CPG) dealing with PCT. They included 17 CPG, most of them dealing with patients affected by either LRTI or sepsis [31].

In the context of septic or critically ill patients, two CPG take PCT in consideration: the Surviving Sepsis Campaign [32] and the Antibiotic Stewardship Program of the Infectious Diseases Society of America (IDSA) [33]. Both guidelines state that PCT is useful to stop antibiotic therapy but do not provide specific cut-offs. The "International Guidelines for Management of Sepsis and Septic Shock" published by Surviving Sepsis Campaign in 2016 confirm the usefulness of low PCT levels to guide antibiotics discontinuation, already suggested in 2012. In particular, the use of PCT levels is suggested to support the reduction of antimicrobial therapy duration in septic patients as well as the discontinuation of empiric antibiotics in patients who initially appeared to have sepsis, but subsequently have limited clinical evidence of infection (weak recommendation, low quality of evidence) [32]. The guidelines do not set a defined cut-off, highlighting that there are no evidences about which of the proposed algorithms performs best. It is also stressed that PCT, as any other biomarker, can provide only supportive and supplemental data to clinical assessment [32]. Similarly, in the Guidelines to Implement an Antibiotic Stewardship Program (ASP), the IDSA suggests to use PCT levels to decrease antibiotic use in adult ICU patients with suspected infection (weak recommendation, moderate-quality evidence) [33].

In patients with respiratory infection, guidelines are even more cautious. The IDSA guidelines suggest to use PCT levels plus clinical criteria to discontinue antibiotic therapy in patients with hospital/ventilator acquired pneumonia (HAP/VAP). The panel questions the potential benefits of using PCT monitoring in contexts where standard antibiotic therapy for VAP is already 7 days or less. Moreover, IDSA guidelines suggest the use of clinical criteria alone rather than clinical criteria associated with PCT levels to decide whether to initiate antibiotic therapy. This recommendation is based on accuracy studies, according to which serum PCT plus clinical criteria can diagnose HAP/VAP with a sensitivity and specificity of 67% and 83%, respectively, leading to a high false negative and false positive rate. Both of these recommendations are weak and based on low quality evidence [34].

Concerning COPD, both the German Respiratory Society and the U.S. Department of Veterans Affairs state that there is insufficient evidence to recommend for or against PCT-guided antibiotic use for patients with acute COPD exacerbations [35, 36].

Despite the lack of official guidelines, an international expert consensus on PCT-guided antibiotic stewardship has recently been published [2]. In this opinion paper, Schuetz et al. propose a shared algorithm in which the likelihood of bacterial infection is evaluated combining initial clinical assessment (including microbiology) with PCT results (see Table 15.1). A high probability of bacterial infection is associated with PCT $\geq$ 0.25 µg/L (or $\geq$ 0.5 µg/L in ICU patients). The subsequent antibiotic strategy is suggested according to the probability of bacterial infection and the severity of clinical presentation. It is suggested to withhold antibiotic therapy when both clinical suspicion and PCT levels are low, only if patients have mild symptoms. In this case, a second PCT test may be done to confirm the diagnosis. Otherwise, antibiotic therapy should always be started according to clinical judgment. However, if PCT levels are low, other diagnostic tests should be considered to investigate differential diagnosis.

When the overall likelihood of bacterial infection is low, a second PCT test below the cut-off levels may be used to stop empiric therapy. Otherwise, when bacterial infection is likely and PCT levels are high, monitoring PCT levels every 24–48 h can help monitoring antibiotics efficacy and suggests discontinuation when PCT levels are lower than defined cut-offs or drop by 80% of the peak value. Specific populations excluded by this algorithm are patients with immunosuppression, cystic fibrosis, pancreatitis, high volume transfusion, malaria, and chronic infections (e.g., osteomyelitis or endocarditis) [2].

15.5 Conclusions

Procalcitonin-guided antibiotic discontinuation in critically ill patients is a useful tool to decrease antibiotic therapy duration, with a good safety profile in terms of reinfection, mortality, and prolonged ICU/hospital stay. However, available evidence does not confirm reduction in the emergence of MDR pathogens, which is the final aim of antimicrobial stewardship programs. Moreover, the sparing effect is less evident in contexts where other antimicrobial stewardship programs have already been implemented.

Table 15.1 PCT use in patients with mild, moderate and severe illness, as suggested by the international consensus, modified from Schuetz P, 2019 [2]

Bacterial infection likelihood			Severity of illness		
			Mild	Moderate	Severe in ICU
	Unlikely				
	Bacterial infection *uncertain* according to initial clinical evaluation	PCT < 0.25 µg/L (or < 0.5 µg/L in ICU pts)	No Abx, consider other diagnostic tests. Consider second PCT test within 6–24 h before sending home	Use empiric Abx according to clinical judgment, consider other diagnostic tests. Use repeated PCT test within 6–24 h to early stop Abx to if PCT still < 0.25 µg/L	Use empiric Abx according to clinical judgment, consider other diagnostic tests. Consider second PCT test within 24 h to stop Abx if PCT still < 0.5 µg/L
	Possible				
	Bacterial infection *highly suspected* according to initial clinical evaluation	PCT < 0.25 µg/L (or < 0.5 µg/L in ICU pts)	Use empiric Abx according to clinical judgment, consider other diagnostic tests. Consider second PCT test within 24 h to stop Abx if PCT still < 0.25 µg/L	Use empiric Abx according to clinical judgment, consider other diagnostic tests. Consider second PCT test within 24 h to stop Abx if PCT still < 0.25 µg/L	Use empiric Abx according to clinical judgment, consider other diagnostic tests. Use PCT within 24–48 h for monitoring and discontinuation of Abx if PCT still < 0.5 µg/L
	Likely				
	Bacterial infection *uncertain* according to initial clinical evaluation	PCT ≥ 0.25 µg/L (or ≥ 0.5 µg/L in ICU pts)	Use Abx according to clinical judgment. Use PCT every 24–48 h for monitoring and discontinuation of Abx if PCT < 0.25 µg/L or drop by 80%	Use Abx according to clinical judgment. Use PCT every 24–48 h for monitoring and discontinuation of Abx if PCT < 0.25 µg/L or drop by 80%	Use Abx according to clinical judgment. Use PCT every 24–48 h for monitoring and discontinuation of Abx if PCT < 0.5 µg/L or drop by 80%
	Highly likely				
	Bacterial infection *highly suspected* according to initial clinical evaluation	PCT ≥ 0.25 µg/L (or ≥ 0.5 µg/L in ICU pts)	Use Abx according to clinical judgment. Use PCT every 24–48 h for monitoring and discontinuation of Abx if PCT < 0.25 µg/L or drop by 80%	Use Abx according to clinical judgment. Use PCT every 24–48 h for monitoring and discontinuation of Abx if PCT < 0.25 µg/L or drop by 80%	Use Abx according to clinical judgment. Use PCT every 24–48 h for monitoring and discontinuation of Abx if PCT < 0.5 µg/L or drop by 80%

PCT procalcitonin, *ICU* intensive care unit, *Abx* antibiotics

Two multicenter RCTs show conflicting results on mortality. Daubin et al. [5] showed an increased mortality risk in the subgroup of patients who were not receiving antibiotics at baseline. This RCT focused on a very limited population (i.e., patients with acute exacerbations of COPD admitted to ICU) and implemented a PCT-guided protocol where PCT values were used not only to stop but also to start antibiotic therapy. Because of these features, it is not appropriate to generalize the results of this trial to the whole critically ill population and an increase in mortality due to PCT-guided antibiotic discontinuation seems unlikely. On the opposite, de Jong et al. showed a survival benefit with PCT-guided antibiotic discontinuation [4]. This study is not at low risk of bias, due to lack of blinding and incomplete outcome data. Moreover, low adherence to PCT protocol and risk of type I error are present. Subsequent meta-analyses confirmed a survival benefit with the use of PCT, but the effect is lost without the results of the trial by de Jong et al. Further large, specifically designed and adequately powered multicenter RCTs are needed in order to assess the potential survival benefit of PCT-guided antibiotic discontinuation in critically ill patients.

References

1. US Food and Drugs Administration (2017) FDA Press releas. FDA clears test to help manage antibiotic treatment for lower respiratory tract infections and sepsis. https://www.fda.gov/news-events/press-announcements/fda-clears-test-help-manage-antibiotic-treatment-lower-respiratory-tract-infections-and-sepsis. Accessed Mar 2020.
2. Schuetz P, Beishuizen A, Broyles M, Ferrer R, Gavazzi G, Gluck EH, González Del Castillo J, Jensen J, Kanizsai PL, Kwa ALH, Krueger S, Luyt C, Oppert M, Plebani M, Shlyapnikov SA, Toccafondi G, Townsend J, Welte T, Saeed K. Procalcitonin (PCT)-guided antibiotic stewardship: an international experts consensus on optimized clinical use. Clin Chem Lab Med. 2019;57:1308–18.
3. Hamade B, Huang DT. Procalcitonin: Where are we now? Crit Care Clin. 2020;36:23–40.
4. de Jong E, van Oers JA, Beishuizen A, Vos P, Vermeijden WJ, Haas LE, Loef BG, Dormans T, van Melsen GC, Kluiters YC, Kemperman H, van den Elsen MJ, Schouten JA, Streefkerk J, Krabbe HG, Kieft H, Kluge GH, van Dam VC, van Pelt J, Bormans L, Otten MB. Efficacy and safety of procalcitonin guidance in reducing the duration of antibiotic treatment in critically ill patients: a randomised, controlled, open-label trial. Lancet Infect Dis. 2016;16:819–27.
5. Daubin C, Valette X, Thiollière F, Mira J, Hazera P, Annane D, Labbe V, Floccard B, Fournel F, Terzi N, Du Cheyron D, Parienti J. Procalcitonin algorithm to guide initial antibiotic therapy in acute exacerbations of COPD admitted to the ICU: a randomized multicenter study. Intensive Care Med. 2018;44:428–37.
6. Ridgeon EE, Young PJ, Bellomo R, Mucchetti M, Lembo R, Landoni G. The fragility index in multicenter randomized controlled critical care trials. Crit Care Med. 2016;44:1278–84.
7. Iankova I, Thompson-Leduc P, Kirson NY, Rice B, Hey J, Krause A, Schonfeld SA, DeBrase CR, Bozzette S, Schuetz P. Efficacy and safety of Procalcitonin guidance in patients with suspected or confirmed Sepsis: a systematic review and meta-analysis. Crit Care Med. 2018;46:691–8.
8. Wirz Y, Meier MA, Bouadma L, Luyt CE, Wolff M, Chastre J, Tubach F, Schroeder S, Nobre V, Annane D, Reinhart K, Damas P, Nijsten M, Shajiei A, de Lange DW, Deliberato RO, Oliveira CF, Shehabi Y, van Oers JAH, Beishuizen A, ARJ G. Effect of procalcitonin-guided antibiotic treatment on clinical outcomes in intensive care unit patients with infection and sepsis patients: a patient-level meta-analysis of randomized trials. Crit Care. 2018;22:191.

9. Pepper DJ, Sun J, Rhee C, Welsh J, Powers JH, Danner RL, Kadri SS. Procalcitonin-guided antibiotic discontinuation and mortality in critically ill adults: a systematic review and meta-analysis. Chest. 2019;155:1109–18.

10. Bloos F, Trips E, Nierhaus A, Briegel J, Heyland DK, Jaschinski U, Moerer O, Weyland A, Marx G, Gründling M, Kluge S, Kaufmann I, Ott K, Quintel M, Jelschen F, Meybohm P, Rademacher S, Meier-Hellmann A, Utzolino S, Kaisers UX, Putensen C. Effect of sodium selenite administration and Procalcitonin-guided therapy on mortality in patients with severe Sepsis or septic shock: a randomized clinical trial. JAMA Intern Med. 2016;176:1266–76.

11. Jensen JU, Hein L, Lundgren B, Bestle MH, Mohr TT, Andersen MH, Thornberg KJ, Løken J, Steensen M, Fox Z, Tousi H, Søe-Jensen P, Lauritsen AØ, Strange D, Petersen PL, Reiter N, Hestad S, Thormar K, Fjeldborg P, Larsen KM, Drenck NE. Procalcitonin-guided interventions against infections to increase early appropriate antibiotics and improve survival in the intensive care unit: a randomized trial. Crit Care Med. 2011;39:2048–58.

12. Bouadma L, Luyt C, Tubach F, Cracco C, Alvarez A, Schwebel C, Schortgen F, Lasocki S, Veber B, Dehoux M, Bernard M, Pasquet B, Régnier B, Brun-Buisson C, Chastre J, Wolff M. Use of procalcitonin to reduce patients' exposure to antibiotics in intensive care units (PRORATA trial): a multicentre randomised controlled trial. Lancet. 2010;375:463–74.

13. Shehabi Y, Sterba M, Garrett PM, Rachakonda KS, Stephens D, Harrigan P, Walker A, Bailey MJ, Johnson B, Millis D, Ding G, Peake S, Wong H, Thomas J, Smith K, Forbes L, Hardie M, Micallef S, Fraser JF. Procalcitonin algorithm in critically ill adults with undifferentiated infection or suspected sepsis. A randomized controlled trial. Am J Respir Crit Care Med. 2014;190:1102–10.

14. Schuetz P, Wirz Y, Sager R, Christ-Crain M, Stolz D, Tamm M, Bouadma L, Luyt CE, Wolff M, Chastre J, Tubach F, Kristoffersen KB, Burkhardt O, Welte T, Schroeder S, Nobre V, Wei L, Bucher HC, Annane D, Reinhart K, Falsey AR. Effect of procalcitonin-guided antibiotic treatment on mortality in acute respiratory infections: a patient level meta-analysis. Lancet Infect Dis. 2018;18:95–107.

15. Li Z, Yuan X, Yu L, Wang B, Gao F, Ma J. Procalcitonin-guided antibiotic therapy in acute exacerbation of chronic obstructive pulmonary disease: an updated meta-analysis. Medicine. 2019;98:e16775.

16. Hey J, Thompson-Leduc P, Kirson NY, Zimmer L, Wilkins D, Rice B, Iankova I, Krause A, Schonfeld SA, DeBrase CR, Bozzette S, Schuetz P. Procalcitonin guidance in patients with lower respiratory tract infections: a systematic review and meta-analysis. Clin Chem Lab Med. 2018;56:1200–9.

17. Sager R, Kutz A, Mueller B, Schuetz P. Procalcitonin-guided diagnosis and antibiotic stewardship revisited. BMC Med. 2017;15:15.

18. Dusemund F, Bucher B, Meyer S, Thomann R, Kühn F, Bassetti S, Sprenger M, Baechli E, Sigrist T, Schwietert M, Amin D, Hausfater P, Carre E, Schuetz P, Gaillat J, Regez K, Bossart R, Schild U, Müller B, Albrich WC. Influence of procalcitonin on decision to start antibiotic treatment in patients with a lower respiratory tract infection: insight from the observational multicentric ProREAL surveillance. Eur J Clin Microbiol Infect Dis. 2013;32:51–60.

19. Schuetz P, Christ-Crain M, Thomann R, Falconnier C, Wolbers M, Widmer I, Neidert S, Fricker T, Blum C, Schild U, Regez K, Schoenenberger R, Henzen C, Bregenzer T, Hoess C, Krause M, Bucher HC, Zimmerli W, Mueller B. Effect of procalcitonin-based guidelines vs standard guidelines on antibiotic use in lower respiratory tract infections: the ProHOSP randomized controlled trial. JAMA. 2009;302:1059–66.

20. Huang DT, Yealy DM, Filbin MR, Brown AM, Chang CH, Doi Y, Donnino MW, Fine J, Fine MJ, Fischer MA, Holst JM, Hou PC, Kellum JA, Khan F, Kurz MC, Lotfipour S, LoVecchio F, Peck-Palmer O, Pike F, Prunty H, Sherwin RL. Procalcitonin-guided use of antibiotics for lower respiratory tract infection. N Engl J Med. 2018;379:236–49.

21. Huang H, Peng J, Weng L, Wang C, Jiang W, Du B. Procalcitonin-guided antibiotic therapy in intensive care unit patients: a systematic review and meta-analysis. Ann Intensive Care. 2017;7:114.

22. Woodhead M, Blasi F, Ewig S, Garau J, Huchon G, Ieven M, Ortqvist A, Schaberg T, Torres A, van der Heijden G, Read R, Verheij TJM. Guidelines for the management of adult lower respiratory tract infections--full version. Clin Microbiol Infect. 2011;17(Suppl6):E1–59.
23. Thomas-Rüddel DO, Poidinger B, Kott M, Weiss M, Reinhart K, Bloos F. Influence of pathogen and focus of infection on procalcitonin values in sepsis patients with bacteremia or candidemia. Crit Care. 2018;22:128.
24. Lippi G, Sanchis-Gomar F. Procalcitonin in inflammatory bowel disease: drawbacks and opportunities. World J Gastroenterol. 2017;23:8283–90.
25. Becker KL, Nylén ES, White JC, Müller B, Snider RH. Clinical review 167: Procalcitonin and the calcitonin gene family of peptides in inflammation, infection, and sepsis: a journey from calcitonin back to its precursors. J Clin Endocrinol Metabol. 2004;89:1512–25.
26. Schuetz P, Albrich W, Mueller B. Procalcitonin for diagnosis of infection and guide to antibiotic decisions: past, present and future. BMC Med. 2011;9:107.
27. Nylén ES, Alarifi AA. Humoral markers of severity and prognosis of critical illness. Best Pract Res Clin Endocrinol Metab. 2001;15:553–73.
28. Meisner M. Update on procalcitonin measurements. Ann Lab Med. 2014;2014(34):263–73.
29. Wacker C, Prkno A, Brunkhorst FM, Schlattmann P. Procalcitonin as a diagnostic marker for sepsis: a systematic review and meta-analysis. Lancet Infect Dis. 2013;13:426–35.
30. Laukemann S, Kasper N, Kulkarni P, Steiner D, Rast AC, Kutz A, Felder S, Haubitz S, Faessler L, Huber A, Fux CA, Mueller B, Schuetz P. Can we reduce negative blood cultures with clinical scores and blood markers? Results from an observational cohort study. Medicine. 2015;94:e2264.
31. Tujula B, Hämäläinen S, Kokki H, Pulkki K, Kokki M. Review of clinical practice guidelines on the use of procalcitonin in infections. Infect Dis. 2020;52:227–34.
32. Rhodes A, Evans LE, Alhazzani W, Levy MM, Antonelli M, Ferrer R, Kumar A, Sevransky JE, Sprung CL, Nunnally ME, Rochwerg B, Rubenfeld GD, Angus DC, Annane D, Beale RJ, Bellinghan GJ, Bernard GR, Chiche J, Coopersmith C, De Backer DP, French CJ. Surviving Sepsis campaign: international guidelines for Management of Sepsis and Septic Shock: 2016. Intensive Care Med. 2017;43:304–77.
33. Barlam TF, Cosgrove SE, Abbo LM, MacDougall C, Schuetz AN, Septimus EJ, Srinivasan A, Dellit TH, Falck-Ytter Y, Fishman NO, Hamilton CW, Jenkins TC, Lipsett PA, Malani PN, May LS, Moran GJ, Neuhauser MM, Newland JG, Ohl CA, Samore MH, Seo SK. Implementing an antibiotic stewardship program: guidelines by the Infectious Diseases Society of America and the Society for Healthcare Epidemiology of America. Clin Infect Dis. 2016;62:e51–77.
34. Kalil AC, Metersky ML, Klompas M, Muscedere J, Sweeney DA, Palmer LB, Napolitano LM, O'Grady NP, Bartlett JG, Carratalà J, El Solh AA, Ewig S, Fey PD, File TM, Restrepo MI, Roberts JA, Waterer GW, Cruse P, Knight SL, Brozek JL. Management of Adults with Hospital-acquired and Ventilator-associated Pneumonia: 2016 clinical practice guidelines by the Infectious Diseases Society of America and the American Thoracic Society. Clin Infect Dis. 2016;63:e61–e111.
35. The Management of Chronic Obstructive Pulmonary Disease Working Group (2014) VA/DoD Clinical practice guideline for the management of chronic obstructive pulmonary disease. https://www.guidelinecentral.com/share/summary/5559e91f5fc99#section-society. Accessed 20 Mar 2020.
36. Vogelmeier C, Buhl R, Burghuber O, Criée C, Ewig S, Godnic-Cvar J, Hartl S, Herth F, Kardos P, Kenn K, Nowak D, Rabe KF, Studnicka M, Watz H, Welte T, Windisch W, Worth H. Guideline for the diagnosis and treatment of COPD patients - issued by the German Respiratory Society and the German Atemwegsliga in Cooperation with the Austrian Society of Pneumology. Pneumologie. 2018;72:253–308.

Selective Decontamination of the Digestive Tract

16

Luciano Silvestri and Hendrick K. F. van Saene

Contents

16.1   General Principles

Selective decontamination of the digestive tract (SDD) is an antimicrobial prophylaxis using parenteral (e.g., third-generation cephalosporin) and enteral antimicrobials (e.g., polymyxin E, tobramycin, and amphotericin B) for the control of severe infections in critically ill patients [1].

SDD is based on the observation that critical illness profoundly affects the body flora, both qualitatively and quantitatively, promoting a shift from normal to abnormal carriage, and from low to high carriage (overgrowth) of normal and abnormal flora [1]. The efficacy of SDD in controlling infections and in reducing mortality is based on the ability of the chosen antimicrobials to clear the carriage of potentially pathogenic microorganisms (PPMs) in overgrowth concentration.

L. Silvestri (✉)
Unit of Biostatistics, Epidemiology and Public Health, Department of Cardiological, Thoracic, Vascular Sciences and Public Health, University of Padova, Padova, Italy

H. K. F. van Saene
Institute of Ageing and Chronic Diseases, University of Liverpool, Liverpool, UK

© Springer Nature Switzerland AG 2021   149
G. Landoni et al. (eds.), *Reducing Mortality in Critically Ill Patients*,
https://doi.org/10.1007/978-3-030-71917-3_16

16.2   Main Evidence

There have been 75 randomized controlled trials (RCTs) of SDD in about 36,000 critically ill patients and several meta-analyses, over a period of more than 35 years of clinical research. However, most RCTs were designed to detect morbidity, i.e., infection of the lower airways and the bloodstream, and were under powered to detect a survival benefit. The full protocol of parenteral and enteral antimicrobials significantly reduced lower airway infection by 72% (odds ratio [OR] 0.28, 95% confidence interval [CI], 0.20–0.38) [2], and bloodstream infection by 27% (OR 0.73, 95% CI, 0.59–0.90) [3]. Mortality reduction ranged from 16% (OR 0.84, 95% CI, 0.73–0.97) [4] to 27% (OR, 0.73, 95% CI, 0.64–0.84) [5] and 29% (OR, 0.71, 95% CI, 0.61–0.82) [6].

The largest RCTs on SDD with the endpoint of mortality were performed in the Netherlands [7–9]. The first Dutch trial included 934 patients and showed a 35% reduction of intensive care unit (ICU) mortality (relative risk [RR] 0.65, 95% CI, 0.49–0.85) in the overall population, and a significant reduction of ICU mortality in the subset of surgical patients who underwent emergency surgery (RR 0.48, 95% CI, 0.26–0.87) [7]. The second Dutch study included about 6000 patients, and compared SDD, selective oropharyngeal decontamination (SOD), a regimen without intestinal and parenteral components, and standard care [8]. SDD reduced ICU mortality compared to standard care [OR 0.81, 95% CI, 0.69–0.94]. A post hoc analysis in surgical patients showed that SDD reduced 28-day mortality, albeit not significantly (OR 0.86, 95% CI, 0.69–1.09) [10]. Oostdijk et al. [9] compared the effects of SOD and SDD and demonstrated a 28-day mortality of 25.7% and 23.8% in SOD and SDD group, respectively (adjusted OR 0.85, 95% CI, 0.77–0.93). Additionally, a German RCT in 546 surgical patients [11] although not designed to detect a survival benefit, showed a significant mortality reduction in patients with mid-range APACHE II score of 10–29 (RR 0.51, 95% CI, 0.29–0.87). Finally, a European RCT in ICUs with moderate to high level of antibiotic resistance, and including 8665 patients, compared the efficacy of SDD (although without the parenteral component), SOD, and standard care on bloodstream infection [12]. Bloodstream infections due to multidrug-resistant microorganisms were reduced, albeit not significantly, by SDD and SOD compared to standard care.

In surgical patients, pneumonia, postoperative infections, and anastomotic leakage were reduced by SDD, mainly in gastrointestinal surgery [13, 14]. There are three meta-analyses in liver transplant recipients receiving SDD [15–17]. Two of them [15, 16] found a significantly reduced infection due to aerobic Gram-negative bacilli (AGNB) and yeasts (OR 0.16, 95% CI, 0.07–0.37, and OR 0.41, 95% CI, 0.23–0.73, respectively) although the mortality reduction was not significant due to the small sample size (OR 0.82, 95% CI, 0.22–2.45) [15]. SDD has been studied in cardiac surgical patients. All RCTs showed a reduction in rates of infections and reduced levels of endotoxin and inflammation mediators in the postoperative period [17]. Three meta-analyses exploring the efficacy of SDD in critically ill surgical patients showed a significant reduction in morbidity and mortality [4, 17, 18]. Remarkably, SDD reduced mortality in surgical population by 36% (OR 0.64, 95 CI, 0.53–0.79) and was superior to SOD (OR 0.80, 95% CI, 0.69–0.93) [4].

Based on evidence from RCTs and meta-analyses, SDD has been included among the non-surgical interventions that may reduce mortality in the perioperative period [19–21]. Additionally, the Dutch working party on antibiotic policy advised to use SDD in patients with an ICU stay of more than 48 h [22].

16.3   Pharmacological Properties

The mechanism of action of SDD is the control of critical illness-related carriage in overgrowth state [1]. Low-grade carriage is defined as $<10^5$ PPMs per gram of digestive tract secretions. High-grade carriage (i.e., overgrowth) is defined as $\geq 10^5$ PPMs per gram of digestive tract secretions. Overgrowth is a risk factor for developing endogenous infection and resistance [1].

The majority of infections developing in ICU patients are endogenous (85%), i.e., they are preceded by overgrowth in throat and/or gut [1]. Oropharyngeal carriage of PPMs in overgrowth concentrations is the first step in the pathogenesis of lower airway infections. Similarly, gut carriage of PPMs in overgrowth concentrations is the first stage in the pathogenesis of bloodstream infections. Normal PPMs are the etiological agents in previously healthy individuals requiring intensive care following an acute event, such as trauma, surgery, pancreatitis, acute hepatic failure, and burns. They are *Streptococcus pneumoniae, Haemophilus influenzae, Moraxella catarrhalis, Escherichia coli*, methicillin-sensitive *Staphylococcus aureus* and *Candida albicans*. There are nine abnormal PPMs carried by individuals with underlying diseases: eight aerobic Gram-negative bacilli (AGNB), e.g., *Klebsiella, Enterobacter, Citrobacter, Proteus, Morganella, Serratia, Acinetobacter,* and *Pseudomonas* species, and methicillin-resistant *S. aureus* (MRSA) [1].

There is a qualitative and quantitative relationship between surveillance cultures of the throat and gut and diagnostic samples of lower airways and blood, i.e., when the potential pathogen reaches overgrowth concentrations in the throat and gut, lower airway secretions and blood may become positive for the same potential pathogen.

Exogenous infections (15%) are not preceded by overgrowth in throat and/or gut; they are usually caused by abnormal bacteria and may occur anytime during ICU stay. A high level of hygiene is the controlling maneuver and, in tracheostomized patients, may be combined with topical SDD antimicrobials onto the tracheostoma to prevent lower airway infections.

16.4   Therapeutic Use

The full protocol of SDD is based on the following four pillars [1] [Table 16.1]:

1. Parenteral antibiotics given immediately on admission for 4 days to control primary endogenous infections due to PPMs already present in the patient's admission flora. Healthy patients with normal flora can be treated with cefotaxime

Table 16.1 The four-component protocol of SDD

Target PPM, antimicrobials, maneuvers	Total daily dose[a]		
	<5 years	5–12 years	>12 years
1. Parenteral antimicrobials for the first 4 days, e.g., cefotaxime, mg	100–150/ kg/day	75–100/ kg/day	4000/day
2. Enteral antimicrobials			
a. Oropharynx			
(1) AGNB: Polymyxin E with tobramycin	2 g of 2% paste or gel		
(2) Yeasts: Amphotericin B or nystatin	2 g of 2% paste or gel		
b. Gut			
(1) AGNB: Polymyxin E, mg	100	200	400
With tobramycin, mg	80	160	320
(2) Yeasts: Amphotericin B, mg	500	1000	2000
Or nystatin units	2×10^6	4×10^6	8×10^6
3. High levels of hygiene			
4. Surveillance samples of throat and rectum taken on admission, and Monday and Thursday, thereafter			

SDD selective decontamination of the digestive tract, *PPM* potentially pathogenic microorganisms, *AGNB* aerobic Gram-negative bacilli, *MRSA* methicillin-resistant *Staphylococcus aureus*, *mg* milligram, *g* gram, *kg* kilogram
[a]Total daily dose must be divided into four doses

    80–100 mg/kg/day. Patients with a chronic underlying disease or patients transferred from other ICUs or general wards may carry both normal and abnormal flora in throat and gut, and they may require an antipseudomonas cephalosporin, or a glycopeptide if MRSA carriage is expected.

2. Enteral non-absorbable antimicrobials, i.e., polymyxin E (colistin), tobramycin, and amphotericin B (PTA), given throughout the treatment in the ICU, to control secondary carriage and subsequent secondary endogenous infections due to PPMs acquired in the ICU. Half a gram of gel or paste containing 2% PTA is applied to the oropharyngeal mucosa with a spatula or a gloved finger four times a day; additionally, 10 mL of a suspension containing 100 mg of polymyxin E, 80 mg of tobramycin and 500 mg of amphotericin B is administered into the gut through the nasogastric tube four times a day. In properly decontaminated patients, surveillance samples of throat and rectum are free from AGNB, *S. aureus* and yeasts.

3. High standards of hygiene are needed to control exogenous infections due to transmission of ICU-associated microorganisms. Identical antimicrobials of PTA and/or vancomycin as gel/paste are indicated for topical use on the tracheostomy in tracheostomized patients to control exogenous lower airway infections.

4. Surveillance cultures of throat and rectum on admission and, afterwards, twice weekly are required to monitor the efficacy of SDD and to detect the emergence of resistance at early stage.

The combination of polymyxin and tobramycin was chosen because it covers most abnormal AGNB including *Pseudomonas* species, and it is synergic in vitro. The use of a polyene, such as amphotericin B or nystatin, eradicates fungal overgrowth. However, the SDD concept is not a mere implementation of the three antimicrobials, and in settings with moderate-to-high prevalence of antibiotic resistance requires an adaptation of the antimicrobials based on the resistance patterns. For instance, in case of MRSA endemicity, half a gram of a 4% vancomycin gel/paste in the oropharynx and/or 500 mg of vancomycin solution in the gut can be added to the classical PTA regimen four times a day, or in case of multidrug-resistant AGNB paromomycin might be required [23].

Experts are concerned that SDD may lead to an ecological catastrophe. In contrast, the best evidence is that the use of SDD is generally safe, and resistance is under control [24]. This is mainly due to the control of gut overgrowth reducing spontaneous mutations, polyclonality, and resistance [1, 24]. Three large RCTs had resistance as endpoint [7–9]. These RCTs showed less resistance in patients receiving SDD than in those receiving standard care. Additionally, the incidence of bacteremia and lower respiratory tract colonization due to highly resistant AGNB was significantly reduced by SDD compared to standard care [24, 25]. Two meta-analyses explored the impact of SDD on resistance [26, 27]. In the first meta-analysis, including only RCTs, resistance was reduced in patients receiving SDD compared with controls (OR 0.56, 95% CI, 0.41–0.76) [26]. Another systematic review showed a reduction in polymyxin and third-generation cephalosporin resistance to AGNB in patients receiving SDD compared with those who received no intervention [27]. These data are confirmed by long-term ecological studies showing a reduction in resistance rates in patients receiving SDD [24].

The enteral antimicrobials of SDD are usually poorly absorbed. However, critical illness may determine a gut barrier failure. Therefore, serum tobramycin levels should be routinely checked in critically ill patients with renal failure and/or receiving renal replacement therapy [28].

Few small studies assessed the impact of SDD on the gut microbiota. Compared with healthy subjects, the microbiota of ICU patients receiving SDD is characterized by a lower microbial diversity, lower levels of *E. coli* and butyrate-producing bacteria, and higher levels of *Bacteroidetes* and enterococci [24, 29].

16.5 Conclusions

SDD, including parenteral and enteral antimicrobials, controls gut overgrowth of potential pathogenic microorganisms, reduces infection of the lower airways and the bloodstream, and provides a survival benefit in critically ill patients. SDD is a safe maneuver with regard to the emergence of resistance.

Clinical summary

Drug	Indications	Cautions	Side-effects	Dosage	Notes
Selective decontamination of the digestive tract (SDD)	• Critically ill patients requiring mechanical ventilation for ≥72 h • Surgical patients scheduled for esophageal, gastric, intestinal surgery, and radical cystectomy with urinary diversion • Transplant recipients • Other conditions (apart from mechanical ventilation) in which a critical illness-related overgrowth of potentially pathogenic microorganisms is present (e.g., pancreatitis, burns, neurological impairment)	• Critically ill patients with renal failure and/or receiving renal replacement therapy should be routinely checked for serum tobramycin levels • *Proteus* species are intrinsically resistant to polymyxin E. In this case, the efficacy of tobramycin should be checked, and in case of tobramycin resistance another aminoglycoside should be used (e.g., amikacin, paromomycin)	• SDD has not been designed to cover methicillin-resistant *S. aureus* (MRSA). In case of MRSA, endemicity SDD may select this pathogen and vancomycin should be added to the SDD protocol (see next column) • Resistance: present data show that SDD does not increase resistance; it may reduce the resistance problem, if present • Gut microbiota may change during SDD showing a low microbial diversity, a decrease in *E. coli* and butyrate-producing bacteria and an increase in *Bacteroidetes* and enterococci.	• Parenteral antibiotic (e.g., cefotaxime 80–100 mg/kg/day for 4 days) • 0.5 g of 2% polymyxin E/ tobramycin/ amphotericin B paste or gel four times a day in the oral cavity • 100 mg polymyxin E + 80 mg tobramycin + 500 mg amphotericin B in the gut four times a day • 0.5 g of 4% vancomycin paste or gel four times a day in the oral cavity and/or 500 mg vancomycin in the gut four times a day (only in case of MRSA endemicity)	• Surveillance cultures of throat and rectum are part of the technique and should be taken on admission and afterwards twice a week to monitor the efficacy of SDD, and to detect resistance in an early stage • High levels of hygiene are required to control exogenous infections • In tracheostomized patients identical antimicrobials of PTA and/or vancomycin as gel/paste are indicated for topical use on the tracheostomy to control exogenous lower airway infections

References

1. Silvestri L, de la Cal MA, van Saene HKF. Selective decontamination of the digestive tract: the mechanism of action is control of gut overgrowth. Intensive Care Med. 2012;38:1738–50.
2. Liberati A, D'Amico R, Pifferi S, et al. Antibiotic prophylaxis to reduce respiratory tract infections and mortality in adults receiving intensive care. Cochrane Database Syst Rev. 2009;2009:CD000022.
3. Silvestri L, van Saene HKF, Milanese M, Gregori D, Gullo A. Selective decontamination of the digestive tract reduces bloodstream infections and mortality in critically ill patients: a systematic review of randomised controlled trials. J Hosp Infect. 2007;65:187–203.
4. Plantinga NL, de Smet AMGA, Oostdijk EAN, et al. Selective digestive and oropharyngeal decontamination in medical and surgical ICU patients: individual patient data meta-analysis. Clin Microbiol Infect. 2018;24(5):505–13.
5. Silvestri L, van Saene HKF, Weir I, Gullo A. Survival benefit of the full selective digestive decontamination regimen. J Crit Care. 2009;24:474e7–474e14.
6. Price R, MacLennan G, Glen J, on behalf of the SuDDICU collaboration. Selective digestive or oropharyngeal decontamination and topical oropharyngeal chlorhexidine for prevention of death in general intensive care: systematic review and network meta-analysis. BMJ. 2014;348:g2197.
7. de Jonge E, Schultz MJ, Spanjaard L, et al. Effects of selective decontamination of digestive tract on mortality and acquisition of resistant bacteria in intensive care: a randomised controlled trial. Lancet. 2003;362:1011–6.
8. deSmet AM, Kluytmans JA, Cooper BS, et al. Decontamination of the digestive tract and oropharynx in ICU patients. N Engl J Med. 2009;360:20–31.
9. Oostdijk EA, Kesecioglu J, Schultz MJ, et al. Effects of decontamination of the oropharynx and intestinal tract on antibiotic resistance in ICUs: a randomized clinical trial. JAMA. 2014;312(14):1429–37. Retraction in JAMA 2017;317:1583–1584
10. Melsen WG, de Smet AMGA, Kluytmans JAJW, et al. Selective decontamination of the oral and digestive tract in surgical versus non-surgical patients in intensive care in a cluster-randomized trial. Br J Surg. 2012;99:232–7.
11. Krueger WA, Lenhart F-P, Neeser G, et al. Influence of combined intravenous and topical antibiotic prophylaxis on the incidence of infections, organ dysfunctions, and mortality in critically ill surgical patients. Am J Respir Crit Care Med. 2002;166:1029–37.
12. Wittekamp BH, Plantinga NL, Cooper BS, et al. Decontamination strategies and bloodstream infections with antibiotic-resistant microorganisms in ventilated patients: a randomized clinical trial. JAMA. 2018;320(20):2087–98.
13. Abis GSA, Stockman HBAC, Bonjer HJ, et al. Randomised clinical trial of selective decontamination of the digestive tract in elective colorectal cancer surgery (SELECT trial). Br J Surg. 2019;106:355–63.
14. Roos D, Dijksman LM, Oudemans-van Straaten HM, et al. Randomized clinical trial of perioperative selective decontamination of the digestive tract versus placebo in elective gastrointestinal surgery. Br J Surg. 2011;98:1365–72.
15. Safdar N, Said A, Lucey MR. The role of selective decontamination for reducing infection in patients undergoing liver transplantation: a systematic review and meta-analysis. Liver Transpl. 2004;10:817–27.
16. van der Voort PHJ, van Saene HKF. The role of SDD in liver transplantation: a meta-analysis. In: van der Voort PHJ, van Saene HKF, editors. Selective digestive tract decontamination in intensive care medicine. Milan: Springer; 2008. p. 165–72.
17. Nathens AB, Marshall JC. Selective decontamination of the digestive tract in surgical patients: a systematic review of the evidence. Arch Surg. 1999;134:170–6.
18. D'Amico R, Pifferi S, Leonetti C, et al. Effectiveness of antibiotic prophylaxis in critically ill adult patients: systematic review of randomised controlled trials. BMJ. 1998;316:1275–85.

19. Landoni G, Rodseth RN, Santini F, et al. Randomized evidence for reduction of perioperative mortality. J Cardiothorac Vasc Anesth. 2012;26:764–72.
20. Landoni G, Augoustides JG, Guarracino F, et al. Mortality reduction in cardiac anesthesia and intensive care: results of the first international consensus conference. HSR Proc Intensive Care Cardiovasc Anesth. 2011;3:9–19.
21. Landoni G, Pisano A, Lomivorotov V, et al. Randomized evidence for reduction of perioperative mortality: an updated consensus process. J Cardiothorac Vasc Anesth. 2017;31(2):719–30.
22. Oostdijk EAN. Selective decontamination: SWAB guidelines revised. Neth J Crit Care. 2019;27:26–7.
23. van der Voort PHJ, Spronk PE. Insufficient implementation of the SDD concept may yield invalid conclusions. Neth J Crit Care. 2019;27:91.
24. Silvestri L, van Saene HKF, Bion J. Antipathy against SDD is justified: no. Intensive Care Med. 2018;44:1169–73.
25. Oostdijk EA, de Smet AM, Kesecioglu J, et al. Decontamination of cephalosporin-resistant Enterobacteriaceae during selective digestive tract decontamination in intensive care units. J Antimicrob Chemother. 2012;67:2250–3.
26. Taylor N, Cortes-Puch I, Silvestri L, et al. Antimicrobial resistance. In: van Saene HKF, Silvestri L, de la Cal MA, Gullo A, editors. Infection control in the intensive care unit. 3rd ed. Cham: Springer; 2012. p. 451–68.
27. Daneman N, Sarwar S, Fowler RA, Cuthbertson BH, on behalf of the SuDDICU Canadian Study Group. Effect of selective decontamination on antimicrobial resistance in intensive care units: a systematic review and meta-analysis. Lancet Infect Dis. 2013;13:328–41.
28. Mohlmann JE, van Luin M, Mascini EM, et al. Monitoring of tobramycin serum concentrations in selected critically ill patients receiving selective decontamination of the digestive tract: a retrospective evaluation. Eur J Clin Pharmacol. 2019;75:831–6.
29. Buelow E, Bello González TDJ, Fuentes S, et al. Comparative gut microbiota and resistome profiling of intensive care patients receiving selective digestive tract decontamination and healthy subjects. Microbiome. 2017;5:88.

Nutrition

17

Gianluca Paternoster, Giuseppina Opramolla,
and Juan Carlos Lopez-Delgado

Contents

17.1 General Principles of the Nutrition Therapy in the Critical Care Patient

The critical illness is associated with a complex metabolic response, which includes catabolic stress and protein mass loss among other processes that are closely related with inflammation [1, 2]. At the same time, many patients suffer from nutritional

G. Paternoster (✉) · G. Opramolla
Cardiovascular Anesthesia and ICU Department, San Carlo Regional Hospital, Potenza, Italy
e-mail: gianluca.paternoster@ospedalesancarlo.it

J. C. Lopez-Delgado
Intensive Care Department, Hospital Universitari de Bellvitge, L'Hospitalet de Llobregat, Barcelona, Spain

Bellvitge Biomedical Research Institute (IDIBELL), L'Hospitalet de Llobregat, Barcelona, Spain

© Springer Nature Switzerland AG 2021
G. Landoni et al. (eds.), *Reducing Mortality in Critically Ill Patients*,
https://doi.org/10.1007/978-3-030-71917-3_17

deficiencies on Intensive Care Unit (ICU) admission that may contribute to enhance inflammation and worsen illness severity [2, 3].

Nutrition is not simply an adjunctive therapy designed to provide exogenous nutrients; it may also help to preserve lean body mass during the stress response and prevent sarcopenia and myopathy, which ultimately can contribute to improve recovery and length of stay (LOS) [2]. Nutrition therapy itself may help to modulate metabolic response to stress, prevent oxidative cell injury, and stimulate an adequate immune response [3]. Indeed, an inadequate nutrition therapy may cause more complications (e.g., infections, prolonged LOS, prolonged weaning from mechanical ventilation) and worst survival in ICU patients. Increased delivery (i.e., overnutrition) of nutrients and also higher nutritional debt (i.e., malnutrition) may both cause worst outcomes [4]. Thus, providing early and adequate nutrition based on guidelines recommendationsis a proactive therapeutic strategy that may help to reduce disease severity, complications, improve LOS, and affect patient survival [4, 5].

Enteral and parenteral nutrition are both provided in ICU patients for nutritional therapy with the aim to reduce lean body mass loss and improve outcomes [4]. Enteral nutrition (EN) is the main route for artificial nutritional therapy in the ICU. However, it is essential to implement all strategies to optimize delivery of EN and EN tolerance (e.g., avoiding inappropriate interruptions, use of prokinetics, and use of post-pyloric access when it is not possible to use the gastric route) [4–6].

Nowadays, parenteral nutrition (PN), which was introduced in clinical practice over 25 years ago, is a standard tool in the management of ICU patients. PN is mainly indicated in selected patients, mostly in those whom EN is contraindicated and/or those in whom oral intake is inadequate, but it can be used to complete nutritional demands if those are not completely achieved by means of EN (i.e, supplementary or complementary PN) [4–6]. The use of PN has been largely controversial and physicians have been reluctant to use early PN. However, as we discuss below, PN represents a safe way to nourish the critically ill.

17.2 Evidence in the General Principles of the Nutrition Therapy

There are several published randomized clinical trials (RCTs) that have shown metabolic and nutrition-related therapies that may help to reduce mortality (see Table 17.1 [2, 7–14]). However, all these reported therapeutical approaches, even if sustained by an important scientific evidence, are not yet so widespread among clinicians and currently used in clinical practice. Indeed, some of them showed contradictory results that challenged scientific rationale and common sense [11]. In the following paragraphs, we discuss these different nutrition-related therapies that may reduce mortality in critically ill, together an insight with the general principles for adequate nutrition therapy that may help to improve outcome of critically ill.

Table 17.1 Main randomized controlled trials focused on mortality reduction with nutrition therapy in ICU patients [2, 7–14]

Authors	Year	Journal	No. patients	Type of study	Primary outcome	Secondary outcome	Mortality influence	Recommendation[a]
Zhu et al. [7]	2018	Crit Care Med	474	Post hoc subgroup analyses of mRCT	90-day mortality	Organ dysfunction, ICU and hospital discharge mortality, physical function	90-day mortality reduction in patients with normal kidney function	Increase **protein intake** (2 g/kg/day)
Zhang et al. [8]	2017	Clin Nutr	312	RCT	Postoperative recovery,complications, and duration of hospital LOS	Surgical mortality within 30 days postoperatively	Reduction of 30-day mortality postoperatively	Administrate **n-3 fatty acid-based** together with PN for cirrhotic patients with liver cancer following hepatectomy
Hall et al. [9]	2015	JPENur	60	RCT	Reduction of SOFA score	28-day mortality, LOS, mean C-reactive protein, and organ failure free days	Mortality reduction in patients with less severe sepsis	Administrate parenteral fish oil (**n-3 fatty acid-based**) in critically ill septic patients
van Zanten et al. [10]	2014	JAMA	301	mRCT 14 ICUs (Netherlands, Gemany, France, Belgium)	Incidence of new infection	Mortality, SOFA Score, MV duration, ICU and hospital LOS, subtypes of infection	Increased mortality at 6 months for immune-modulating high protein group vs standard high protein in medical subgroup	High protein EN enriched with **immune-modulating nutrients (glutamine, n-3 fatty acid, and antioxidant)** is not superior to standard EN high protein alone

(continued)

Table 17.1 (continued)

Authors	Year	Journal	No. patients	Type of study	Primary outcome	Secondary outcome	Mortality influence	Recommendation[a]
Heyland et al. [11]	2013	N Engl J Med	1223	mRCT 40 ICUs (Canada, the USA,Europe)	28-day mortality	In in-hospital and 6-month mortality	Increased mortality in the intervention group	Administration of higher doses of **glutamine** and **antioxidants** (Oral and IV) is not indicated in critically ill patients with multiorgan failure
Wernerman et al. [12]	2011	Acta Anaest Scand	418	mRCT—11 ICUs (Sweden, Finland, Norway)	Change in the SOFA score from day 1 to day 7	The change in the SOFA score from day 1 to day 10, length of ICU LOS, ICU mortality, and all-cause 6-month mortality	Reduction of ICU mortality	IV **glutamine** supplementation may be indicated in ICU patients
Pontes Arruda et al. [13]	2006	Crit Care Med	165	RCT	28-day mortality	Changes in oxygenation status, time receiving MV, development of new organ dysfunctions	Reduction of ICU and hospital mortality	EN with **n-3 fatty acids** (eicosapentaenoic acid, γ-linolenic acid) and **antioxidants** in patients receiving MV with severe sepsis and septic shock is feasible and may be indicated
Crimi et al. [3]	2004	Anesth Analg	216	RCT	28-day mortality	Reduction in oxidative stress	Reduction of ICU and hospital mortality	**Antioxidant** (Vitamin C and E) supplementation with EN

Bertolini et al. [14]	2003	*Int Care Med*	237	mRCT 33 Italian ICUs	ICU mortality	28-day mortality	Increased mortality in patients with severe sepsis treated with enteral immunonutrition	Enteral **immunonutrition** (**Arginine, n-3 fatty acids,** and **antioxidants**) is not indicated in patients with severe sepsis or septic shock when PN is indicated

Abreviations: IV: Intravenous; ICU: Intensive Care Unit; EN: Enteral Nutrition; PN: Parenteral Nutrition; MV: Mechanical Ventilation; SOFA: Sequential Organ Failure Assessment; mRCT: Multicenter Randomized Controlled Trial; LOS: Length of Stay

[a]In bold are the metabolic and nutrition-related therapies that may help to reduce mortality

17.2.1 Caloric Intake: Focus on Progressive Feeding and Prevent Refeeding Syndrome, Underfeeding and Overfeeding

The initial catabolic response of the critically ill is mainly caused by the systemic inflammatory response to medical illness, major surgery or trauma. It does markedly increase metabolic demands and enhances proteolysis of muscle tissue, resulting in a reduction of lean body mass, which ultimately may cause myopathy. This may negatively impact during ICU recovery [1, 2]. However, there is not a complete agreement on optimal timing, route, type, and amount of nutrition therapy in critically ill patients.

Progressive feeding is a restrictive strategy recommended during the initial/acute phase of ICU LOS (i.e., first 3–4 days). After this phase, full caloric dose should be provided, preferably based on indirect calorimetry [4]. However, some patients who are at nutritional risk or already suffer from a degree of malnutrition when admitted at the ICU, do not tolerate complete energy delivery and develop refeeding syndrome, which is associaded with worst outcomes (e.g., weaning failure from ventilator, arrhythmias, nosocomial infections, higher mortality). Refeeding syndrome is a potentially life-threatening condition induced by initiation of feeding after a period of starvation and hypophosphatemia is the main sign of its presence [15, 16].

In an RCT, Doig et al. enrolled 339 adult critically ill patients who developed refeeding syndrome within 72 h of commencing nutritional therapy in the ICU. The patients enrolled were allocated to receive standard or protocolized caloric restriction when refeeding syndrome was developed. They demonstrated that caloric restriction (i.e., 50% reduction during at least 48 h) was associated with improvement in overall survival time and mortality at day 60 of follow-up. Moreover, caloric restriction also significantly reduced the incidence of major infections [17]. Thus, caloric restriction may be a suitable therapeutic option for adult critically ill patients suffering from refeeding syndrome [15–17].

Overfeeding is energy administration of 110% above the defined target. Underfeeding is defined as an energy administration below 70% of the defined target. Both represent a risk for adverse outcomes in critically ill. However, Arabi et al. in an RCT demonstrated that permissive underfeeding (i.e., 50% of energy needs approximately) was associated with lower mortality and morbidity [18]. This strategy is controversial and it may be recommended to patients with severely ill with previous nutritional reserve; it cannot be recommended in patients at nutritional risk or those who suffer from malnutrition [4–6].

In critically ill patients, especially those who develop refeeding synbdrome, a standardized and multidisciplinary care plan can reduce complication rates and overall mortality. This has been shown in several recent studies that also reported lower mortality rates with low caloric intake compared with full nutritional support [16, 17]. This is probably explained by the avoidance of overfeeding and refeeding syndrome with low caloric intake. Thus, an individualized nutrition therapy strategy should be made based on the occurrence of nutritional complications, such as refeeding syndrome, and the nutritional status of the patient [4–6].

17.2.2 The Route of Nutrition Therapy: Enteral Vs Parenteral

There has been over the past years a debate on the best type of nutrition and route of administration in critically ill patients. As we mentioned above, EN is reccomended by many authors and scientific societies as the main and first route for nutrition therapy. However, supporting evidence comes from elective surgery and trauma patients [4–6]. Early initiation of EN is recommended in hemodynamically stable patients who are unable to maintain oral intake within 48 h, or even within 24 h, if there is no reason to delay EN [3, 4]. Indeed, early EN, even when TROPHIC EN is administered (i.e., <25% nutritional needs via enteral route), is associated with lower risk of infections and preserves structure and function of the gut (i.e., immunity and absorptive capacity) [4, 18].

PN is indicated when the delivery of nutrients via the gastrointestinal tract is contraindicated or insufficient for the needs of the patient. PN can be provided either as a full source of nutrition (exclusive PN) or as an additional nutrition source when full requirements are not able to be met by oral intake or EN (supplemental or complementary PN). PN is easy to be administered and managed, but its benefits were counterbalanced by complications related to central venous catheter infections and gut bacteria translocation. Improvements in catheter-related nosocomial infections and PN technology, together with the recent reported safety of PN compared with EN in contemporary studies, have both overcome the reluctance to the early use of PN in patients witn malnutrition (or at risk) [1, 2, 4–6].

17.2.3 Appropriate Caloric and Protein Target

In critically ill patients, it is difficult to estabilish the exact caloric needs and it is recommended to gradually achieve caloric and protein target particularly in the early/acute phase of ICU LOS. Recommended caloric and protein target are 20-25 Kcal/kg/day and 1.3 g/kg/day, respectively, when indirect calorimetry is not available [3–5]. Caloric and protein requirements must be considered separately, especially due to the importance of protein for the prevention of higher loss of muscle mass, which is caused by the remarkable proteolysis during the acute phase of illness. A significative mortality reduction in patients with normal kidney function may be achieved if patients receive higher dose of protein intake (i.e., 2 g/Kg/day) [7].

In total PN, the protein source can be administrated by means of specific type of aminoacids, which may be helpful to design formulas enriched with aminoacids that have beneficial propierties for some type of patients. Indeed, Garcia deLorenzo et al. demonstrated in a multicenter RCT a mortality reduction in septic patients receiving high branch-chain aminoacids [19]. This study showed for the first time the importance of early protein administration in ICU patients.

ICU patients during EN frequently do not receive the prescribed energy and protein dose. The reasons for this are multifactorial, including interruptions for diagnostic or therapeutical procedures, delayed initiation of EN, and gastrointestinal intolerance, among others. Standard operating procedures may be helpful to avoid caloric and proteic debt. An analysis of data from a prospective, international study evaluating more than 7000 mechanically ventilated patients found a significant inverse association between the administered calories and the risk of mortality. Based on the findings, the authors proposed that patients should receive a minimum of 80% of prescribed calories and protein and suggested that this measure could serve as a quality indicator [20]. A subsequent retrospective cohort study assessed the relationship between nutritional adequacy and long-term outcomes in 475 critically ill patients requiring prolonged mechanical ventilation. Nutritional efficacy was defined depending on the percentage of prescribed calories received during the first week in the ICU as low (<50%), moderate (50–<80%), or high (≥80%). Higher caloric and protein delivery during the first week in the ICU was associated with longer survival time and enhanced recovery after ICU discharge in critically ill who required prolonged mechanical ventilation [21]. In view of those studies, underfeeding is not recommended as nutritional therapy strategy in the most severe ICU patients.

17.2.4 Nutrition Monitoring

Nutrition monitoring represents a real challenge in ICU. Anthropometric and biochemical markers are traditionally used as monitoring tools to evaluate nutritional status, but their use in critical illness is not appropriate due to many confounding factors (e.g., volume overload, inflammation). It is necessary to realize locally adapted standard operating procedures (SOPs) for follow-up of EN and/ or PN administration. Clinical observations, laboratory parameters (e.g., blood glucose levels, electrolytes, triglycerides, liver tests), and monitoring of energy expenditure and body composition have to be addressed daily, focusing on prevention, and early detection of nutrition-related complications. In consequence, understanding and defining risks and developing local SOPs are critical to reduce those complications that eventually may prolong ICU LOS and cause death [22].

17.3   Evidence in Immunonutrition Enteral Formulas

The main purpose of immunonutrition (IMN) EN formulas or the supplementation of higher doses of immunonutrients (combined or alone) was to protect patients from infections and improve ICU LOS. Indeed, some formulas enriched with specific immune-modulating nutrients are actually in the market for clinical use. Such nutrients include Omega-3 (n-3) polyunsaturated fatty acids (PUFAs), arginine, glutamine, and nucleotides. Despite the strong rationale for their use based on the biological propierties (i.e., modulate inflammatory response) of the different components of IMN formulas, due to the great variety of their composition and the lack of strong results, the use of these formulas is controversial [23].

The PUFAs have anti-inflammatory effects by blocking eicosanoid production. Arginine performs several actions, in particular it has an anabolic effect (e.g., increases growth hormone production), improves immune function (e.g., increases the number of T-helper lymphocytes), and modulates vasoplegia (e.g., stimulates nitric oxide synthesis). Nucleotides, which are usually associated with arginine in IMN formulas, could have important effects upon T cell function [24].

Several meta-analyses suggest that immunonutrient mixtures, which contain one or more of the PUFAs, glutamine, arginine, and nucleotides, are useful perioperative use in trauma and surgical patients by determining a reduction in hospital LOS and infection rates, but not in mortality [23]. In septic ICU patients, IMN has shown a reduction mortality and infection rate, especially in less severe patients [24].

Glutamine plays an important role in immune response as it is the fundamental energy substrate for lymphocytes and macrophages, the gut mucosa, and it also improves the antioxidant status by enhancing glutathione production. Low plasma glutamine concentration is a condition linked to unfavorable outcomes in ICU patients [11, 12]. In an mRCT, intravenous glutamine was administered within 3 days after ICU admission, which showed a reduced ICU mortality with the use of glutamine group, even if this result was not sustained at 6 months [11]. Heyland et al. in a blinded 2-by-2 factorial trial with 1223 patients, demonstrated that early provision of glutamine or antioxidant or both did not improve clinical outcomes, and glutamine was associated with an increase in mortality in patients with multiple organ failure. However, results were conflicting because major part of the patients did not receive appropriate protein intake [12].

In the last 10 years, various RCT evaluated the potential benefits of specific IMN formulas in major oncologic surgery due to the significant role of the immune system in cancer physiopathology. The inflammation produced by a surgical insult may be modulated by IMN which is of special importance due to the impaired immune response in cancer patients [8]. IMN may reduce overall complications, postoperative infections, and hospital LOS, and it represents an emerging possibility in oncology and further research is needed.

Agreement is still lacking about the value of individual immune-modulating substrates for specific patient populations. However, in critical illness, it is difficult to draw any conclusion on the effect of IMN at the present moment due to different factors and their use is not strongly recommended in medical patients.

17.4 Evidence in Micronutrients and Antioxidants

Several studies evaluated the benefits of micronutrients (i.e., vitamins, electrolytes, and specific substrates) and antioxidant supplementation in various clinical settings of ICU patients. An early RCT featured by Crimi et al., antioxidant vitamins C and E supplementation were evaluated in critically ill who were fed by EN. In this study, 216 patients were enrolled and they received at least 10 days of EN: 105 patients received EN supplemented with antioxidants and 111 control patients received an isocaloric formula. This study showed that antioxidants supplementation reduced oxidative stress and 28-day mortality [3]. In a recent RCT of patients with sepsis and Acute Respiratory Distress Syndrome, the administration of high doses of IV vitamin C during the first 96 h of ICU admission showed a reduction in 28-day all-cause mortality [25]. The beneficial effects of antioxidants in RCTs are mainly explained due to their anti-inflammatory effects against Reactive Oxygen Species (ROS).

There are other several examples of RCTs aiming to evaluate micronutrients in terms of survival. Selenium, which is essential for normal antioxidant function, showed a reduction in 28-day mortality when administered (1 mg once daily during 2 weeks) in septic patients at the ICU [26]. Magnesium administration, which deficit is associated with weaning failure and cardiac arrhythmias, has been recently associated with lactate clearance and a potential for improving outcomes in septic patients [27]. High-dose of vitamin D (300,000 IU), which seems to have immuno-modulatory properties and reduce the risk of infections, has also shown a trend towards a reduction in the needs of mechanical ventilation [28]. Preliminary data of an RCT has shown a better survival in sepsis with the admistration of L-carnitine infusion, a micronutrient that is involved in mitochondrial metabolism [29]. Administration of higher doses of Vitamin B1 (200 mg of IV Thiamine twice daily), which is important for metabolic cell function and plays a role in lactate clearance, has shown survival benefit in septic patients with thiamine deficiency on ICU admission [30]. Indeed, ESPEN guidelines on clinical nutrition in ICU, recommend daily supplementation with multivitamins and trace elements, especially for PN prescriptions [6]. However, there is not still a strongly evidence for the general use of micronutrients in all critically ill. Despite this, their use in patients may be recommeneded due to their low adverse side-effects profile.

17.5   Nutritional Management in ICU Patients Infected with SARS-COV-2

Emerging evidence shows that the COVID-19 infection is associated with negative outcomes in older, comorbid and hypoalbuminemic patients, characteristics which are associated with nutritional risk [31]. The emerging literature on COVID-19 indirectly exhibits the importance of nutrition in improving their outcomes. Older age and the presence of comorbid conditions are almost invariably associated with impaired nutritional status and sarcopenia, independently of body mass index (BMI) [32]. High BMI is also related to poor prognosis in comorbid COVID-19 patients due to a possible role of sarcopenic obesity in influencing outcome. In addition, lymphopenia, a marker of malnutrition, is a negative prognostic factor in COVID-19 patients [33]. Finally, the timing of nutritional therapy proves to be critical since most patients rapidly progress from cough to dyspnea, and then to respiratory failure and ICU admission for mechanical ventilation [31–33].

In COVID-19 non-intubated ICU patients when the energy target is not possible with an oral diet, oral nutritional supplements (ONS) should be considered before initiate EN support. If there are limitations for achieving caloric and protein targets by means of the enteral route, it could be advised to prescribe supplementary PN. Prescribe EN in patients under non-invasive ventilation (NIV) can be difficult due to the difficulty in placing nasal gastric (NG) tube. Stomach dilatation may both compromise the effectiveness of NIV and delivery of EN. PN may be therefore considered under these conditions to avoid the risk of patient starvation and development of malnutrition, especially in the first 48 h of ICU stay, and also for reducing higher risk of related complications with EN, such as aspiration [34].

Regarding patients oxygenated through high-flow nasal cannula (HFNC), it may be generally considered appropriate to resume oral feeding. However, limited evidence indicates that caloric and protein intake may remain low and inadequate to prevent or treat malnutrition in HFNC patients [35]. For this reason, adequate assessment of nutrient intake is recommended with the ONS administration or with EN if oral route is insufficient.

In the management of patients infected with SARS-COV-2 when HFNC or NIV have been applied for more than 2 h without successful oxygenation, it is recommended to intubate and ventilate the patient. In COVID-19 intubated and ventilated ICU patients, EN should be started through an NG tube (10–12 Fr); post-pyloric feeding should be provided in patients with gastric intolerance after prokinetic treatment or in patients at high risk for aspiration; the prone position is not a limitation or an absolute contraindication for EN. When EN is introduced in prone position, it is recommended to hold the head of the bed elevated (reverse Trendelenburg) to least 10 to 30 degrees to reduce the risk of aspiration of gastric contents, facial edema, and intra-abdominal hypertension [36].

As in other critical patients, hypocaloric nutrition (not exceeding 70% of energy expenditure) should be administered in the early phase of acute illness with increments up to 80–100% after day 3. In those patients who do not tolerate full dose of EN during the first week in the ICU, PN should not be started until all strategies to optimize EN tolerance have been tried. However, PN should be performed as soon as possible in patients who suffer malnutrition or are at risk of malnutrition if EN is not tolerated or contraindicated [4–6, 36].

In summary, nutrition therapy should be considered as an integral part of the approach to patient's victim of SARS-CoV-2 infection, with stronger focus on older, frail, and comorbid individuals. There is still need to develop and implement a protocol based on the clinical practice with the aim of identifying the best nutritional approach and identifying optimal care in this population of patients.

17.6 Conclusions

The results achieved by recent large-scale trials in heterogeneous groups of patients showed no clear benefit of intensive feeding protocols compared to underfeeding during the acute phase of critical illness. However, this is probably mainly related with the occurrence of overnutrition with intensive therapy. A progressive and invidualized nutritional approach should be performed, especially in patients already suffering malnutrition or at risk of malnutrition on ICU admission, in order to avoid higher caloric and protein debts. The use of PN should be strongly considered, even early when patient is at risk.

It remains uncertain the impact of specific nutrition interventions, such as IMN enteral formulas, has in the acute and recovery phase of illness. Specific subgroups (e.g., septic patients) respond differently to nutrition interventions, with the need of regular evaluation of nutrition requirements and constant monitoring, in particular patients admitted to the ICU more than a week. The effect of nutrition delivery on other clinically meaningful outcomes, such as muscle health and physical function, is also insufficiently studied. However, administration of higher amounts of protein during nutrition therapy, parenteral PUFAs, and higher doses of antioxidants and vitamins, may exert beneficial effects over critically ill, even in terms of mortality, with lower risk of side-effects.

Despite the effort of many trials to evaluate how to improve nutritional assessment, nutrition therapy remains a challenge. Therefore, it remains essential to examine the effects of nutrition therapy on other important outcomes, such as reduced loss of lean mass, muscle health and physical function, poorly studied until now.

References

1. Marik PE, Zaloga GP. Early enteral nutrition in acutely ill patients: a systematic review. Crit Care Med. 2001;29:2264–70. https://doi.org/10.1097/00003246-200112000-00005.
2. van Zanten AR, De Waele E, Wischmeyer PE. Nutrition therapy and critical illness: practical guidance for the ICU, post-ICU, and long-term convalescence phases. Crit Care. 2019;23:368. https://doi.org/10.1186/s13054-019-2657-5.
3. Crimi E, Liguori A, Condorelli M, et al. The beneficial effects of antioxidant supplementation in enteral feeding in critically ill patients: a prospective, randomized, double-blind, placebo-controlled trial. Anesth Analg. 2004;99:857–63. https://doi.org/10.1213/01. ANE.0000133144.60584.F6.
4. Herrero-Meseguer JI, Lopez-Delgado JC, Martínez-García MP. Recommendations for specialized nutritional-metabolic management of the critical patient: indications, timing and access routes. Metabolism and Nutrition Working Group of the Spanish Society of Intensive and Critical Care Medicine and Coronary Units (SEMICYUC). Med Intensiva. 2020;44(Suppl 1):33–8. https://doi.org/10.1016/j.medin.2019.12.017.
5. Taylor BE, McClave SA, Martindale RG, et al. Guidelines for the provision and assessment of nutrition support therapy in the adult critically ill patient: Society of Critical Care Medicine (SCCM) and American Society for Parenteral and Enteral Nutrition (A.S.P.E.N.). Crit Care Med. 2016;44:390–438. https://doi.org/10.1097/CCM.0000000000001525.
6. Singer P, Blaser AR, Berger MM, et al. ESPEN guideline on clinical nutrition in the intensive care unit. Clin Nutr. 2019;38:48–79. https://doi.org/10.1016/j.clnu.2018.08.037.
7. Zhu R, Allingstrup MJ, Perner A, Doig GS, Nephro-Protective Trial Investigators Group. The effect of IV amino acid supplementation on mortality in ICU patients may be dependent on kidney function: post hoc subgroup analyses of a multicenter randomized trial. Crit Care Med. 2018;46:1293–301. https://doi.org/10.1097/CCM.0000000000003221.
8. Zhang B, Wei G, Li R, et al. n-3 fatty acid-based parenteral nutrition improves postoperative recovery for cirrhotic patients with liver cancer: a randomized controlled clinical trial. Clin Nutr. 2017;36:1239–44. https://doi.org/10.1016/j.clnu.2016.08.002.

9. Hall TC, Bilku DK, Al-Leswas D, et al. A randomized controlled trial investigating the effects of parenteral fish oil on survival outcomes in critically ill patients with sepsis: a pilot study. J Parenter Enter Nutr. 2015;39:301–12. https://doi.org/10.1177/0148607113518945.
10. van Zanten AR, Sztark F, Kaisers UX, et al. High-protein enteral nutrition enriched with immune-modulating nutrients vs standard high-protein enteral nutrition and nosocomial infections in the ICU: a randomized clinical trial. JAMA. 2014;312:514–24. https://doi.org/10.1001/jama.2014.7698.
11. Heyland D, Muscedere J, Wischmeyer PE, et al. A randomized trial of glutamine and antioxidants in critically ill patients. N Engl J Med. 2013;368:1489–97. https://doi.org/10.1056/NEJMoa1212722.
12. Wernerman J, Kirketeig T, Andersson B, Berthelson H, et al. Scandinavian glutamine trial: a pragmatic multi-Centre randomised clinical trial of intensive care unit patients. Acta Anaesthesiol Scand. 2011;55:812–8. https://doi.org/10.1111/j.1399-6576.2011.02453.x.
13. Pontes-Arruda A, Albuquerque-Aragão AM, Deusdará-Albuquerque J. Effects of enteral feeding with eicosapentaenoic acid, gamma-linolenic acid, and antioxidants in mechanically ventilated patients with severe sepsis and septic shock. Crit Care Med. 2006;34:2325–33. https://doi.org/10.1097/01.CCM.0000234033.65657.B6.
14. Radrizzani D, Bertolini G, Facchini R, et al. Early enteral immunonutrition vs. parenteral nutrition in critically ill patients without severe sepsis: a randomized clinical trial. Intensive Care Med. 2006;32:1191–8. https://doi.org/10.1007/s00134-006-0238-y.
15. Van Zanten AR. Nutritional support and refeeding syndrome in critical illness. Lancet Respir Med. 2015;3:904–5. https://doi.org/10.1016/S2213-2600(15)00433-6.
16. Olthof LE, Koekkoek WACK, van Setten C, Kars JCN, van Blokland D, van Zanten ARH. Impact of caloric intake in critically ill patients with, and without, refeeding syndrome: a retrospective study. Clin Nutr. 2018;37:1609–17. https://doi.org/10.1016/j.clnu.2017.08.001.
17. Doig GS, Simpson F, Heighes PT, Bellomo R, Chesher D, Caterson ID, Reade MC, Harrigan PW, Refeeding Syndrome Trial Investigators Group. Restricted versus continued standard caloric intake during the management of refeeding syndrome in critically ill adults: a randomized, parallel group, multicentre, single-blind controlled trial. Lancet Respir Med. 2015;3:943–52. https://doi.org/10.1016/S2213-2600(15)00418-X.
18. Arabi YM, Tamim HM, Dhar GS, et al. Permissive underfeeding and intensive insulin therapy in critically ill patients: a randomized controlled trial. Am J Clin Nutr. 2011;93:569–77. https://doi.org/10.3945/ajcn.110.005074.
19. García-de-Lorenzo A, Ortíz-Leyba C, Planas M, Montejo JC, Núñez R, Ordóñez FJ, Aragón C, Jiménez FJ. Parenteral administration of different amounts of branch-chain amino acids in septic patients: clinical and metabolic aspects. Crit Care Med. 1997;25:418–24. https://doi.org/10.1097/00003246-199703000-00008.
20. Heyland DK, Murch L, Cahill N, et al. Enhanced protein-energy provision via the enteral route feeding protocol in critically ill patients: results of a cluster randomized trial. Crit Care Med. 2013;41:2743–53. https://doi.org/10.1097/CCM.0b013e31829efef5.
21. Wei X, Andrew GD, Ouellette-Kuntz H, Heyland DK. The association between nutritional adequacy and long-term outcomes in critically ill patients requiring prolonged mechanical ventilation: a multicenter cohort study. Crit Care Med. 2015;43:1569–79. https://doi.org/10.1097/CCM.0000000000001000.
22. Berger MM, Reintam-Blaser A, Calder PC, et al. Monitoring nutrition in the ICU. Clin Nutr. 2019;38:584–93. https://doi.org/10.1016/j.clnu.2018.07.009.
23. Dushianthan A, Cusack R, Burgess VA, Grocott MP, Calder P. Immunonutrition for adults with ARDS: results from a Cochrane systematic review and meta-analysis. Respir Care. 2020;65:99–110. https://doi.org/10.4187/respcare.06965.
24. Galbán C, Montejo JC, Mesejo A, et al. An immune-enhancing enteral diet reduces mortality rate and episodes of bacteremia in septic intensive care unit patients. Crit Care Med. 2000;28:643–8. https://doi.org/10.1097/00003246-200003000-00007.

25. Fowler AA 3rd, Truwit JD, Hite RD, et al. Effect of vitamin C infusion on organ failure and biomarkers of inflammation and vascular injury in patients with Sepsis and severe acute respiratory failure: the CITRIS-ALI randomized clinical trial. JAMA. 2019;322:1261–70. https://doi.org/10.1001/jama.2019.11825.

26. Angstwurm MW, Engelmann L, Zimmermann T, et al. Selenium in intensive care (SIC): results of a prospective randomized, placebo-controlled, multiple-center study in patients with severe systemic inflammatory response syndrome, sepsis, and septic shock. Crit Care Med. 2007;35:118–26. https://doi.org/10.1097/01.CCM.0000251124.83436.0E.

27. Noormandi A, Khalili H, Mohammadi M, Abdollahi A. Effect of magnesium supplementation on lactate clearance in critically ill patients with severe sepsis: a randomized clinical trial. Eur J Clin Pharmacol. 2020;76:175–84. https://doi.org/10.1007/s00228-019-02788-w.

28. Miri M, Kouchek M, Dahmardeh AR, Sistanizad M. Effect of high-dose vitamin D on duration of mechanical ventilation in ICU patients. Iran J Pharm Res. 2019;18:1067–72. https://doi.org/10.22037/ijpr.2019.1100647.

29. Puskarich MA, Kline JA, Krabill V, Claremont H, Jones AE. Preliminary safety and efficacy of L-carnitine infusion for the treatment of vasopressor-dependent septic shock: a randomized control trial. J Parenter Enter Nutr. 2014;38:736–43. https://doi.org/10.1177/0148607113495414.

30. Donnino MW, Andersen LW, Chase M, Berg KM, et al. Randomized, double-blind, placebo-controlled trial of thiamine as a metabolic resuscitator in septic shock: a pilot study. Crit Care Med. 2016;44:360–7. https://doi.org/10.1097/CCM.0000000000001572.

31. Zhou F, Yu T, Du R, et al. Clinical course and risk factors for mortality of adult inpatients with COVID-19 in Wuhan, China: a retrospective cohort study. Lancet. 2020;395:1054–62. https://doi.org/10.1016/S0140-6736(20)30566-3.

32. Laviano A, Koverech A, Michela ZM. Nutrition support in the time of SARS-CoV 2 (COVID-19). Nutrition. 2020;74:110834. https://doi.org/10.1016/j.nut.2020.110834.

33. Peng YD, Meng K, Guan HQ, et al. Clinical characteristics and outcomes of 112 cardio-vascular disease patients infected by 2019-nCoV. Zhonghua Xin Xue Guan Bing Za Zhi. 2020;48:E004. https://doi.org/10.3760/cma.j.cn112148-20200220-00105.

34. Terzi N, Darmon M, Reignier J, et al. OUTCOMEREA study group. Initial nutritional man-agementduring noninvasive ventilation and outcomes: a retrospective cohort study. Crit Care. 2017;21:293. https://doi.org/10.1186/s13054-017-1867-y.

35. Frat JP, Thille AW, Mercat A, et al. High-flow oxygen through nasal cannula in acute hypoxemic respiratory failure. N Engl J Med. 2015;372:2185–96. https://doi.org/10.1056/NEJMoa1503326.

36. Barazzoni R, Bischoff SC, Breda J, et al. ESPEN expert statements and practical guid-ance for nutritional management of individuals with SARS-CoV-2 infection. Clin Nutr. 2020;39:1631–8. https://doi.org/10.1016/j.clnu.2020.03.022.

ECMO and Survival

18

Marina Pieri and Anna Mara Scandroglio

Contents

18.1 General Principles

Extracorporeal membrane oxygenation (ECMO) is a technology capable of providing short-term mechanical support to the heart, lungs, or both. Despite being employed clinically first in the 1970s [1], the more widespread use of ECMO in critically ill adult patients is a recent phenomenon [2], and the number of centers offering ECMO has grown rapidly. During the same period, the indications for ECMO in adults have expanded from refractory severe respiratory and cardiac failure [3] to extracorporeal cardiopulmonary resuscitation (ECPR) [4] and as a bridge to lung transplantation [5]. Furthermore, the use of ECMO is strongly established in neonatal and pediatrics populations [6].

ECMO treatment has therefore represented a crucial improvement in the treatment of patients with refractory organ failure. There are two types of ECMO—venoarterial (VA) and venovenous (VV), used for cardiogenic shock and respiratory failure, respectively. Indeed, both provide respiratory support, but only VA ECMO provides hemodynamic support.

M. Pieri (✉) · A. M. Scandroglio
Department of Anesthesia and Intensive Care, IRCCS San Raffaele Scientific Institute, Milan, Italy
e-mail: pieri.marina@hsr.it; scandroglio.mara@hsr.it

© Springer Nature Switzerland AG 2021   171
G. Landoni et al. (eds.), *Reducing Mortality in Critically Ill Patients*,
https://doi.org/10.1007/978-3-030-71917-3_18

Technological and clinical improvements have made them a fundamental resource in the therapeutic armamentarium of critical care specialists, and they have helped in saving thousands of lives in the last decades.

Randomized evidence on survival benefits on such treatments however is lacking, and this has several explanations. First, the clinical setting in which ECMO treatment is performed makes randomization extremely challenging: indeed ECMO is performed 7/7 days and 24/24 days with almost no time for randomization. At the same time, a valuable alternative strategy is often not available, and it would be unethical to deny ECMO treatment when standard therapy has already failed. Furthermore, patients candidate to ECMO treatment are not ideal patients for an RCT, since they are very sick, generally present concomitant pathological conditions and acute critical organ failures, and this makes very difficult to interpret the results of ECMO treatment by itself on major clinical outcomes. For all these reasons, evidence from RCTs is few and not solid, but we think that stronger evidence is going to be produced in the next few years.

18.2   VV ECMO for Respiratory Failure

Several observational studies and uncontrolled clinical trials have evaluated the effect of ECMO on mortality in patients with severe acute respiratory failure. They reported survival rates from 50 to 71% among patients who received ECMO compared with historical control rates [7–18].

Notably, only two randomized studies have assessed the benefits of VV ECMO on major clinical outcomes.

The Conventional ventilatory support versus Extracorporeal membrane oxygenation for Severe Acute Respiratory failure (CESAR; 2009) [19] trial randomly assigned 180 patients with severe acute respiratory failure to either be referred to a single ECMO center or undergo continued conventional management. Referral to ECMO center was associated with increased survival without disability at 6 months compared to conventional management (63 versus 47 percent). The conclusion of this trial was that adults with severe acute respiratory failure should be referred to an ECMO center for evaluation for ECMO.

This trial has the extraordinary merit to be the first randomized trial ever performed on ECMO treatment although it didn't actually show any survival benefit of ECMO treatment. On the contrary, it was referral to a tertiary care center that resulted associated with survival benefit. Furthermore, this trial was criticized for the heterogeneous ventilation strategies in the control group and the large number of patients transferred for ECMO that never received it (due to improvement with standard low-volume ventilation).

The second randomized trial on VV ECMO was performed almost 10 years later (EOLIA; 2018) [20] In the EOLIA trial, 249 patients with severe ARDS were randomized (partial arterial pressure of oxygen: fraction of inspired oxygen ratio [PaO_2:FiO_2] <50 mmHg >3 h or PaO_2:FiO_2 <80 mmHg for >6 h) to receive early VV

ECMO or conventional protective ventilation. In this second arm, late ECMO was however possible as a rescue therapy [20]. ECMO resulted in improved oxygenation, more days free of renal failure (46 versus 21%), and fewer patients with ischemic stroke (0 versus 5%). Although the study was stopped early by the data safety and monitoring board for interim results that were in favor of ECMO [21], after the final analysis, the difference in 60-day mortality, although in favor of ECMO (35 versus 46%) was not significant. Furthermore, survival was higher in those who received early (2 days after onset; 65%) compared with late (6 days after onset, i.e., rescue) ECMO (43%). As for complications and adverse effects, ECMO was associated with higher rates of bleeding requiring transfusion (46 versus 28%) and severe thrombocytopenia (27 versus 16%) compared with conventional therapy. These results may however have been biased in favor of conventional care by several factors including the high percentage of very sick patients that crossed over from the conventional treatment group to the ECMO group for rescue therapy (28%; median PaO_2 was 51 mmHg compared with 73 mmHg at study entry), and the high utilization in the control group of ARDS therapies associated with improved outcome or oxygenation including prone positioning (90%), inhaled pulmonary vasodilators (83%), and neuromuscular blockade (100%). Therefore, this study overall supports the consideration that patients with ARDS refractory optimal treatment should be managed with ECMO promptly rather than later as a rescue treatment.

Stronger evidence on effects of VV ECMO treatment on survival has been provided by meta-analysis, which included the results of randomized evidence. A meta-analysis of the two randomized trials [19, 20] and three observational studies reported the 60-day mortality rate was lower in patients receiving venovenous ECMO (34 versus 47%; relative risk 0.73, 95% CI 0.58–0.92) [22]. Furthermore, a network meta-analysis that compared several interventions in patients with ARDS on low tidal volume ventilation reported that ECMO was associated with a reduced 28-day mortality [23].

18.3 VA ECMO for Cardiogenic Shock

Venoarterial (VA) ECMO can provide acute support in cardiogenic shock or cardiac arrest in adults. VA ECMO is provided until the patient recovers or receives a long-term ventricular assist device as a bridge to cardiac transplantation. Unlike ECMO for respiratory failure, it is almost impossible to perform a controlled trial of ECMO for cardiac failure because assignment to a control group is not justified. In an extracorporeal life support organization registry, among 9000 adults who underwent ECMO, 41% survived to hospital discharge [24]. It is reasonable that this survival rate will continuously increase due to improved expertise and evolution of technology. Furthermore, cardiogenic shock patients represent a very heterogeneous group, which includes patients with arrhythmia, acute myocardial infarction-related shock, post-cardiotomic shock, sudden cardiac arrest, etc.; different outcomes are therefore also to be expected according to the cause of cardiogenic shock itself.

18.4 Key Points

- Few randomized studies exist on VV ECMO for respiratory failure: no effect on mortality has been shown by a single RCT although a survival benefit in patients treated with VV ECMO compared to optimal medical therapy has been shown in meta-analysis of RCTs.
- VA ECMO for cardiogenic shock represents a crucial clinical improvement to treat a heterogeneous population of patients with different cardiac diseases: it is almost impossible to perform RCT in this setting due to ethical reason in this high-risk setting.

References

1. Hill JD, O'Brien TG, Murray JJ, Dontigny L, Bramson ML, Osborn JJ, Gerbode F. Prolonged extracorporeal oxygenation for acute post-traumatic respiratory failure (shock-lung syndrome). Use of the Bramson membrane lung. N Engl J Med. 1972;286(12):629–34.
2. Sauer CM, Yuh DD, Bonde P. Extracorporeal membrane oxygenation use has increased by 433% in adults in the United States from 2006 to 2011. ASAIO J. 2015;61(1):31–6.
3. Shekar K, Mullany DV, Thomson B, Ziegenfuss M, Platts DG, Fraser JF. Extracorporeal life support devices and strategies for management of acute cardiorespiratory failure in adult patients: a comprehensive review. Crit Care. 2014;18(3):219.
4. Mosier JM, Kelsey M, Raz Y, Gunnerson KJ, Meyer R, Hypes CD, Malo J, Whitmore SP, Spaite DW. Extracorporeal membrane oxygenation (ECMO) for critically ill adults in the emergency department: history, current applications, and future directions. Crit Care. 2015;19:431.
5. Schechter MA, Ganapathi AM, Englum BR, Speicher PJ, Daneshmand MA, Davis RD, Hartwig MG. Spontaneously breathing extracorporeal membrane oxygenation support provides the optimal bridge to lung transplantation. Transplantation. 2016;100(2):2699–704.
6. Robinson S, Peek G. The role of ECMO in neonatal and paediatric patients. Paediatr Child Health. 2015;25(5):222–7.
7. Hemmila MR, Rowe SA, Boules TN, et al. Extracorporeal life support for severe acute respiratory distress syndrome in adults. Ann Surg. 2004;240:595.
8. Peek GJ, Moore HM, Moore N, et al. Extracorporeal membrane oxygenation for adult respiratory failure. Chest. 1997;112:759.
9. Lewandowski K, Rossaint R, Pappert D, et al. High survival rate in 122 ARDS patients managed according to a clinical algorithm including extracorporeal membrane oxygenation. Intensive Care Med. 1997;23:819.
10. Ullrich R, Lorber C, Röder G, et al. Controlled airway pressure therapy, nitric oxide inhalation, prone position, and extracorporeal membrane oxygenation (ECMO) as components of an integrated approach to ARDS. Anesthesiology. 1999;91:1577.
11. Rich PB, Awad SS, Kolla S, et al. An approach to the treatment of severe adult respiratory failure. J Crit Care. 1998;13:26.
12. Kolla S, Awad SS, Rich PB, et al. Extracorporeal life support for 100 adult patients with severe respiratory failure. Ann Surg. 1997;226:544.
13. Australia and New Zealand Extracorporeal Membrane Oxygenation (ANZ ECMO) Influenza Investigators, Davies A, Jones D, et al. Extracorporeal membrane oxygenation for 2009 influenza A (H1N1) acute respiratory distress syndrome. JAMA. 2009;302:1888.
14. Brogan TV, Thiagarajan RR, Rycus PT, et al. Extracorporeal membrane oxygenation in adults with severe respiratory failure: a multi-center database. Intensive Care Med. 2009;35:2105.

15. Noah MA, Peek GJ, Finney SJ, et al. Referral to an extracorporeal membrane oxygenation center and mortality among patients with severe 2009 influenza A (H1N1). JAMA. 2011;306:1659.
16. Posluszny J, Rycus PT, Bartlett RH, et al. Outcome of adult respiratory failure patients receiving prolonged (≥14 days) ECMO. Ann Surg. 2016;263:573.
17. Robba C, Ortu A, Bilotta F, et al. Extracorporeal membrane oxygenation for adult respiratory distress syndrome in trauma patients: a case series and systematic literature review. J Trauma Acute Care Surg. 2017;82:165.
18. Boissier F, Bagate F, Schmidt M, et al. Extracorporeal life support for severe acute chest syndrome in adult sickle cell disease: a preliminary report. Crit Care Med. 2019;47:e263.
19. Peek GJ, Mugford M, Tiruvoipati R, et al. Efficacy and economic assessment of conventional ventilatory support versus extracorporeal membrane oxygenation for severe adult respiratory failure (CESAR): a multicentre randomised controlled trial. Lancet. 2009;374:1351.
20. Combes A, Hajage D, Capellier G, et al. Extracorporeal membrane oxygenation for severe acute respiratory distress syndrome. N Engl J Med. 2018;378:1965.
21. Harrington D, Drazen JM. Learning from a trial stopped by a data and safety monitoring board. N Engl J Med. 2018;378:2031.
22. Munshi L, Walkey A, Goligher E, et al. Venovenous extracorporeal membrane oxygenation for acute respiratory distress syndrome: a systematic review and meta-analysis. Lancet Respir Med. 2019;7:163.
23. Aoyama H, Uchida K, Aoyama K, et al. Assessment of therapeutic interventions and lung protective ventilation in patients with moderate to severe acute respiratory distress syndrome: a systematic review and network meta-analysis. JAMA Netw Open. 2019;2:e198116.
24. Thiagarajan RR, Barbaro RP, Rycus PT, et al. Extracorporeal life support organization registry international report 2016. ASAIO J. 2017;63:60.

Ultrasounds

19

Francesco Corradi, Ludovica Tecchi, and Francesco Forfori

Contents

19.1 General Principles

With the word POCUS, we refer to a bedside examination conducted by an expert physician in order to add information to clinical evaluation. Owing to its unstructured physical approach based on multidistrict visual, problem-focused analysis, and functional rather than anatomical evaluation, POCUS is largely different from other kinds of ultrasonography [1]. This approach provides simple answers to simple questions, the most valuables being those with yes/no responses, and leads to the so-called early gold-directed therapy.

F. Corradi (✉) · L. Tecchi · F. Forfori
Department of Surgical, Medical and Molecular Pathology and Critical Care Medicine,
University of Pisa, Pisa, Italy
e-mail: Francesco.corradi@unipi.it; francesco.forfori@unipi.it

© Springer Nature Switzerland AG 2021 177
G. Landoni et al. (eds.), *Reducing Mortality in Critically Ill Patients*,
https://doi.org/10.1007/978-3-030-71917-3_19

In emergency and critical care, POCUS can empower a common sequence of echo-enhanced advanced life support by analyzing airways first, then breathing, and finally circulation.

19.2   Main Evidences

Numerous studies have provided support to the use of ultrasonography in various clinical applications, including upper airways procedures such as intubation and tracheostomy, evaluation of lower respiratory tract diseases, and emergency medicine and intensive care.

19.2.1 Ultrasonography in Upper Airways Procedures

The analysis of upper airways can confirm the correct placement of an endotracheal tube, by its direct visualization within the trachea, and check the cuff position [2]. Bilateral ventilation can be confirmed by bilateral lung sliding, whereas esophageal intubation is easily identified from the appearance of the double-tract sign [3] or excluded by tracheal rapid ultrasound examination [4]. Ultrasonographic evaluation of neck anatomy and vessels before percutaneous dilatational tracheostomy can predict the success of procedure [5–9]. Besides, some authors decided to modify the planned puncture location in around 50% of their patients after ultrasound evaluations [6, 8, 10].

Moreover, it has been recently demonstrated that percutaneous dilatational tracheostomy under ultrasound guidance is, compared to endoscopic procedure, not associated with remarkable hypercapnia or intracranial pressure increase, which are harmful complications in neurosurgical patients [11].

19.2.2 Ultrasonography in the Assessments of Lower Respiratory Tract

For diagnostic purposes, lung ultrasonography allows detecting pneumonia consolidations [12], pneumothorax [13], pleural effusions [14], and the so-called ultrasonographic interstitial syndrome associated with increased extravascular lung water [15], thus differentiating between "dry" and "wet" lung. In these applications, lung ultrasonography resulted to be superior not only to auscultation [16] but also to chest X-ray [17].

For mechanical ventilation, ultrasonography can help guide lung recruitment maneuvers and adjust positive end expiratory pressure [18].

19.2.3 Ultrasonography in Intensive Care

In emergency settings, ultrasonography allows investigating the hemodynamic status by epigastric or apical heart scanning. These simple views can provide information on pericardium, left and right ventricles, valves, inferior cava vein, aorta and position of central venous lines. Table 19.1 shows a summary of the main applications of POCUS in emergency and intensive care settings.

In addition, by investigating kidneys and spleen perfusion, POCUS can give information on splanchnic perfusion, tissue hypoxemia [19–21] and hemodynamic status [22] that cannot be usually detected by physical examination [16, 23]. Thus, point-of-care ultrasound is considered a precious method for the evaluation of undistinguished shock, resuscitation guide [24, 25], preoperative assessment of patients undergoing surgery [26, 27].

19.3 Randomized-Controlled Studies of POCUS

The characteristics of the available randomized-controlled studies of POCUS in different settings are summarized in Table 19.2.

19.3.1 POCUS in Percutaneous Dilatational Tracheostomy

In a single-center randomized clinical trial, Rudas and co-workers [28] studied whether the use of ultrasound can improve its safety and efficacy. In comparison with the reference method, the ultrasound-based technique tended to be better in terms of appropriate midline punctures and reduced complications though the differences did not achieve statistical significance.

19.3.2 POCUS in Respiratory Patients

A single-center randomized clinical trial study [29] showed that the bedside evaluation of heart and lungs, in addition to the diagnostic methods currently used, increased by 24% the number of correct diagnoses and by 21% the choice of appropriate treatment in patients with respiratory symptoms within 4 h after accessing the emergency room.

19.3.3 POCUS Impact on Mortality and Complication Rates in Hip Fracture Patients

A pilot study conducted by Canty et al. [30] showed that targeted echocardiography (FOCUS) is feasible in patients undergoing hip fracture surgery leading to a

Table 19.1 Main applications of point of care ultra sound (POCUS) in emergency and intensive care settings

Targets	Diagnoses					Interventions
Trachea and vocal cords	ET tube position	Esophageal intubation	Unilateral intubation	Cord palsy	Stridor and edema	Tracheostomy
Pleura	Pleural effusions	Pneumothorax	Lung sliding	Lung pulse	Lung point	Thoracentesis
Lung	Interstitial syndrome	Consolidations	ARDS	Pulmonary edema	Pulmonary embolism	PEEP titration and recruitment maneuvers
Vessels	Thrombosis	ICV collapsibility	ICV distensibility	Vascular filling	Aortic dissection	CVC cannulation
Heart and pericardium	Tamponade	Pneumopericardium	Ventricular strain	Monitoring volumes	Valve diseases	Pericardiocentesis
Diaphragm	Thickening fraction	Thickness	Excursion	Diaphragmatic dysfunction	Work of breathing	Weaning from MV

Abbreviations: ET: endotracheal tube; IVC: inferior vena cava; CVC: central venous catheter; ARDS: acute respiratory distress syndrome; PEEP: positive end expiratory pressure; MV mechanical ventilation

Table 19.2 Characteristics of randomized trials that evaluate POCUS

First author	Year	No. centers	Setting	Application	No. patients POCUS group	No. patients CONTROL group	Outcomes
Lanspa MJ	2018	1	ICU	Early septic shock	15	15	Mortality 5 pts. (33%) vs 3 pts. (20%) p = 0.68
Rudas M	2014	2	ICU	Percutaneous dilatational tracheostomy (PDT)	23	24	First-pass success rate 20 pts. (87%) vs 14 pts. (58%) p = 0.028
Laursen CB	2014	1	ED	Respiratory symptoms	158	157	Correct presumptive diagnosis 4 h 139 pts. (88%) vs 100 pts. (63.7%) p = <0,0001
Pontet J	2019	2	Polyvalent ICUs	Critical care	40	40	Better characterization of ICU admission diagnosis 14 pts. (35%); change in clinical management 24 pts. (60%)
Canty DJ	2019	Multicenter [14]	Preoperative medicine	Cardiac mortality in orthopedic surgery	49	51	Mortality reduction 7 vs 12 pts. with relative group separation of 39%
Pallesen J	2020	2	Perioperative care	Cardiopulmonary complications in abdominal and orthopedic surgery	400	400	Mortality within 30 days or admission >10 days (study to be concluded ongoing study, recruiting patients)
Cid X	2020	1	Internal medicine	Length of stay at the hospital (LOS)	122	122	LOS; diagnosis and management change; 30 days readmission (study to be concluded ongoing study, recruiting patients)

reduction in complications and mortality at 30 days and 12 months. A prospective multicenter study to confirm these data is advisable.

19.3.4 Impact of Ultrasound Protocol in Early ICU Stay

In a prospective randomized clinical trial conducted in two polyvalent ICUs [31], patients were assigned to two groups: one underwent ultrasound examination of optic nerve, lungs, pleura and venous district, the other only clinical evaluation. The result showed a better diagnostic definition (35%) and clinical management (60%) in patients evaluated with ultrasound technique, in terms of accurate administration of fluid administration, reduced mechanical ventilation, as well as a more contained use of conventional imaging resources in the first week of hospitalization.

19.3.5 Echocardiography in the Treatment of Septic Shock

A study conducted by Lanspa et al. [32] assigned patients with septic shock to two groups: one first evaluated with a resuscitation protocol under echocardiographic guidance, the other directly treated with early gold-directed therapy in the first hours of onset. The results showed no significant differences in outcomes, namely, organ failure, number of days out of intensive care, weaning from mechanical ventilation at 28 days, and changes in mortality. However, the study missed feasibility outcomes, namely, fluid and dobutamine administration and time to lactate clearance, for patients had been resuscitated before entering the randomization. Moreover, because of the small sample size the study was prone to type-2 error, thus making any conclusion on non-inferiority unconvincing.

19.4   Conclusions

Only few randomized clinical trials showed that POCUS could have a beneficial effect on survival. It may reduce mortality in elderly and frail traumatic patients submitted to a multiorgan approach, if by trained intensivists [31]. POCUS should be considered to treat critical care patients, especially during emergency in unstable hemodynamic conditions and cardiac arrest at an early stage since it is capable of identifying individuals who have a higher survival rate after discharge since it can recognize patients with higher likelihood of survival to hospital discharge and recognize interventions that go beyond the ACLS algorithm.

Hence, POCUS has to be considered an invaluable tool among physicians since it is the only method available, safe and rapid, and has proven to be able to enormously increase the diagnostic capacity of the clinician and to modify the treatment in terms of therapeutic attitude. Although, it is likely that both the definition of correct diagnoses and the change in patient management can improve the clinical approach and, therefore, modify the workload, as well as reduce hospitalization times.

Further research is warranted to evaluate POCUS in other fields and in controversial areas.

References

1. Ball L, Corradi F, Pelosi P. Ultrasonography in critical care medicine: the WAMS approach. ICU Manag. 2012;12(2):30–3.
2. Bin OA, Chuan TW, Manikam R. A feasibility study on bedside upper airway ultrasonography compared to waveform capnography for verifying endotracheal tube location after intubation. Crit Ultrasound J. 2013;5(1):1.
3. Gottlieb M, Bailitz JM, Christian E, Russell FM, Ehrman RR, Khishfe B, et al. Accuracy of a novel ultrasound technique for confirmation of endotracheal intubation by expert and novice emergency physicians. West J Emerg Med. 2014;15(7):834–9.
4. Chou HC, Tseng WP, Wang CH, Ma MHM, Wang HP, Huang PC, et al. Tracheal rapid ultrasound exam (T.R.U.E.) for confirming endotracheal tube placement during emergency intubation. Resuscitation. 2011;82(10):1279–84.
5. Bertram S, Emshoff R, Norer B. Ultrasonographic anatomy of the anterior neck: implications for tracheostomy. J Oral Maxillofac Surg. 1995;53(12):1420–4.
6. Bonde J, Nørgaard N, Antonsen K, Faber T. Implementation of percutaneous dilation tracheotomy - value of preincisional ultrasonic examination? Acta Anaesthesiol Scand. 1999;43(2):163–6.
7. Muhammad JK, Major E, Wood A, Patton DW. Percutaneous dilatational tracheostomy: Haemorrhagic complications and the vascular anatomy of the anterior neck. A review based on 497 cases. Int J Oral Maxillofac Surg. 2000;29(3):217–22.
8. Kollig E, Heydenreich U, Roetman B, Hopf F, Muhr G. Ultrasound and bronchoscopic controlled percutaneous tracheostomy on trauma ICU. Injury. 2000;31(9):663–8.
9. Flint AC, Midde R, Rao VA, Lasman TE, Ho PT. Bedside ultrasound screening for pretracheal vascular structures may minimize the risks of percutaneous dilatational tracheostomy. Neurocrit Care. 2009;11(3):372–6.
10. Guinot PG, Zogheib E, Petiot S, Marienne JP, Guerin AM, Monet P, et al. Ultrasound-guided percutaneous tracheostomy in critically ill obese patients. Crit Care. 2012;16(2):R40.
11. Kerwin AJ, Croce MA, Timmons SD, Maxwell RA, Malhotra AK, Fabian TC. Effects of fiberoptic bronchoscopy on in patients with brain injury: a prospective clinical study. J Trauma Inj Infect Crit Care. 2000;48(5):878–83.
12. Corradi F, Brusasco C, Garlaschi A, Paparo F, Ball L, Santori G, et al. Quantitative analysis of lung ultrasonography for the detection of community-acquired pneumonia: a pilot study. Biomed Res Int. 2015;2015:868707.
13. Vezzani A, Brusasco C, Palermo S, Launo C, Mergoni M, Corradi F. Ultrasound localization of central vein catheter and detection of postprocedural pneumothorax: an alternative to chest radiography. Crit Care Med. 2010;38(2):533–8.
14. Xirouchaki N, Magkanas E, Vaporidi K, Kondili E, Plataki M, Patrianakos A, et al. Lung ultrasound in critically ill patients: comparison with bedside chest radiography. Intensive Care Med. 2011;37(9):1488–93.
15. Corradi F. Computer-aided quantitative ultrasonography for detection of pulmonary edema in mechanicall ventilated cardiac surgery patients. Chest. 2016;150:640–51.
16. Vezzani A, Manca T, Brusasco C, Santori G, Valentino M, Nicolini F, et al. Diagnostic value of chest ultrasound after cardiac surgery: a comparison with chest X-ray and auscultation. J Cardiothorac Vasc Anesth. 2014;28(6):1527–32.

17. Xirouchaki N, Magkanas E, Vaporidi K, et al. Lung ultrasound in critically ill patients: comparison with bedside chest radiography. Intensive Care Med. 2011;37(9):1488–93.

18. Luecke T, Corradi F, Pelosi P. Lung imaging for titration of mechanical ventilation. Curr Opin Anaesthesiol. 2012;25(2):131–40.

19. Corradi F, Brusasco C, Vezzani A, Palermo S, Altomonte F, Moscatelli P, et al. Hemorrhagic shock in polytrauma patients: early detection with renal Doppler resistive index measurements. Radiology. 2011;260(1):112–8.

20. Brusasco C, Tavazzi G, Robba C, Santori G, Vezzani A, Manca T, et al. Splenic doppler resistive index variation mirrors cardiac responsiveness and systemic hemodynamics upon fluid challenge resuscitation in postoperative mechanically ventilated patients. Biomed Res Int. 2018;2018:1978968.

21. Corradi F, Via G, Tavazzi G. What's new in ultrasound-based assessment of organ perfusion in the critically ill: expanding the bedside clinical monitoring window for hypoperfusion in shock. Intensive Care Med. 2020;46:775–9.

22. Shokoohi H, Boniface KS, Pourmand A, Liu YT, Davison DL, Hawkins KD, et al. Bedside ultrasound reduces diagnostic uncertainty and guides resuscitation in patients with undifferentiated hypotension. Crit Care Med. 2015;43(12):2562–9.

23. Manno E, Navarra M, Faccio L, Motevallian M, Bertolaccini L, Mfochivè A, et al. Deep impact of ultrasound in the intensive care unit: the "iCU-sound" protocol. Anesthesiology. 2012;117(4):801–9.

24. Pelosi P, Corradi F. Ultrasonography in the intensive care unit. Anesthesiology. 2012;117(4):696–8.

25. Gaspari R, Weekes A, Adhikari S, Noble VE, Nomura JT, Theodoro D, et al. Emergency department point-of-care ultrasound in out-of-hospital and in-ED cardiac arrest. Resuscitation. 2016;109:33–9.

26. Heiberg J, El-Ansary D, Canty DJ, Royse AG, Royse CF. Focused echocardiography: a systematic review of diagnostic and clinical decision-making in anaesthesia and critical care. Anaesthesia. 2016;71(9):1091–100.

27. Haji DL, Royse A, Royse CF. Review article: clinical impact of non-cardiologist-performed transthoracic echocardiography in emergency medicine, intensive care medicine and anaesthesia. Emerg Med Australas. 2013;25(1):4–12.

28. Rudas M, Seppelt I, Herkes R, Hislop R, Rajbhandari D, Weisbrodt L. Traditional landmark versus ultrasound guided tracheal puncture during percutaneous dilatational tracheostomy in adult intensive care patients: a randomised controlled trial. Crit Care. 2014;18(5):1–10.

29. Laursen CB, Sloth E, Lassen AT, Christensen R, Lambrechtsen J, Madsen PH, et al. Point-of-care ultrasonography in patients admitted with respiratory symptoms: a single-blind, randomised controlled trial. Lancet Respir Med. 2014;2(8):638–46.

30. Canty DJ, Heiberg J, Yang Y, Royse AG, Margale S, Nanjappa N, et al. Pilot multi-centre randomised trial of the impact of pre-operative focused cardiac ultrasound on mortality and morbidity in patients having surgery for femoral neck fractures (ECHONOF-2 pilot). Anaesthesia. 2018;73(4):428–37.

31. Pontet J, Yic C, Díaz-Gómez JL, Rodriguez P, Sviridenko I, Méndez D, et al. Impact of an ultrasound-driven diagnostic protocol at early intensive-care stay: a randomized-controlled trial. Ultrasound J. 2019;11(1):24.

32. Lanspa MJ, Burk RE, Wilson EL, Hirshberg EL, Grissom CK, Brown SM. Echocardiogram-guided resuscitation versus early goal-directed therapy in the treatment of septic shock: a randomized, controlled, feasibility trial. J Intensive Care. 2018;6(1):1–8.

Alternative Medicine

20

Antonio Pisano, Manuela Angelone, and Diana Di Fraja

Contents

20.1 Introduction

The Pubmed search strategy used during the last update of previous "Democracy-based" international consensus conferences [1, 2] to identify all randomized controlled trials (RCTs) dealing with nonsurgical interventions which were found to affect mortality in the perioperative and critical care settings returned, among others, two RCTs investigating the use of acupuncture and an herbal preparation, respectively, as an adjunctive therapy in patients with sepsis [3, 4]. These topics, regarded to as a whole with the term "alternative medicine," were excluded from the consensus process before the web poll according to pre-specified criteria (individual small single-center RCTs without other supportive evidence) [1]. However, the number of RCTs reporting a significant survival benefit with the use of Traditional

A. Pisano (✉) · M. Angelone · D. Di Fraja
Cardiac Anesthesia and Intensive Care Unit, A.O.R.N. "Dei Colli", Monaldi Hospital, Naples, Italy
e-mail: antonio.pisano@ospedalideicolli.it; manuela.angelone@ospedalideicolli.it; dianadifraja@libero.it

© Springer Nature Switzerland AG 2021
G. Landoni et al. (eds.), *Reducing Mortality in Critically Ill Patients*,
https://doi.org/10.1007/978-3-030-71917-3_20

Chinese Medicine (TCM), particularly intravenous herbal remedies, as an adjunct to standard therapy in critically ill patients has increased in the last few years and, as discussed below, also includes a couple of relatively large investigations published in a top-rating international journal [5, 6]. Moreover, although acupuncture and, especially, herbal intravenous injections are regarded as "alternative" in western countries, they represent two cornerstones of Traditional Medicine (including TCM as well as Japanese and Korean Traditional Medicines) [7], a set of practices with a thousand-year-old tradition, some of which are often still used, in addition to conventional care, in the intensive care units (ICUs) of East Asian countries [5, 6, 8, 9].

Considering the international scope of the consensus conference whose findings are discussed in details in the book, this chapter briefly summarizes the main evidences about the potential role of alternative medicine in reducing mortality among critically ill patients although for Western clinicians (including the authors of the present chapter) any interpretation of such evidences is very difficult and the implications for clinical practice are virtually absent (at least in the short term).

20.2   Alternative Medicine and Mortality in the ICU Setting: Main Evidences

As discussed in the following paragraphs, a reduced mortality has been reported in patients with sepsis or septic shock receiving either various TCM remedies (including acupuncture, herbal intravenous injections, or decoctions administered by nasogastric tube or enteroclysis) [3, 10–13] or other herbal preparations available in some Middle Eastern countries [4, 14], in patients with return of spontaneous circulation (ROSC) after in-hospital cardiac arrest (IHCA) receiving *Shenfu* infusions [5], and in patients with community-acquired pneumonia receiving *XueBiJing* infusions [6].

20.2.1 Traditional Chinese Medicine in Patients with Sepsis

TCM includes acupuncture, herbal remedies, moxibustion, cupping, and manual therapies (Tuina) [7]. In a small RCT, 90 patients with sepsis (of unknown severity since the article is in Chinese) were randomized to receive either acupuncture or thymosin alpha-1 (an endogenous immunomodulatory peptide with a potential role in the treatment of cancer, sepsis, and viral diseases) [15] in addition to standard care, or standard care alone: 28-day mortality was significantly lower in both the acupuncture and thymosin groups as compared with the standard care group (16.7 vs 20 vs 30%, respectively, $p = 0.01$) [3]. Moreover, ICU length of stay (LOS) was shorter and both CD3$^+$, CD4$^+$, and CD8$^+$ T-cell subtypes and immunoglobulin levels increased to a greater extent in the acupuncture and thymosin groups as compared with the standard care group. However, a subsequent small RCT, although confirming a possible immunomodulatory effect of acupuncture, failed to show a significant difference in 28-day mortality among 58 septic patients randomized to receive or not electro-acupuncture in addition to usual care [16].

The most often used TCM remedy in Chinese ICUs is intravenous herbal injection [10]. Two RCTs [10, 11] and a couple of meta-analyses [12, 17] suggested a possible favorable impact on mortality of this type of TCM treatments in patients with sepsis. However, the largest RCT of intravenous herbal injection in septic patients ever performed [10] failed to show any difference in outcomes (including, among others, 7-day and 28-day mortality, ICU and hospital LOS, lactate levels, and use of vasopressors) in 199 patients with septic shock randomized to either *Shenfu* injections or saline, with the exception of a reduction in 7-day mortality in the *Shenfu* group (83.3 vs 54.5%, $p = 0.034$) when considering only patients with arterial lactate levels ≥4.5 mmol/L. Another RCT found a significant reduction in ICU LOS and 28-day mortality among 167 septic patients randomized to conventional (Western) medicine in association or not with *Qishen Huoxue Granule* (a preparation of Astragalus membranaceus, Salvia miltiorrhiza, Flos carthami, Angelicae sinensis, and other herbs) [11].

Finally, a recent multicenter RCT of 302 patients with sepsis-associated acute gastrointestinal injury found a significantly reduced 28-day mortality in patients treated with a TCM bundle (including acupuncture and herbal decoctions administered by nasogastric tube or enteroclysis) in addition to conventional care as compared with conventional care alone (35.3 vs 48.3%, $p = 0.01$) [13].

20.2.2 Septimeb™ in Patients with Sepsis

Septimeb™ is an herbal remedy containing extracts of Tanacetum vulgare, Rosa canina, and Urtica dioica (see Fig. 20.1) in addition to selenium, carotenes, and flavonoids which is approved in Iran as an immunomodulatory agent. A very small (multicenter) RCT of 29 septic ICU patients found a dramatic reduction in 14-day mortality in patients receiving Septimeb™ as an adjunct to usual care as compared with usual care alone (18.8 vs 53.8%, $p = 0.048$) [4]. A subsequent RCT of 51

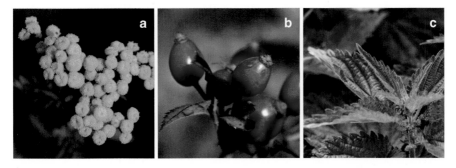

Fig. 20.1 Septimeb™ is an herbal remedy containing extracts of Tanacetum vulgare (**a**), Rosa canina (**b**) and Urtica dioica (**c**) in addition to selenium, carotenes, and flavonoids

patients with "severe sepsis" admitted to the ICU or a medical ward of a single hospital found a similar decrease in 90-day mortality (8.3 vs 25%) in those receiving adjunctive Septimeb™ as compared with usual care alone [14]. Of note, none of these two trials was placebo-controlled. Moreover, the lack of clear inclusion criteria, the reported baseline vital signs and laboratory tests (as well as the missing data about baseline illness severity and organ injury scores), the inclusion of non-ICU patients, and the relatively low mortality rate in the control group raise some doubt that all patients in the second study really had "severe sepsis" (or sepsis according to current definition).

20.2.3 *Shenfu* Injection After In-Hospital Cardiac Arrest

Shenfu is a well-known herbal preparation containing red ginseng roots and aconite roots (see Fig. 20.2) which, according to TCM, is indicated for shock and is often still used in Chinese emergency departments [5, 12]. In a recently published multicenter RCT involving 50 hospitals in China, Zhang et al. [5] randomly assigned 978 patients with ROSC after IHCA to either intravenous *Shenfu* injection as an adjunct to a standardized post-resuscitation bundle (including early percutaneous coronary revascularization if indicated, therapeutic hypothermia, targeted ventilatory and hemodynamic management, seizures prevention, etc.) or to the post-resuscitation bundle alone. Both 28-day mortality and 90-day mortality were significantly lower in the *Shenfu* group as compared with the control group (hazard ratio [HR] 0.61, 95% confidence interval [CI] 0.43–0.89, $p = 0.009$ and HR 0.55, 95% CI 0.38–0.79, $p = 0.002$, respectively). Moreover, duration of mechanical ventilation and hospital LOS were significantly reduced in the *Shenfu* group as

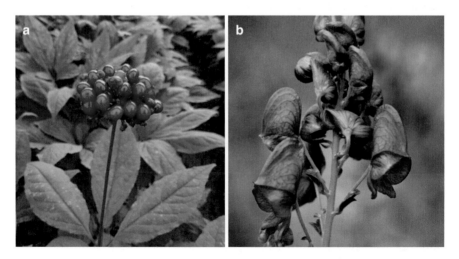

Fig. 20.2 *Shenfu* is a well-known herbal Traditional Chinese Medicine remedy prepared from roots of red ginseng (**a**) and aconite (**b**)

compared with the control group. In addition to possible immunomodulation and inhibition of inflammatory response [5, 12, 18], *Shenfu* is thought to increase systemic arterial pressure, improve microcirculation, and attenuate post-resuscitation myocardial dysfunction through mechanisms such as scavenging of reactive oxygen species, reduction of calcium overload, and restoration of Na^+-K^+-ATPase and Ca^{2+}-ATPase activities [5, 12].

20.2.4 *XueBiJing* Injection in Patients with Severe Community-Acquired Pneumonia

XueBiJing is a TCM herbal remedy containing more than a hundred substances from different herbs (such as Carthamus tinctorius flowers, Paeonia lactiflora roots, Ligusticum chuanxiong rhizomes, Angelica sinensis roots, and Salvia miltiorrhiza roots); it is approved and commonly used in China for the treatment of sepsis in critically ill patients and is believed to antagonize endotoxin, attenuate inflammatory cytokines, modulate coagulation and immune response, and improve microcirculation [6]. In a large RCT published in 2019, 710 adult patients with severe community-acquired pneumonia were randomized in 33 Chinese hospitals to receive either intravenous *XueBiJing* or placebo in addition to usual care [6]. The authors found a reduced 28-day mortality in the *XueBiJing* group as compared with the placebo group (15.87 vs 24.63%, between-group difference 8.8%, 95% CI2.4–15.2%, $p = 0.006$). Moreover, duration of mechanical ventilation and ICU LOS were significantly shorter, and improvement in the pneumonia severity index was greater, in the *XueBiJing* group as compared with the placebo group.

20.3 Relevance to Clinical Practice: A Brief Comment

As mentioned, the enormous cultural distance between the world of Traditional Medicines and that of "official" medicine makes it very difficult to interpret and comment the abovementioned evidences. Beyond the small and mostly non-blinded and not placebo-controlled investigations which appear to have little more than anecdotal value according to our evidence-based medicine standards, the findings of the two seemingly high-quality large multicenter RCTs [5, 6] leave us at least perplexed. It is possible that, as suggested for acupuncture [19], also the beneficial effects observed with the use of herbal remedies may be attributable to neurophysiological mechanisms as well as to the deep trust of both clinicians and patients in a strongly rooted tradition. On the other hand, a direct pharmacological action (e.g., on the molecular mechanisms of inflammation and immune response) of some among the multitude of substances which are present in these preparations cannot be excluded, as well as the potential toxicity of these substances is poorly known (in this regard, a recent retrospective investigation reported 30 cases of acute liver failure caused by TCM remedies [20]).

Also considering the difficult availability of these preparations and, above all, the lack of regulation about their use in Western countries, it is clear that there is currently no clinical application for these "alternative" treatments in ICU patients in our latitudes, unless after possible isolation of some active substance (which would first undergo all the stages of drug testing).

References

1. Sartini C, Lomivorotov V, Pieri M, et al. A systematic review and international web-based survey of randomized controlled trials in the perioperative and critical care setting: interventions reducing mortality. J Cardiothorac Vasc Anesth. 2019;33(5):1430–9.
2. Sartini C, Lomivorotov V, Pisano A, et al. A systematic review and international web-based survey of randomized controlled trials in the perioperative and critical care setting: interventions increasing mortality. J Cardiothorac Vasc Anesth. 2019;33(10):2685–94.
3. Xiao QS, Ma MY, Zhang XS, et al. Effect of acupuncture on prognosis and immune function of sepsis patients. Zhongguo Zhong Xi Yi Jie He Za Zhi. 2015;35(7):783–6. Article in Chinese
4. Eslami K, Mahmoodpoor A, Ahmadi A, et al. Positive effect of septimeb™ on mortality rate in severe sepsis: a novel non antibiotic strategy. Daru. 2012;20(1):40.
5. Zhang Q, Li C, Shao F, et al. Efficacy and safety of combination therapy of Shenfu injection and post-resuscitation bundle in patients with return of spontaneous circulation after in-hospital cardiac arrest: a randomized, assessor-blinded, controlled trial. Crit Care Med. 2017;45(10):1587–95.
6. Song Y, Yao C, Yao Y, et al. XueBiJing injection versus placebo for critically ill patients with severe community-acquired pneumonia: a randomized controlled trial. Crit Care Med. 2019;47(9):e735–43.
7. Park HL, Lee HS, Shin BC, et al. Traditional medicine in China, Korea, and Japan: a brief introduction and comparison. Evid Based Complement Alternat Med. 2012;2012:429103.
8. China Association Of Integrative Medicine Emergency Medicine Committee, Editorial Committee Of Chinese Journal Of Integrated Traditional And Western Medicine, Li Z, Wang D, Li Y. Expert consensus on diagnosis and treatment of septic shock with integrated traditional Chinese and Western medicine. Zhonghua Wei Zhong Bing JiJiu Yi Xue. 2019;31(11):1317–23. Article in Chinese
9. Matsumoto-Miyazaki J, Ushikoshi H, Miyata S, et al. Acupuncture and traditional herbal medicine therapy prevent Deliriumin patients with cardiovascular disease in intensive care units. Am J Chin Med. 2017;45(2):255–68.
10. Li Y, Zhang X, Lin P, et al. Effects of Shenfu injection in the treatment of septic shock patients: a multicenter, controlled, randomized, open-label trial. Evid Based Complement Alternat Med. 2016;2016:2565169.
11. Su YL, Wang H, Zhang SW. Effect of Qishen Huoxue granule in treating severe sepsis. Zhongguo Zhong Xi Yi Jie He Za Zhi. 2008;28(3):209–11. Article in Chinese
12. Mou Z, Lv Z, Li Y, et al. Clinical effect of Shenfu injection in patients with septic shock: a meta-analysis and systematic review. Evid Based Complement Alternat Med. 2015;2015:863149.
13. Xing X, Zhi Y, Lu J, et al. Traditional Chinese medicine bundle therapy for septic acute gastrointestinal injury: a multicenter randomized controlled trial. Complement Ther Med. 2019;47:102194.
14. Pourdast A, Sanaei M, Jafari S, et al. Effect of Septimeb™ as a new natural extract on severe sepsis: a randomized clinical trial. Caspian J Intern Med. 2017;8(1):35–43.
15. Li C, Bo L, Liu Q, Jin F. Thymosin alpha1 based immunomodulatory therapy for sepsis: a systematic review and meta-analysis. Int J Infect Dis. 2015;33:90–6.
16. Yang G, Hu RY, Deng AJ, et al. Effects of electro-acupuncture at Zusanli, Guanyuan for Sepsis patients and its mechanism through immune regulation. Chin J Integr Med. 2016;22(3):219–24.

17. Liang X, Zhou M, Ge XY, et al. Efficacy of traditional Chinese medicine on sepsis: a systematic review and meta-analysis. Int J Clin Exp Med. 2015;8(11):20024–34.
18. Xia ZY, Liu XY, Zhan LY, et al. Ginsenosides compound (shen-fu) attenuates gastrointestinal injury and inhibits inflammatory response after cardiopulmonary bypass in patients with congenital heart disease. J Thorac Cardiovasc Surg. 2005;130(2):258–64.
19. Karst M, Li C. Acupuncture-a question of culture. JAMA Netw Open. 2019;2(12):e1916929.
20. Zhao P, Wang C, Liu W, Wang F. Acute liver failure associated with traditional Chinese medicine: report of 30 cases from seventertiary hospitals in China. Crit Care Med. 2014;42(4):e296–9.

Interventions Increasing Mortality

21

Laura Pasin, Nicolò Sella, and Annalisa Boscolo

Contents

L. Pasin (✉) · N. Sella · A. Boscolo
Department of Anesthesia and Intensive Care, University Hospital of Padua, Padua, Italy
e-mail: laura.pasin@aopd.veneto.it; nicolo.sella@aopd.veneto.it;
annalisa.boscolobozza@aopd.veneto.it

© Springer Nature Switzerland AG 2021
G. Landoni et al. (eds.), *Reducing Mortality in Critically Ill Patients*,
https://doi.org/10.1007/978-3-030-71917-3_21

According to already published randomized controlled trials (RCTs), several interventions significantly increase mortality in critically ill and perioperative settings. Most evidences are supported by multicenter RCTs, while others are sustained by one single-center RCT.

All the identified drugs or interventions negatively affecting patients' survival will be briefly discussed below.

21.1   Patients with Acute Kidney Injury (AKI)

One intervention has shown to negatively affect survival of critically ill patients with AKI.

21.1.1 Thyroxine

Thyroid hormones have both pre-renal and intrinsic renal effects that increase the renal blood flow and the glomerular filtration rate (GFR). In fact, hypothyroidism is commonly associated with reduced GFR, while hyperthyroidism results in both increased GFR and renin—angiotensin—aldosterone system's activation. Moreover, patients with chronic kidney disease are often affected by primary and subclinical hypothyroidism [1]. Preclinical studies showed that the administration of thyroid hormone in the early phases of acute renal failure improved recovery in different ischemic and toxic models of kidney injury. On the contrary, one single-center, double-blind, placebo-controlled trial performed on 59 critically ill patients with AKI showed increased mortality in patients treated with thyroxine (43% vs 13%). In addition, thyroxine administration resulted in a progressive and severe suppression of thyroid-stimulating hormone (TSH) levels, without affecting the severity of renal failure [2].

21.2   Sepsis and Infectious Disease

Six interventions have shown to increase mortality in critically ill patients with sepsis or infectious diseases: protein C zymogen, nitric oxide synthase inhibitor 546C88, methylprednisolone at high doses, hypothermia in severe bacterial meningitis, cytokine hemoadsorption device on IL-6 and early resuscitation protocol.

21.2.1 Protein C Zymogen

Protein C plays a fundamental role in the host response to infection since it participates in the immunomodulatory and inflammatory processes. It is a modulator of the coagulation system synthesized by the liver as a vitamin K-dependent proenzyme. In blood, it is activated by the endothelial and platelet thrombin–thrombomodulin complexes and by an endothelial receptor thus acquiring anticoagulant effect. In conditions associated with acquired protein C zymogen deficit, such as severe sepsis, the use of this plasma-derived drug suggested improved outcomes in different observational studies [3, 4].On the contrary, Pappalardo et al., in one single-center, randomized, double-blind, placebo-controlled, parallel-group trial on 37 patient with severe sepsis or septic shock showed that intensive care unit (ICU) mortality was increased in the group who received protein C zymogen (79% vs 39%), as was in-hospital mortality (84% vs 44%) [5]. No difference in mortality was reported in longer follow-up (30-day). The trial planned to enroll 120 patients but was stopped earlier in a situation of futility for the composite outcome of prolonged ICU stay and/or 30-day mortality.

21.2.2 Nitric Oxide Synthase Inhibitor 546C88

Sepsis is associated with an increased production of nitric oxide (NO), leading to hypotension and decreased responsiveness to vasoconstrictors. Limiting the overproduction of NO by administrating different kind of inhibitors of nitric oxide synthase (NOS) in septic patients showed to restore vascular responsiveness to vasoconstrictive therapy and improved hemodynamics, without clinical relevant adverse events [6, 7]. On the contrary, in an international, multicentric, double-blind, placebo-controlled trial on the use of the NOS inhibitor 546C88 in patients with septic shock, Lopez et al. found an increased 28-day mortality in the treatment group (59% vs 49%) and the trial was stopped for safety reasons. In the 546C88 group, a higher proportion of vascular death and a lower incidence of deaths caused by multiple organ failure were observed [8].

21.2.3 High-Dose Methylprednisolone

The use of corticosteroids in infectious diseases and sepsis is still a debated subject. The rationale for their use in this setting is that this class of drugs downregulates the proinflammatory response, thereby limiting the inflammatory response while preserving innate immunity. Moreover, it is well known that critical illness induces a state of absolute or relative adrenal insufficiency that may contribute to hemodynamic instability and shock. A very old single-center, double-blind, placebo-controlled trial on the use of high-dose methylprednisolone (30 mg/kg) in 382 patients with severe sepsis or septic shock showed no difference in the prevention and reversal of shock and in the overall mortality between groups. Nonetheless, it showed a 14-days increased mortality in the subgroup of patients with elevated serum creatinine levels (>2 mg/dL) at enrollment (59% vs 29%). The increased number of deaths in the high-dose corticosteroids group was related to occurrence of secondary infections [9]. The topic remained debated in the following decades [10].

21.2.4 Hypothermia in Meningitis

Hypothermia was widely applied in different setting, such as global cerebral hypoxemia post-cardiac-arrest and traumatic brain injury (TBI), sometimes with conflicting results. In preclinical models of meningitis, moderate hypothermia showed positive effects by lowering intracranial pressure, preventing cellular apoptosis and modulating nuclear factor-kB, therefore concurring to reduce brain injury [11–15].Moreover, experimental studies and case reports suggested that hypothermia improved outcome of most severe cases [13, 14].

One multicentric, open-label RCT performed in 49 ICUs in France in patients with severe bacterial meningitis was stopped after the inclusion of the first 98 patients because mortality rate in patients treated with hypothermia was significantly higher than mortality in the control group (51% vs 31%) [15].

21.2.5 Cytokine Hemoadsorption Device on IL-6

Sepsis is characterized by an overwhelming production of proinflammatory cytokines. Trying to block this overproduction was suggested as a possible strategy to improve patients' outcome. One possibility is the use of therapeutic monoclonal antibodies against specific cytokines, but clinical trials on this topic did not confirm the benefits observed in preclinical studies and the recombinant-activated protein C (Xigris®) was withdrawn from the market in 2011 after the results of the PROWESS-SHOCK trial [16]. Another possibility is the use of extracorporeal blood purification to reduce cytokines' level. One meta-analysis on the various techniques of blood purification showed that only plasma exchange and hemoadsorption appeared to be potentially effective in septic patients [17]. CytoSorb (Cytosorbents, Corporation, New Jersey, USA) is a hemoadsorption device containing a porous polymeric beads able to remove cytokines and other toxins from blood and showed promising results in preclinical studies. One open label, multicentric RCT was conducted in ten German ICUs and enrolled 100 patients to be treated with standard of care and CytoSorb hemoperfusion for 6 h per day, up to 7 consecutive days or to standard of care therapy alone [18]. Unfortunately, the 60-day unadjusted mortality rate of patients treated with Cytosorb resulted to be significantly higher than mortality in the standard of care group (44.7% vs 26%). Nonetheless, after adjustment for baseline patients' morbidity and imbalances, no association of hemoperfusion with mortality was found.

21.2.6 Early Resuscitation Protocol on Septic Patients with Hypotension

While mortality of septic patients in developed countries has declined in the last decades, it remains extremely high in low-income countries. Different studies tried to determine if early resuscitation protocols could improve outcome in septic patients in resource-limited countries and results were conflicting [19, 20]. From October 2012 to November 2013, a monocentric RCT on 212 Zambian adult patients with sepsis and hypotension was performed to determine whether an early resuscitation protocol with administration of intravenous fluids, vasopressors, and blood transfusion could affect in-hospital mortality when compared with usual care [21]. The primary outcome of in-hospital mortality occurred in 48.1% of patients in the intervention group compared with 33.0% of patients in the usual care group.

21.3 Acute Respiratory Distress Syndrome (ARDS)

Six interventions have shown to increase mortality of critically ill patients with ALI or ARDS: intravenous salbutamol, keratinocyte growth factor, cysteine prodrug (L-2-oxothiazolidine-4-carboxylic acid), intensive nutrition, methylprednisolone, and high-frequency oscillation ventilation.

21.3.1 Intravenous Salbutamol

One of the main targets in patients with ARDS is the reduction of inflammatory pulmonary edema. In preclinical studies, stimulation of β_2 adrenergic receptors led to an increase in the transport of sodium across the alveolar epithelium and facilitated edema clearance. Nonetheless, several studies failed to demonstrate that intravenous infusion or inhalation of short- and long-acting β_2-agonists were effective in improving outcome of ARDS patients and their routinely use is not recommended. The Beta-Agonist Lung injury TrIal-2 (BALTI-2) enrolled 326 mechanically ventilated ARDS patients and randomized them to receive either intravenous infusion of albuterol or placebo [22]. The study was prematurely stopped for safety reasons because it showed an increase in 28-day mortality in the group of patients treated with albuterol (34% vs. 23%).

21.3.2 Keratinocyte Growth Factor

The National Heart, Lung and Blood Institute Working Group emphasized the lung epithelium as an important target for future research and new therapies for patients with ARDS. Keratinocyte growth factor (KGF) modulates several mechanisms involved in the epithelial repair and, therefore, could be potentially effective in the treatment of patients with ARDS. Recombinant human KGF (palifermin) is a

23 N-terminal aminoacid truncated version of endogenous KGF, which showed to decrease the incidence, duration, and severity of oral mucositis in patients with hematological malignancies. This efficacy in the repairment of the epithelium led to study its potential use in the treatment of epithelial injury in ARDS. Beneficial effects of KGF have been shown in preclinical studies. A double-blind trial undertaken in two adult general ICUs in the United Kingdom randomized 60 mechanically ventilated patients with severe ARDS to receive either recombinant KGF (palifermin) or placebo. 28-day mortality of patients who received palifermin was significantly higher than mortality in control group (31% vs 10%) [23].

21.3.3 Cysteine Prodrug (L-2-Oxothiazolidine-4-Carboxylic Acid)

Reactive oxygen species play an important role in the pathogenesis of ARDS. Ion superoxide produced by neutrophils can be metabolized to hydroxyl radicals, hydrogen peroxide, and hypochlorous acid. This process may also be the result of an antioxidant defense system overwhelmed. In fact, a decrease in glutathione was associated with the development of lung injury. Synthesis of glutathione can be limited by the supply of intracellular cysteine. Therefore, improving the availability of cysteine can be considered a therapeutic approach in patients with ARDS. L-2-oxothiazolidine-4 carboxylic acid (OTZ) is a cysteine prodrug and is metabolized to cysteine within the cells. Different preclinical and one clinical study showed an increased level of glutathione with the use of OTZ [24]. In a double-blind multicentric RCT, patients with ARDS were randomized to receive OTZ or placebo. 30-day mortality in the OTZ group was significantly higher than in the placebo group (29.7% vs 15.8%) [25].The study was stopped prematurely for safety reasons after enrolling 215 of the planned 352 patients.

21.3.4 Intensive Nutrition in Acute Lung Injury

Both enteral and parenteral nutrition support are always provided to ICU patients to avoid the loss of lean body mass and improve outcome. Nonetheless, evidence to support their efficacy is still limited. Braunschweig et al., in 2013, performed one high-quality single-center RCT to determine if a comprehensive nutrition program improved outcome in 78 normal and malnourished ICU patients with ALI [26]. According to study protocol, the control group received standard care, while the intervention group received early enteral nutrition (within 6 h of hemodynamic stability), with close monitoring in order to achieve estimated daily needs. Feedings were prescribed during a 24-hour period, eliminating bolus or intermittent feeding prescriptions. Actually, the only significant clinical difference between the groups was the higher energy and protein received in those randomized to intensive nutrition. The trial was stopped prematurely due to greater mortality in the intensive nutrition group (40%v s 15.8%).

21.3.5 High-Frequency Oscillation Ventilation (HFOV)

In patients with ARDS, lung protective mechanical ventilation with low tidal volumes is considered the standard of care. Prone positioning, extracorporeal membrane oxygenation, and HFOV were suggested as potential strategies for improving oxygenation in life-threatening severe hypoxemia.

HFOV was developed by Lunkenheimer et al. in 1972 and is characterized by a very low tidal volume (frequently less than anatomical dead space), delivered at a very high-frequency rate. It theoretically avoids volutrauma and atelectotrauma of the lung and, therefore, was studied in the last decade in severe ARDS patients. Different observational studies and a small number of RCTs supported the safety of HFOV and its role in improving oxygenation in ARDS patients [27].On the contrary, a large multicenter RCT on patients with moderate to severe ARDS, proved that early application of HFOV was associated with higher mortality rate (47% vs 35%) when compared with a ventilation strategy that used small tidal volumes, high positive end-expiratory pressure (PEEP) levels, and HFOV only in the subgroup of patients with severe refractory hypoxemia [28].

21.4 Perioperative Setting

Three interventions have proven to negatively affect survival in the perioperative setting: metoprolol retard in non-cardiac surgery, aprotinin, and prophylactic bicarbonate to prevent AKI in cardiac surgery.

21.4.1 Metoprolol Retard in Non-cardiac Surgery

Surgical stress causes a rise in catecholamine concentrations that results in an increase in blood pressure, heart rate, and free fatty acid concentrations leading to an increased myocardial oxygen demand. β blockers attenuate the effects of increased catecholamine levels and might theoretically prevent perioperative cardiovascular complications in non-cardiac surgery. Several RCTs were performed on this topic, suggesting that β blockers could prevent the occurrence of major cardiovascular events but increase the risk of hypotension and bradycardia [29].

The POISE trial, a large multicentric, double-blind, placebo-controlled trial, showed that patients randomized to metoprolol had increased mortality when compared to the placebo group (3.1% vs 2.3%]. Moreover, in the metoprolol group a significant increase in the number of strokes was observed (1% vs 0.5%) [30].

21.4.2 Aprotinin in Cardiac Surgery

Different pharmacological strategies were used to minimize bleeding and reduce the perioperative need for transfusion. In particular, three antifibrinolytic agents were largely used in cardiac surgery: aprotinin, tranexamic acid, and aminocaproic acid. Aprotinin is a naturally occurring serine protease inhibitor (thus counteracts fibrinolysis), while tranexamic acid and aminocaproic acid are lysine analogues. Different trials and meta-analyses were performed on these drugs. In 2005, a Cochrane review of 20 head-to-head comparisons of RCTs concluded that data were not enough to definitively recommend one drug over another [31]. Therefore, a large, double-blind, multicenter RCT was performed to determine whether aprotinin was superior to either tranexamic acid or aminocaproic acid in decreasing massive postoperative bleeding and other clinically relevant outcomes [32]. The trial was early stopped because of a higher rate of death in patients receiving aprotinin (3.2% in the aprotinin group vs 1.3% and 1.7% in the tranexamic acid and aminocaproic acid group, respectively).

21.4.3 Prophylactic Bicarbonate to Prevent Acute Kidney Injury in Cardiac Surgery

The pathophysiology of the development of AKI in cardiac surgery is extremely complex. A pilot RCT reported that perioperative urinary alkalinization in patients undergoing cardiac surgery resulted in a reduction in postoperative AKI (from 52% to 32%) and postoperative acute tubular damage, with no significant side effects [33]. These protective effects of bicarbonate may be due to its ability to alkalinize the urine and slow the Haber-Weiss reaction, reducing the generation of reactive oxygen species [34]. These hypothesis were supported by two other studies: a large meta-analysis on the contrast-related nephropathy (another form of AKI related to oxidative stress) and a systematic review that identified urinary alkalinization as the single most important drug-based intervention to prevent AKI [35]. Therefore, a large multicenter, double-blind RCT was performed to test whether prophylactic perioperative bicarbonate infusion was efficient to reduce the incidence of AKI in patients undergoing open heart surgery with the use of cardiopulmonary bypass. The study was stopped early because an interim analysis showed that hospital mortality was increased in patients receiving sodium bicarbonate compared with control group (6.3% vs 1.7%) [36].

21.5   Nutrition and Supplementation

Three nutritions/supplementations were proven to negatively affect survival of critically ill patients: growth hormone, glutamine supplementation, and high-protein enteral nutrition enriched with immune-modulating nutrients.

21.5.1 Growth Hormone (GH)

Negative nitrogen balance due to an increase in protein turnover is commonly observed in critically ill patients. This results in skeletal muscle wasting, difficult weaning from mechanical ventilation, and delayed return to full mobility. Small RCTs on the use of GH supplementation in patients receiving adequate nutrition support showed positive effects. Therefore, in 1999, a large, double-blind RCT in patients who were expected to remain in ICU for at least 10 days was performed to confirm those promising findings [37]. The published report of the trial combined two studies conducted in parallel (the Finnish study and the European study), recruiting a total of 532 patients. In both trials, the in-hospital mortality was higher in the patients receiving GH (39% vs 20% in the Finnish study; 44% vs 18% in the European study).

21.5.2 Glutamine

Malnourishment is frequently observed in critically ill patients and different specialized nutrition therapies are often used to prevent malnutrition since it is associated with increased morbidity and mortality [38, 39]. Different RCTs were published on this topic [40]. Among them, the potential benefit of glutamine supplementation in critical care setting was extensively studied.

Glutamine is the most abundant essential amino acid and is mostly stored in skeletal muscle tissue. It is a precursor of glutathione and plays a crucial role in different stress-response pathways by modulating inflammatory response and metabolism of glucose, by preventing organ injury, and by inducing cellular protection pathways in critical ill patients [41]. Low serum glutamine levels have shown to be independent predictors of mortality in ICU [42, 43].

In 2013, Heyland et al. in a large, high-quality, multicentric RCT from 40 different ICUs in Canada, the United States, and Europe provided evidence that glutamine supplementation increases 28-day mortality in critically ill mechanically ventilated patients with multiorgan failure (32.4% vs.

27.2%) [44]. On the contrary, previous meta-analysis suggested that glutamine and antioxidant supplementation were associated with improved outcome in this population [45, 46]. Later, RCTs and meta-analyses did not confirm such beneficial effects [47–49].

21.5.3 High-Protein Enteral Nutrition Enriched with Immune-Modulating Nutrients

Different immune-modulating nutrients (i.e., arginine, glutamine, selenium, nucleic acids, omega-3 fatty acids, and antioxidants) may modulate inflammatory and oxidative stress responses. Several meta-analyses reported that the use of artificial enteral nutrition with immune-modulating nutrients was associated with reductions in infectious morbidity and improved outcome in critically ill patients when compared with standard enteral nutrition [50–52].

Scientific societies guidelines are contradictory on the use of immune-modulating nutrients in severely ill patients. While the European Society for Clinical Nutrition and Metabolism did not recommend it, the Society of Critical Care Medicine and the American Society for Parenteral and Enteral Nutrition suggested that immune-modulating supplementation should be used only in appropriate patients, with caution in severe sepsis, with grade A recommendations for surgical and grade B recommendations for medical ICU patients. Both guidelines recommend use of high-protein enteral nutrition (1.2–2.0 g/kg/die), supported by observational studies showing improved survival in patients reaching higher protein targets [53, 54]. The MetaPlus trial was a randomized, multicenter, international, double-blind trial performed in 14 ICUs in Europe. A total of 301 patients requiring mechanical ventilation for more than 72 h were randomized to receive immune-modulating nutrients or standard high-protein enteral nutrition. Six-month mortality rate in the subgroup of medical patients who received immune-modulating nutrients was significantly higher than mortality rate of medical patients who received standard high-protein enteral nutrition (54% vs 35%) [55].

21.6 Trauma and Shock

Six interventions have shown to increase mortality in patients with trauma or shock: stress ulcer prophylaxis with antacids in ventilated trauma patients, systematic ICU admission for older patients, albumin in patients with traumatic brain injury (TBI), dopamine versus noradrenaline as first-choice vasopressor in patients with shock, diaspirin cross-linked hemoglobin (DCLHb), and methylprednisolone in TBI.

21.6.1 Stress Ulcer Prophylaxis in Ventilated Trauma Patients

Different drugs such as sucralfate, antacids, or histamine-2 (H_2) antagonists were used to prevent stress ulcer bleeding in mechanically ventilated patients. Results on the potential role of H_2 antagonist to increase the risk of nosocomial pneumonia, by augmenting the gastric pH and allowing the colonization with Gram-bacilli, were conflicting. Therefore, a randomized clinical trial on mechanically ventilated injured patients randomized to one of three distinct stress ulcer prophylaxis regimens (sucralfate, antacid, or ranitidine) was performed. Between November 1990 and May 1994, 424 patients were randomized to receive one of the three prophylaxis regimens. The mortality rate of patients treated with antacids was significantly higher compared with patients given sucralfate or ranitidine (23.2% vs 12.5% vs 10%, respectively) [56]. In the last decade, research mainly focused on the role of proton pump inhibitors in preventing stress ulcer in critically ill patients. In a post hoc analysis of patients with high disease severity included in the SUP-ICU trial [57], higher 90-day mortality and fewer days alive without life support with pantoprazole vs placebo were observed [58].

21.6.2 Systematic ICU Admission for Older Patients

According to the World Health Organization, older people are a rapidly growing proportion of the world's entire population. In fact, in 2015, this population rose by 55 million and the proportion of the older people reached 8.5% of the total population. This trend unavoidably leads to an increasing demand for health care resources, including ICU beds. Moreover, ICU costs in this population are substantial. These limitations pose great challenges to the ICU triage decision-making process.

Observational studies reported conflicting results on the benefits of ICU admission in the elderly and triage guidelines adapted to these patients are still lacking, leading to wide heterogeneity in the ICU triage decision-making process [59–62]. In 2017, The Intensive Care for Elderly–CUB-Réa 2 (ICE-CUB 2) trial, a large multicentric cluster-RCT performed in 24 French hospitals, tried to determine whether a recommendation for systematic ICU admission in critically ill elderly patients (>75 years old) could reduce 6-month mortality compared with usual practice [63]. Six-month mortality of patients randomized to the systematic strategy group was significantly higher than mortality of patients in the standard practice group (45% vs 39%). No further RCTs were published on this topic so far.

21.6.3 Albumin in Patients with Traumatic Brain Injury

The best fluid strategy to maintain systemic and cerebral perfusion in patients with TBI is still debated and both crystalloids and colloids were used in the past.

The Saline versus Albumin Fluid Evaluation (SAFE) study evaluated the effect of fluid resuscitation with 4% albumin or saline on mortality in ICU patients [64]. No difference was found between groups. On the contrary, a post hoc follow-up study of patients from the SAFE study who had traumatic brain injury (the SAFE–TBI study), showed an increased 24-month mortality among patients in the albumin group (33.2%), as compared with patients in the saline group (20.4%).

21.6.4 Dopamine Versus Noradrenaline as First-Choice Vasopressor in Patients with Shock

Both norepinephrine and dopamine are used as a first-choice vasopressor in patients with shock. However, different studies suggested that the administration of dopamine was associated with worst outcome [65, 66]. Therefore, between December 2003 and October a multicentric RCT was performed in eight centers in Belgium, Austria, and Spain to evaluate whether norepinephrine over dopamine as first-line vasopressor agent could reduce the rate of death among patients in shock. A total of 1679 patients were enrolled. No difference in the overall mortality was find between groups. Nonetheless, the rate of death at 28 days was significantly higher among patients with cardiogenic shock who were treated with dopamine than among those with cardiogenic shock who were treated with norepinephrine [67].A meta-analyses published in 2017 confirmed that norepinephrine, when compared to dopamine as first-line vasopressor in patients with cardiogenic shock was associated with a lower 28-day mortality, a lower risk of arrhythmic events, and gastrointestinal reaction [68].

21.6.5 Diaspirin Cross-Linked Hemoglobin (DCLHb)

In case of reduced cardiac output and/or hypoxemia, hemoglobin (Hb) concentration plays a fundamental role in preventing cellular dysfunction and tissue hypoxia. Over the past decades, different artificial blood solutions (blood substitutes, blood surrogates, artificial Hb, or artificial blood) were synthetized and tested in order to replace blood transfusion. Some of them reached phase III in clinical trials but, unfortunately, many of these products were withdrawn from the market because of severe reported side effects.

Sloan et al., in 1999, tested the addition of 500–1000 mL DCLHb, a purified and chemically modified human Hb solution (HemAssist®, 10 g/dL diaspirin cross-linked human Hb in balanced electrolytes solution) during initial fluid resuscitation in patients with shock [69]. In patients treated with DCLHb, mortality rate was higher than in patients who received standard treatment (46% vs. 17%). A subsequent RCT performed in 2003 did not confirm these findings and was interrupted prematurely for futility after an interim evaluation [70].

21.6.6 Methylprednisolone in Traumatic Brain Injury

Corticosteroids were used to treat head injury for decades. Different small RCTs were performed in the past and an old review and meta-analyses performed in 1997 suggested that the absolute risk of death in the corticosteroid group was about 1–2% lower than in controls although 95% CI ranged from 6% fewer to 2% more deaths [71].

The CRASH trial, a large international multicentric RCT, enrolled 10,008 adults with head injury to receive 48 h infusion of methylprednisolone or placebo [72]. Compared with placebo, 14-days mortality rate of patients allocated to the corticosteroids group resulted significantly higher (21.1% vs 17.9%). Two different meta-analyses published in 2005 confirmed the detrimental effect of corticosteroids on survival of patients with TBI [73, 74].

References

1. Basu G, Mohapatra A. Interactions between thyroid disorders and kidney disease. Indian J Endocrinol Metab. 2012; https://doi.org/10.4103/2230-8210.93737.
2. Acker CG, Singh AR, Flick RP, Bernardini J, Greenberg A, Johnson JP. A trial of thyroxine in acute renal failure. Kidney Int. 2000; https://doi.org/10.1046/j.1523-1755.2000.00827.x.
3. Silvetti S, Crivellari M, Mucchetti M, et al. Administration of protein C concentrates in patients without congenital deficit: a systematic review of the literature. Signa Vitae. 2013; https://doi.org/10.22514/SV82.102013.2.
4. Fourrier F, Leclerc F, Aidan K, et al. Combined antithrombin and protein C supplementation in meningococcal purpura fulminans: a pharmacokinetic study. Intensive Care Med. 2003; https://doi.org/10.1007/s00134-003-1784-1.
5. Pappalardo F, Crivellari M, Di Prima AL, et al. Protein C zymogen in severe sepsis: a double-blinded, placebo-controlled, randomized study. Intensive Care Med. 2016; https://doi.org/10.1007/s00134-016-4405-5.
6. Grover R, Zaccardelli D, Colice G, Guntupalli K, Watson D, Vincent JL. An open-label dose escalation study of the nitric oxide synthase inhibitor, N(G)-methyl-L-arginine hydrochloride (546C88), in patients with septic shock. Crit Care Med. 1999; https://doi.org/10.1097/00003246-199905000-00025.
7. Avontuur JAM, Tutein Nolthenius RP, Van Bodegom JW, Bruining HA. Prolonged inhibition of nitric oxide synthesis in severe septic shock: a clinical study. Crit Care Med. 1998; https://doi.org/10.1097/00003246-199804000-00012.
8. López A, Lorente JA, Steingrub J, et al. Multiple-center, randomized, placebo-controlled, double-blind study of the nitric oxide synthase inhibitor 546C88: effect on survival in patients with septic shock. Crit Care Med. 2004; https://doi.org/10.1097/01.CCM.0000105581.01815.C6.
9. Bone RC, Fisher CJ, Clemmer TP, Slotman GJ, Metz CA, Balk RA. A controlled clinical trial of high-dose methylprednisolone in the treatment of severe Sepsis and septic shock. N Engl J Med. 1987; https://doi.org/10.1056/NEJM198709103171101.
10. Patel GP, Balk RA. Systemic steroids in severe sepsis and septic shock. Am J Respir Crit Care Med. 2012; https://doi.org/10.1164/rccm.201011-1897CI.
11. Irazuzta JE, Pretzlaff RK, Zingarelli B, Xue V, Zemlan F. Modulation of nuclear factor-κB activation and decreased markers of neurological injury associated with hypothermic therapy in experimental bacterial meningitis. Crit Care Med. 2002; https://doi.org/10.1097/00003246-200211000-00025.
12. Xu L, Yenari MA, Steinberg GK, Giffard RG. Mild hypothermia reduces apoptosis of mouse neurons in vitro early in the cascade. J Cereb Blood Flow Metab. 2002; https://doi.org/10.1097/00004647-200201000-00003.
13. Cuthbertson BH, Dickson R, Mackenzie A. Intracranial pressure measurement, induced hypothermia and barbiturate coma in meningitis associated with intractable raised intracranial pressure. Anaesthesia. 2004; https://doi.org/10.1111/j.1365-2044.2004.03748.x.
14. Lepur D, Kutleša M, Baršić B. Induced hypothermia in adult community-acquired bacterial meningitis - more than just a possibility? J Infect. 2011; https://doi.org/10.1016/j.jinf.2010.10.001.
15. Mourvillier B, Tubach F, Van De Beek D, et al. Induced hypothermia in severe bacterial meningitis: a randomized clinical trial. JAMA. 2013; https://doi.org/10.1001/jama.2013.280506.
16. Ranieri VM, Thompson BT, Barie PS, et al. Drotrecogin alfa (activated) in adults with septic shock. N Engl J Med. 2012; https://doi.org/10.1056/NEJMoa1202290.
17. Zhou F, Peng Z, Murugan R, Kellum JA. Blood purification and mortality in sepsis: a meta-analysis of randomized trials. Crit Care Med. 2013; https://doi.org/10.1097/CCM.0b013e31828cf412.

18. Schädler D, Pausch C, Heise D, et al. The effect of a novel extracorporeal cytokine hemoadsorption device on IL-6 elimination in septic patients: a randomized controlled trial. PLoS One. 2017; https://doi.org/10.1371/journal.pone.0187015.

19. Andrews B, Muchemwa L, Kelly P, Lakhi S, Heimburger DC, Bernard GR. Simplified severe sepsis protocol. Crit Care Med. 2014; https://doi.org/10.1097/ccm.0000000000000541.

20. Maitland K, Kiguli S, Opoka RO, et al. Mortality after fluid bolus in African children with severe infection. N Engl J Med. 2011; https://doi.org/10.1056/NEJMoa1101549.

21. Andrews B, Semler MW, Muchemwa L, et al. Effect of an early resuscitation protocol on in-hospital mortality among adults with sepsis and hypotension: a randomized clinical trial. JAMA. 2017; https://doi.org/10.1001/jama.2017.10913.

22. Smith FG, Perkins GD, Gates S, et al. Effect of intravenous β-2 agonist treatment on clinical outcomes in acute respiratory distress syndrome (BALTI-2): a multicentre, randomised controlled trial. Lancet. 2012; https://doi.org/10.1016/S0140-6736(11)61623-1.

23. McAuley DF, Cross LM, Hamid U, et al. Keratinocyte growth factor for the treatment of the acute respiratory distress syndrome (KARE): a randomised, double-blind, placebo-controlled phase 2 trial. Lancet Respir Med. 2017; https://doi.org/10.1016/S2213-2600(17)30171-6.

24. Bernard GR, Wheeler AP, Arons MM, et al. A trial of antioxidants N-acetylcysteine and procysteine in ARDS. Chest. 1997; https://doi.org/10.1378/chest.112.1.164.

25. Morris PE, Papadakos P, Russell JA, et al. A double-blind placebo-controlled study to evaluate the safety and efficacy of L-2-oxothiazolidine-4-carboxylic acid in the treatment of patients with acute respiratory distress syndrome. Crit Care Med. 2008; https://doi.org/10.1097/CCM.0B013E318164E7E4.

26. Braunschweig CA, Sheean PM, Peterson SJ, et al. Intensive nutrition in acute lung injury: a clinical trial (INTACT). J Parenter Enter Nutr. 2015; https://doi.org/10.1177/0148607114528541.

27. Fessler HE, Hess DR. Does high-frequency ventilation offer benefits over conventional ventilation in adult patients with acute respiratory distress syndrome? Respir Care. 2007;52:595–608.

28. Ferguson ND, Cook DJ, Guyatt GH, et al. High-frequency oscillation in early acute respiratory distress syndrome. N Engl J Med. 2013; https://doi.org/10.1056/NEJMoa1215554.

29. Devereaux PJ, Beattie WS, Choi PTL, et al. How strong is the evidence for the use of perioperative β blockers in non-cardiac surgery? Systematic review and meta-analysis of randomised controlled trials. Br Med J. 2005; https://doi.org/10.1136/bmj.38503.623646.8F.

30. Devereaux PJ, Yang H, Yusuf S, et al. Effects of extended-release metoprolol succinate in patients undergoing non-cardiac surgery (POISE trial): a randomised controlled trial. Lancet. 2008; https://doi.org/10.1016/S0140-6736(08)60601-7.

31. Carless PA, Moxey AJ, Stokes BJ, Henry DA. Are antifibrinolytic drugs equivalent in reducing blood loss and transfusion in cardiac surgery? A meta-analysis of randomized head-to-head trials. BMC Cardiovasc Disord. 2005; https://doi.org/10.1186/1471-2261-5-19.

32. Fergusson DA, Hébert PC, Mazer CD, et al. A comparison of aprotinin and lysine analogues in high-risk cardiac surgery. N Engl J Med. 2008; https://doi.org/10.1056/NEJMoa0802395.

33. Haase M, Haase-Fielitz A, Bellomo R, et al. Sodium bicarbonate to prevent increases in serum creatinine after cardiac surgery: a pilot double-blind, randomized controlled trial. Crit Care Med. 2009; https://doi.org/10.1097/CCM.0b013e318193216f.

34. Halliwell B, Gutteridge JMC. Role of free radicals and catalytic metal ions in human disease: an overview. Methods Enzymol. 1990; https://doi.org/10.1016/0076-6879(90)86093-B.

35. Meier P, Ko DT, Tamura A, Tamhane U, Gurm HS. Sodium bicarbonate-based hydration prevents contrast-induced nephropathy: a meta-analysis. BMC Med. 2009; https://doi.org/10.1186/1741-7015-7-23.

36. Haase M, Haase-Fielitz A, Plass M, et al. Prophylactic perioperative sodium bicarbonate to prevent acute kidney injury following open heart surgery: a multicenter double-blinded randomized controlled trial. PLoS Med. 2013; https://doi.org/10.1371/journal.pmed.1001426.

37. Takala J, Ruokonen E, Webster NR, et al. Increased mortality associated with growth hormone treatment in critically ill adults. N Engl J Med. 1999; https://doi.org/10.1056/NEJM199909093411102.

38. Cartin-Ceba R, Afessa B, Gajic O. Low baseline serum creatinine concentration predicts mortality in critically ill patients independent of body mass index. Crit Care Med. 2007; https://doi.org/10.1097/01.CCM.0000281856.78526.F4.

39. Robinson MK, Mogensen KM, Casey JD, et al. The relationship among obesity, nutritional status, and mortality in the critically ill. Crit Care Med. 2015; https://doi.org/10.1097/CCM.0000000000000602.

40. Desai SV, McClave SA, Rice TW. Nutrition in the ICU: an evidence-based approach. Chest. 2014; https://doi.org/10.1378/chest.13-1158.

41. Wischmeyer PE. Glutamine: mode of action in critical illness. Crit Care Med. 2007; https://doi.org/10.1097/01.CCM.0000278064.32780.D3.

42. Rodas PC, Rooyackers O, Hebert C, Norberg Å, Wernerman J. Glutamine and glutathione at ICU admission in relation to outcome. Clin Sci. 2012; https://doi.org/10.1042/CS20110520.

43. Oudemans-van Straaten HM, Bosman RJ, Treskes M, Van der Spoel HJI, Zandstra DF. Plasma glutamine depletion and patient outcome in acute ICU admissions. Intensive Care Med. 2001; https://doi.org/10.1007/s001340000703.

44. Heyland D, Muscedere J, Wischmeyer PE, et al. A randomized trial of glutamine and antioxidants in critically ill patients. N Engl J Med. 2013; https://doi.org/10.1056/NEJMoa1212722.

45. Novak F, Heyland DK, Avenell A, Drover JW, Su X. Glutamine supplementation in serious illness: a systematic review of the evidence. Crit Care Med. 2002; https://doi.org/10.1097/00003246-200209000-00011.

46. Manzanares W, Dhaliwal R, Jiang X, Murch L, Heyland DK. Antioxidant micronutrients in the critically ill: a systematic review and meta-analysis. Crit Care. 2012; https://doi.org/10.1186/cc11316.

47. Wernerman J, Kirketeig T, Andersson B, et al. Scandinavian glutamine trial: A pragmatic multi-centre randomised clinical trial of intensive care unit patients. Acta Anaesthesiol Scand. 2011; https://doi.org/10.1111/j.1399-6576.2011.02453.x.

48. Andrews PJD, Avenell A, Noble DW, et al. Randomised trial of glutamine, selenium, or both, to supplement parenteral nutrition for critically ill patients. BMJ. 2011; https://doi.org/10.1136/bmj.d1542.

49. Pasin L, Nardelli P, Piras D. Glutamine supplementation in critically ill patients. In: Reducing mortality in critically ill patients. Cham: Springer; 2015. https://doi.org/10.1007/978-3-319-17515-7_15.

50. Beale RJ, Bryg DJ, Bihari DJ. Immunonutrition in the critically ill: a systematic review of clinical outcome. Crit Care Med. 1999; https://doi.org/10.1097/00003246-199912000-00032.

51. Heyland DK, Novak F, Drover JW, Jain M, Su X, Suchner U. Should immunonutrition become routine in critically III patients? A systematic review of the evidence. J Am Med Assoc. 2001; https://doi.org/10.1001/jama.286.8.944.

52. Montejo JC, Zarazaga A, López-Martínez J, et al. Immunonutrition in the intensive care unit. A systematic review and consensus statement. Clin Nutr. 2003; https://doi.org/10.1016/S0261-5614(03)00007-4.

53. Weijs PJM, Stapel SN, De Groot SDW, et al. Optimal protein and energy nutrition decreases mortality in mechanically ventilated, critically ill patients: a prospective observational cohort study. J Parenter Enter Nutr. 2012; https://doi.org/10.1177/0148607111415109.

54. Allingstrup MJ, Esmailzadeh N, Wilkens Knudsen A, et al. Provision of protein and energy in relation to measured requirements in intensive care patients. Clin Nutr. 2012; https://doi.org/10.1016/j.clnu.2011.12.006.

55. Van Zanten ARH, Sztark F, Kaisers UX, et al. High-protein enteral nutrition enriched with immune-modulating nutrients vs standard high-protein enteral nutrition and nosocomial infections in the ICU: a randomized clinical trial. JAMA. 2014; https://doi.org/10.1001/jama.2014.7698.

56. Thomason MH, Payseur ES, Hakenewerth AM, et al. Nosocomial pneumonia in ventilated trauma patients during stress ulcer prophylaxis with sucralfate, antacid, and ranitidine. J Trauma Inj Infect Crit Care. 1996; https://doi.org/10.1097/00005373-199609000-00020.

57. Krag M, Marker S, Perner A, et al. Pantoprazole in patients at risk for gastrointestinal bleeding in the ICU. N Engl J Med. 2018;379(23):2199–208. https://doi.org/10.1056/NEJMoa1714919.
58. Marker S, Perner A, Wetterslev J, et al. Pantoprazole prophylaxis in ICU patients with high severity of disease: a post hoc analysis of the placebo-controlled SUP-ICU trial. Intensive Care Med. 2019;45(5):609–18. https://doi.org/10.1007/s00134-019-05589-y.
59. Boumendil A, Angus DC, Guitonneau AL, et al. Variability of intensive care admission decisions for the very elderly. PLoS One. 2012; https://doi.org/10.1371/journal.pone.0034387.
60. Sprung CL, Artigas A, Kesecioglu J, et al. The Eldicus prospective, observational study of triage decision making in European intensive care units. Part II: Intensive care benefit for the elderly. Crit Care Med. 2012; https://doi.org/10.1097/CCM.0b013e318232d6b0.
61. Valley TS, Sjoding MW, Ryan AM, Iwashyna TJ, Cooke CR. Association of intensive care unit admission with mortality among older patients with pneumonia. JAMA. 2015; https://doi.org/10.1001/jama.2015.11068.
62. Fuchs L, Novack V, McLennan S, et al. Trends in severity of illness on ICU admission and mortality among the elderly. PLoS One. 2014; https://doi.org/10.1371/journal.pone.0093234.
63. Guidet B, Leblanc G, Simon T, et al. Effect of systematic intensive care unit triage on long-term mortality among critically ill elderly patients in France a randomized clinical trial. JAMA. 2017; https://doi.org/10.1001/jama.2017.13889.
64. Finfer S, Bellomo R, Boyce N, et al. A comparison of albumin and saline for fluid resuscitation in the intensive care unit. N Engl J Med. 2004; https://doi.org/10.1056/NEJMoa040232.
65. Martin C, Viviand X, Leone M, Thirion X. Effect of norepinephrine on the outcome of septic shock. Crit Care Med. 2000; https://doi.org/10.1097/00003246-200008000-00012.
66. Müllner M, Urbanek B, Havel C, Losert H, Gamper G, Herkner H. Vasopressors for shock. Cochrane Database Syst Rev. 2004; https://doi.org/10.1002/14651858.cd003709.pub2.
67. De Backer D, Biston P, Devriendt J, et al. Comparison of dopamine and norepinephrine in the treatment of shock. N Engl J Med. 2010; https://doi.org/10.1056/NEJMoa0907118.
68. Rui Q, Jiang Y, Chen M, Zhang N, Yang H, Zhou Y. Dopamine versus norepinephrine in the treatment of cardiogenic shock. Med (United States). 2017; https://doi.org/10.1097/MD.0000000000008402.
69. Sloan EP, Koenigsberg M, Gens D, et al. Diaspirin cross-linked hemoglobin (DCLHb) in the treatment of severe traumatic hemorrhagic shock: a randomized controlled efficacy trial. J Am Med Assoc. 1999; https://doi.org/10.1001/jama.282.19.1857.
70. Kerner T, Ahlers O, Veit S, Riou B, Saunders M, Pison U. DCL-Hb for trauma patients with severe hemorrhagic shock: the European "on-scene" multicenter study. Intensive Care Med. 2003; https://doi.org/10.1007/s00134-002-1622-x.
71. Alderson P, Roberts I. Corticosteroids in acute traumatic brain injury: systematic review of randomised controlled trials. Br Med J. 1997; https://doi.org/10.1136/bmj.314.7098.1855.
72. Olldashi F, Muzha I, Filipi N, et al. Effect of intravenous corticosteroids on death within 14 days in 10008 adults with clinically significant head injury (MRC CRASH trial): randomised placebo-controlled trial. Lancet. 2004; https://doi.org/10.1016/S0140-6736(04)17188-2.
73. Alderson P, Roberts I. Corticosteroids for acute traumatic brain injury. Cochrane Database Syst Rev. 2005; https://doi.org/10.1002/14651858.cd000196.pub2.
74. Czekajlo MS, Milbrandt EB. Corticosteroids increased short and long-term mortality in adults with traumatic head injury. Crit Care. 2005; https://doi.org/10.1186/cc3813.

Conflicting Evidences

22

Cosimo Chelazzi, Zaccaria Ricci, and Stefano Romagnoli

Contents

C. Chelazzi (✉)
Department of Anesthesiology and Intensive Care, University of Florence,
Azienda Ospedaliero-Universitaria Careggi, Florence, Italy

Z. Ricci
Department of Pediatric Cardiac Surgery, Pediatric Cardiac Intensive Care Unit,
Bambino Gesù Children's Hospital, Rome, Italy

S. Romagnoli
Department of Anesthesiology and Intensive Care, University of Florence,
Azienda Ospedaliero-Universitaria Careggi, Florence, Italy

Department of Health Science, Section of Anesthesia and Intensive Care,
University of Florence, Florence, Italy
e-mail: Stefano.romagnoli@unifi.it

© Springer Nature Switzerland AG 2021
G. Landoni et al. (eds.), *Reducing Mortality in Critically Ill Patients*,
https://doi.org/10.1007/978-3-030-71917-3_22

Evidence-based medicine (EBM) is of utmost importance to drive current clinical practice, and randomized controlled trials (RCTs) represent the beating heart of EBM. However, tight glycemic control and the use of hydroxyethyl starch have conflicting randomized published evidence (showing both increased mortality and increased survival).

22.1 Tight Glycemic Control

22.1.1 Physiology

Stress-induced hyperglycemia is common among critically ill and surgical patients [1–3]. Inflammatory cytokines activate the hypothalamic-pituitary-adrenal axis, enhancing secretion of cortisol, hepatic glycogenolysis, and gluconeogenesis. The inhibited synthesis of glucose-transporter family (GLUT)-4 reduces intracellular insulin-dependent glucose transport in adipocytes and myocytes [4]. This implies hyper-catabolism with peripheral insulin resistance, fostering energy production in acute stress responses cells, e.g., white blood cells [2]. Hepatic glycogenolysis and protein breakdown promote hepatic gluconeogenesis and synthesis of acute phase reactants. Progressive hyperglycemia ensues ("stress hyperglycemia"/"stress diabetes") whose severity is related to severity of underlying acute illness. In prolonged critical illness, this state leads to mitochondrial dysfunction, persistent inflammation, immune-paralysis, anemia, and increased mortality [3].

22.1.2 Stress-Induced Hyperglycemia

It is widely accepted that stress-induced hyperglycemia is associated to increased mortality and morbidity [5–9]. Patients with acute myocardial infarction and stroke are particularly susceptible [5, 7, 8, 10–12]. Hyperglycemic trauma patients shown increased ICU−/hospital length-of-stay and higher mortality rates, possibly related to increased nosocomial infections and duration of mechanical ventilation (MV) [13]. In patients with traumatic brain injury, admission's hyperglycemia was independently related to worse neurological outcomes [14]. After coronary artery bypass hyperglycemia is associated to sternal wound infections, longer ICU length-of-stay, increased risk for stroke, myocardial infarction, sepsis, and mortality [15, 16].

In light of this evidence, strategies to control hyperglycemia in critically ill patients have been implemented.

22.1.3 Tight Glycemic Control: Main Evidence

In 2001, the Leuven trial enrolled 1548 surgical patients to receive intensive insulin therapy (IIT) with continuous intravenous insulin infusion or conventional blood glucose management. Targeted blood glucose for IIT patients was 80–110 mg/dL, while for controls was 180–200 mg/L. There was a significant reduction in ICU (42%) and in-hospital mortality (34%) in the IIT group compared to controls. IIT was associated with reduced incidence of acute renal failure (−41%), blood stream infections (−46%), transfusion requirements, and polyneuropathy. The reduction in mortality was observed mostly among non-diabetic patients. Incidence of hypoglycemia was significantly higher in the IIT group [17, 18]. In 2006, IIT was associated with an absolute 10% reduction in mortality rates for long staying, critically ill patients, as much with reduced ICU- and hospital length-of-stays, duration of MV, and incidence of acute renal failure [19].

In 2008 and 2009, two trials comparing the effects of IIT (blood glucose 80–110 mg/dL) versus conventional therapy (180–200 mg/dL) did not confirm these positive results and raised concerns about hypoglycemia [20, 21]. In the subsequent NICE-SUGAR trial (6104 patients), patients on IIT showed higher rates of hypoglycemia and 90-day mortality [22].

However, in a recent metanalysis on 57 RCTs involving 21,840 critically ill patients, intensive glucose control significantly reduced all-cause mortality, ICU length-of-stay, and rate of secondary infection/sepsis compared to patients treated with the usual care strategy, while the intensive glucose control strategy was associated with higher occurrence of severe hypoglycemic events [23].

22.1.4 The Role of Nutrition and Diabetes

The risk for hypoglycemia is higher in patients undergoing IIT, particularly if diabetic and poorly controlled. In the Leuven trials, a mean non-protein daily caloric intake of 20 kCal/kg was achieved with glucose administration. In the NICE-SUGAR, the median daily caloric intake was 11.04 ± 6.08 kCal/kg. Thus, an appropriate nutrition protocol should be part of IIT [24, 25]. The concomitant infusion of glucose/nutrients and insulin, rather than the sole tight glycemic control, can be beneficial to prevent hypoglycemia and opposing hyper-catabolism [26, 27]. Stress-induced glycogenolysis and hepatic gluconeogenesis are associated with muscle energy depletion and hepatic hypoxic injury. Insulin-mediated increased expression of GLUT-4/GLUT-2 on muscle cells and hepatocytes restores adenosine triphosphate (ATP) levels and inhibits protein wasting [28–32]. Insulin may exert immune-modulator effects, preventing the apoptosis of activated macrophages and promoting a shift towards a T-helper 2-phenotype [33]. These effects may translate in lower rate of muscle weakness, secondary infections, length-of-stay, and mortality.

The blood glucose target is different for non-diabetic and diabetic patients [34–36]. Blood glucose time-in-range during IIT is independently associated with reduced mortality in critically ill, non-diabetic patients [37]. Higher pre- and post-admission glycemic GAP and lower glycosylated hemoglobin are associated to higher mortality in diabetic patients [38, 39]. Tight glycemic control in ICU would bring advantage to previously non-diabetic or diabetic patients with good preadmission glycemic control. For poorly controlled diabetic patients, tight blood glucose is less safe. To date, definite evidence is lacking and general recommendations is to target a glycemia of 140–160 mg/dL, for both non-diabetic and diabetic patients in good pre-ICU control [40, 41].

22.1.5 Continuous Glucose Monitoring and Automated Insulin Infusion

The major safety concern about IIT is hypoglycemia. Poorly controlled diabetic patients are particularly susceptible. Moreover, a glucose variability >20% is associated to increased oxidative stress and worse outcomes alone in critically ill/surgical patients [42], irrespective of hypoglycemia [43–46]. To reduce glucose variability and avoid hypoglycemia, a combination of continuous glucose monitoring and automated infusion of insulin is advised [47]. Though still experimental, this method showed promising results in clinical applications. In cardio-surgical and non-cardiac patients, automated algorithm of insulin infusion resulted in higher rates of time-in-range blood glucose levels compared to paper-based algorithm (49% vs. 27%, respectively) [48, 49]. Subcutaneous continuous monitoring and micro-dialysis methods are promising tool [50]. With recent technology, subcutaneous glucose monitoring probes showed to be more precise than intravascular or blood-gas analysis [51]. Automated systems for insulin therapy include automatic subcutaneous insulin infusers, electronic-medical record-based infusion algorithm and totally automatic glucose management systems. Those tools are under investigation and need to prove cost-effective [52]. Up to date, none is routinely applied to ICU patients.

22.1.6 Conclusions

Stress-related hyperglycemia is associated with adverse outcomes in surgical and non-surgical critically ill patients, particularly non-diabetic and well-controlled diabetic patients. The randomized controlled trials that aimed to achieve a survival benefit towards and tight glucose management found conflicting results. Since hypoglycemia and fluctuations in blood glucose, as well as hyperglycemia, are associated with increased mortality, tools for continuous glucose monitoring and automated insulin infusion are under investigation. Concomitant administration of insulin and nutrition seems beneficial to prevent hypoglycemia and oppose metabolic consequences of prolonged critical illness.

22.2 Hydroxyethyl Starches

22.2.1 General Considerations on Fluid Choice

Hypovolemia impairs oxygen transport to cells and may contribute to multiple organ failure in critical illness [53]. Fluid therapy/volume resuscitation are the most extensively applied therapy in ICUs. In respect to their composition, replacement fluids are divided into crystalloids and colloids; the latter may be natural (e.g., albumin), or semi-synthetic (e.g., gelatins or starches), including hydroxyethyl starch (HES). The debate on which fluid is the best is still ongoing, and the RCTs performed in critically ill patients found conflicting evidences on mortality. The rationale for use of colloids is that their larger molecules will remain at a higher proportion in the intravascular space leading to better hemodynamics with less loss interstitial edema. In a recent metanalysis, accounting for 55 RCTs and more than 27,000 patients, central venous pressure and mean arterial pressure were higher and the overall fluid volume infused was lower with colloids than crystalloids [54]. This is important issue to limit the negative effects of crystalloids accumulation in the critically ill patients, including interstitial edema of gut, lungs, kidneys, and coagulation disorders. Thus, it has been suggested that colloids may be introduced as resuscitation fluid when the total amount of crystalloids infused exceeds 3–4 l [55]. However, the use of HES has been extensively associated to increased mortality when compared to balanced solution of crystalloids [54] and albumin is the only colloid recommended by the Surviving Sepsis Campaign [56]. More so, the evidence supporting the of starches is limited by low quality of trials (limited sample size, short follow-up time, and high risk of bias) [57]. A large proportion of initial data supporting HES was retracted due to scientific misconduct [58]. Indeed, large randomized clinical trials (RCTs) [59–61] and meta-analyses [62–66] should orient the choice of fluid therapy in ICU patients.

22.2.2 Main Lines of Evidence

In the Crystalloid Morbidity Associated with Severe Sepsis (CRYSTMAS) study on 196 septic patients, the hemodynamic stabilization was achieved with less volume of 6% HES 130/0.4 than isotonic saline [67]. Use of HES was associated to increased use of renal replacement therapy (RRT) and risk for mortality [68]. The Scandinavian Starch for Severe Sepsis/Septic Shock (6S) trial included 798 patients in 26 Scandinavian ICUs [59]. At 90 days, patients resuscitated with HES showed increased mortality. More patients in the HES group needed renal replacement therapies and blood products, as they showed more bleeding events as compared to patients resuscitated with Ringer's solution.

The large Crystalloids vs Hydroxyethyl Starch Trial (CHEST) randomized 7000 ICU patients to receive either 6% HES 130/0.4 or normal saline [60]. The trial confirmed an increased HES' associated use of RRT and higher rate of adverse events including need for blood products. No difference in mortality rate was noted. These results were confirmed by other trials, in which HES' use was not associated to increased mortality rate or RRT [61, 69, 70]. Some of the last trials have been criticized for heavy biasing [71].

In a Cochrane review assessing the effect of resuscitation with colloids vs. crystalloids on all-cause mortality in critically ill patients, HES was found to increase mortality compared to crystalloids [65]. Other systematic reviews assessing the effects of the new generation of HES, tetrastarch, excluded any clinical benefit and found increased risk of death and RRT with new starches both in patients with and without sepsis [62, 64].

22.2.3 Physiologic Considerations

The negative effects of colloids on mortality are possibly related to their structure and pharmacokinetics. HES are colloids derived from potatoes or maize solubilized in a crystalloid carrier solution. They are defined by their average molecular weight (MW), their substitution ratio, and pattern of hydroxyl-ethylating ratio (C2/C6 ratio). Several kinds of HES exist; the so-called tetrastarches, with MW around 130 kDa and a substitution ratio between 0.38 and 0.45 are the most commonly used HES. Hydroxyethyl starches are almost entirely excreted by glomerular filtration after hydrolysis by amylase, [72] but tissue uptake is pronounced regardless of subtype [73] and elimination of this part has not been clarified. Plasma and urine HES permanence, may be as high as 40% after 24 h from the end of infusion [73]. Modern 130/0.4–130/0.42 HES seems to be deposited in the tissue to an even larger extent than the older HES solutions. In a systematic review including necropsy and biopsy studies of patients who had received HES formulations, a profound and long-lasting deposition of HES residues in a broad spectrum of cells was evident [74]. The concentration and accumulation in tissues is thought to be linked to their renal toxicity and interaction with coagulation systems.

22.2.4 Therapeutic Use

Due to the above-mentioned issues, the use of HES has been highly restricted to acutely bleeding patients in case crystalloids are insufficient [68, 75]. This is an official statement from the EU and US health authorities. The lower dose must be used and for no more than 24 h. Maximum dosing is 50 ml/kg in adults. In children, HES should be avoided at all. Kidney function should be monitored for at least 90 days after administration due to risk of kidney injury. The use of HES in hypovolemic, not-bleeding, critically ill patients is counter-indicated, i.e., in septic shock. Due to potential side effects, HES should also be avoided in patients with severe liver disease, congestive heart failure, clinical signs of fluid overload and pre-existing renal injury, coagulation, or bleeding disorders.

22.2.5 Conclusions

High-quality RCTs consistently show that HES can quickly restore circulation in hypovolemic patients at expense of renal and hemostatic impairment and, possibly, increased mortality. There is no evidence that differences in molecular weight, substitution ratio or carrier fluid influence clinical outcome. Use of HES is actually strictly limited to low dose in acutely bleeding patients.

References

1. Mazeraud A, Polito A, Annane D, et al. Experimental and clinical evidences for glucose control in intensive care: is infused glucose the key point for study interpretation? Crit Care. 2014;18(4):232.
2. Marik PE, Bellomo R. Stress hyperglycemia: an essential survival response! Crit Care. 2013;17(2):305.
3. Schulman RC, Mechanick JI. Metabolic and nutrition support in the chronic critical illness syndrome. Respir Care. 2012;57(6):958–77.
4. Qi C, Pekala PH. Tumor necrosis factor-alpha-induced insulin resistance in adipocytes. Proc Soc Exp Biol Med. 2000;223(2):128–35.
5. Salim A, Hadjizacharia P, Dubose J, et al. Persistent hyperglycemia in severe traumatic brain injury: an independent predictor of outcome. Am Surg. 2009;75(1):25–9.
6. Finney SJ, Zekveld C, Elia A, et al. Glucose control and mortality in critically ill patients. JAMA. 2003;290(15):2041–7.
7. Baird TA, Parsons MW, Phan T, et al. Persistent poststroke hyperglycemia is independently associated with infarct expansion and worse clinical outcome. Stroke. 2003;34(9):2208–14.
8. Capes SE, Hunt D, Malmberg K, et al. Stress hyperglycaemia and increased risk of death after myocardial infarction in patients with and without diabetes: a systematic overview. Lancet. 2000;355(9206):773–8.
9. Krinsley JS. Association between hyperglycemia and increased hospital mortality in a heterogeneous population of critically ill patients. Mayo Clin Proc. 2003;78(12):1471–8.
10. Capes SE, Hunt D, Malmberg K, et al. Stress hyperglycemia and prognosis of stroke in nondiabetic and diabetic patients: a systematic overview. Stroke. 2001;32(10):2426–32.
11. Parsons MW, Barber PA, Desmond PM, et al. Acute hyperglycemia adversely affects stroke outcome: a magnetic resonance imaging and spectroscopy study. Ann Neurol. 2002;52(1):20–8.
12. Iwakura K, Ito H, Ikushima M, et al. Association between hyperglycemia and the no-reflow phenomenon in patients with acute myocardial infarction. J Am Coll Cardiol. 2003;41(1):1–7.
13. Bochicchio GV, Sung J, Joshi M, et al. Persistent hyperglycemia is predictive of outcome in critically ill trauma patients. J Trauma. 2005;58(5):921–4.
14. Rovlias A, Kotsou S. The influence of hyperglycemia on neurological outcome in patients with severe head injury. Neurosurgery. 2000;46(2):335–42. Discussion 342–3
15. Jones KW, Cain AS, Mitchell JHet al. Hyperglycemia predicts mortality after CABG: postoperative hyperglycemia predicts dramatic increases in mortality after coronary artery bypass graft surgery. J Diabetes Complicat. 2008;22(6):365–70.
16. McAlister FA, Man J, Bistritz L, et al. Diabetes and coronary artery bypass surgery: an examination of perioperative glycemic control and outcomes. Diabetes Care. 2003;26(5):1518–24.
17. Van Den Berghe G. Intensive insuline therapy in critically ill patients. N Engl J Med. 2001;345(19):1359–67.
18. Furnary AP, Gao G, Grunkemeier GL, et al. Continuous insulin infusion reduces mortality in patients with diabetes undergoing coronary artery bypass grafting. J Thorac Cardiovasc Surg. 2003;125(5):1007–21.
19. Van Den Berghe G, Wilmer A. Intensive insulin therapy in the medical ICU. N Engl J Med. 2006;354(5):449–61.
20. Brunkhorst F, Engel C, Bloos F, et al. Intensive insulin therapy and pentastarch resuscitation in severe sepsis. N Engl J Med. 2008;358:125–39.
21. Preiser JC, Devos P, Ruiz-Santana S, et al. A prospective randomised multi-Centre controlled trial on tight glucose control by intensive insulin therapy in adult intensive care units: the Glucontrol study. Intensive Care Med. 2009;35(10):1738–48.
22. NICE-SUGAR Study Investigators, Finfer S, Chittock DR, Su SY, et al. Intensive versus conventional glucose control in critically ill patients. N Engl J Med. 2009;360(13):1283–97.
23. Yao RQ, Ren C, Wu GS, et al. Is intensive glucose control bad for critically ill patients? A systematic review and meta-analysis. Int J Biol Sci. 2020;16(9):1658–75.
24. Marik PE, Preiser J-C. Toward understanding tight glycemic control in the ICU: a systematic review and metaanalysis. Chest. 2010;137(3):544–51.

25. Hermans G, Ph D, Wouters PJ, et al. Early versus late parenteral nutrition in critically ill adults. N Engl J Med. 2011;365:506–17.
26. Chase JG, Shaw G, Le Compte A, et al. Implementation and evaluation of the SPRINT protocol for tight glycaemic control in critically ill patients: a clinical practice change. Crit Care. 2008;12(2):R49.
27. Vanhorebeek I, Langouche L, Van den Berghe G. Glycemic and nonglycemic effects of insulin: how do they contribute to a better outcome of critical illness? Curr Opin Crit Care. 2005;11(4):304–11.
28. Battelino T, Goto M, Krzisnik C, et al. Tissue glucose transport and glucose transporters in suckling rats with endotoxic shock. Shock. 1996;6(4):259–62.
29. Vanhorebeek I, De Vos R, Mesotten D, et al. Protection of hepatocyte mitochondrial ultrastructure and function by strict blood glucose control with insulin in critically ill patients. Lancet. 2005;365(9453):53–9.
30. Carré JE, Orban J-C, Re L, et al. Survival in critical illness is associated with early activation of mitochondrial biogenesis. Am J Respir Crit Care Med. 2010;182(6):745–51.
31. Langouche L, Vander Perre S, Wouters PJ, et al. Effect of intensive insulin therapy on insulin sensitivity in the critically ill. J Clin Endocrinol Metab. 2007;92(10):3890–7.
32. Jeschke MG, Rensing H, Klein Det al. Insulin prevents liver damage and preserves liver function in lipopolysaccharide-induced endotoxemic rats. J Hepatol. 2005;42(6):870–9.
33. Deng HP, Chai JK. The effects and mechanisms of insulin on systemic inflammatory response and immune cells in severe trauma, burn injury, and sepsis. Int Immunopharmacol. 2009;9(11):1251–9.
34. Heller SR. Abnormalities of the electrocardiogram during hypoglycaemia: the cause of the dead in bed syndrome? Int J Clin Pract Suppl. 2002;129:27–32.
35. Lindström T, Jorfeldt L, Tegler L, et al. Hypoglycaemia and cardiac arrhythmias in patients with type 2 diabetes mellitus. Diabet Med. 1992;9(6):536–41.
36. Koivikko ML, Karsikas M, Salmela PIet al. Effects of controlled hypoglycaemia on cardiac repolarisation in patients with type 1 diabetes. Diabetologia. 2008;51(3):426–35.
37. Graham BB, Keniston A, Gajic O, et al. Diabetes mellitus does not adversely affect outcomes from a critical illness. Crit Care Med. 2010;38(1):16–24.
38. Egi M, Bellomo R, Stachowski Eet al. The interaction of chronic and acute glycemia with mortality in critically ill patients with diabetes. Crit Care Med. 2011;39(1):105–11.
39. Krinsley JS. The long and winding road toward personalized Glcyemic control in critically ill. J Diabetes Sci Technol. 2018;12(1):26–32.
40. Abdelmalak BB, Lansang MC. Revisiting tight glycemic control in perioperative and critically ill patients: when one size may not fit all. J Clin Anesth. 2013;25(6):499–507.
41. Mesotten D, Van den Berghe G. Glycemic targets and approaches to management of the patient with critical illness. Curr Diab Rep. 2012;12(1):101–7.
42. Krinsley JS. Glycemic variability: a strong independent predictor of mortality in critically ill patients. Crit Care Med. 2008;36(11):3008–13.
43. Todi S, Bhattacharya M. Glycemic variability and outcome in critically ill. Indian J Crit Care Med. 2014;18(5):285–90.
44. Egi M, Bellomo R, Stachowski E, et al. Variability of blood glucose concentration and short-term mortality in critically ill patients. Anesthesiology. 2006;105(2):244–52.
45. Monnier L, Mas E, Ginet C, et al. Activation of oxidative stress by acute glucose fluctuations compared with sustained chronic hyperglycemia in patients with type 2 diabetes. JAMA. 2006;295(14):1681–7.
46. Farrokhi F, Chandra P, Smiley D, et al. Glucose variability is an independent predictor of mortality in hospitalized patients treated with total parenteral nutrition. Endocr Pract. 2014;20(1):41–5.
47. Krinsley JS, Chase JG, Gunst J, et al. Continuous glucose monitoring in the ICU: clinical considerations and consensus. Crit Care. 2017;21:197–205.

48. Saager L, Collins GL, Burnside Bet al. A randomized study in diabetic patients undergoing cardiac surgery comparing computer-guided glucose management with a standard sliding scale protocol. J Cardiothorac Vasc Anesth. 2008;22(3):377–82.

49. Saur NM, Kongable GL, Holewinski S, et al. Software-guided insulin dosing: tight glycemic control and decreased glycemic derangements in critically ill patients. Mayo Clin Proc. 2013;88(9):920–9.

50. Boom DT, Sechterberger MK, Rijkenberg S, et al. Insulin treatment guided by subcutaneous continuous glucose monitoring compared to frequent point-of-care measurement in critically ill patients: a randomized controlled trial. Crit Care. 2014;18(4):453.

51. Punke MA, Decker C, Reuter DA, et al. Head-to-head comparison of two glucose monitoring systems on a cardio-surgical ICU. J Clin Monit Comput. 2019;33(5):895–901.

52. Okabayashi T, Shima Y. Are closed-loop systems for intensive insulin therapy ready for prime time in the ICU? Curr Opin Clin Nutr Metab Care. 2014;17(2):190–9.

53. Van der Mullen J, Wise R, Vermeulen G, et al. Anesthesiol Intensive Ther. 2018;50:141–9.

54. Martin GS, Basset P. Crystalloids vs. colloids for fluid resuscitation in the intensive care unit: a systematic review and meta-analysis. J Crit Care. 2019;50:144–54.

55. Hahn RG. Adverse effects of crystalloid and colloid fluids. Anaesthesiol Intensive Ther. 2017;49(4):303–8.

56. Rhodes, et al. Surviving sepsis campaign: international guidelines for management of septic shock: 2016. Intensive Care Med. 2017;43(3):304–77.

57. Hartog CS, Kohl M, Reinhart K. A systematic review of third-generation hydroxyethyl starch (HES 130/0.4) in resuscitation: safety not adequately addressed. Anesth Analg. 2011;112:635–45.

58. Wise J. Boldt: the great pretender. BMJ. 2013;346:f1738.

59. Perner A, Haase N, Guttormsen AB, et al. Hydroxyethyl starch 130/0.42 versus Ringer's acetate in severe sepsis. N Engl J Med. 2012;367:124–34.

60. Myburgh JA, Finfer S, Bellomo R, et al. Hydroxyethyl starch or saline for fluid resuscitation in intensive care. N Engl J Med. 2012;367:1901–11.

61. Annane D. Effects of fluid resuscitation with colloids vs crystalloids on mortality in critically ill patients presenting with hypovolemic shock. JAMA. 2013;310(17):1809–17.

62. Haase N, Perner A, Hennings LI, et al. Hydroxyethyl starch 130/0.38-0.45 versus crystalloid or albumin in patients with sepsis: systematic review with meta-analysis and trial sequential analysis. BMJ. 2013;346:f839.

63. Zarychanski R, Abou-Setta AM, Turgeon AF, et al. Association of hydroxyethyl starch administration with mortality and acute kidney injury in critically ill patients requiring volume resuscitation: a systematic review and meta-analysis. JAMA. 2013;309:678–88.

64. Gattas DJ, Dan A, Myburgh J, et al. Fluid resuscitation with 6% hydroxyethyl starch (130/0.4 and 130/0.42) in acutely ill patients: systematic review of effects on mortality and treatment with renal replacement therapy. Intensive Care Med. 2013;39:558–68.

65. Perel P, Roberts I, Ker K. Colloids versus crystalloids for fluid resuscitation in critically ill patients. Cochrane Database Syst Rev. 2013;2:CD000567.

66. Mutter TC, Ruth CA, Dart AB. Hydroxyethyl starch (HES) versus other fluid therapies: effects on kidney function. Cochrane Database Syst Rev. 2013;7:CD007594.

67. Guidet B, Martinet O, Boulain T, Philippart F, Poussel JF, Maizel J, Forceville X, Feissel M, Hasselmann M, Heininger A, Van Aken H. Assessment of hemodynamic efficacy and safety of 6% hydroxyethylstarch 130/0.4 vs. 0.9% NaCl fluid replacement in patients with severe sepsis: the CRYSTMAS study. Crit Care. 2012;16:R94.

68. FDA. Safety Communication: Boxed Warning on increased mortality and severe renal injury, and additional warning on risk of bleeding, for use of hydroxyethyl starch solutions in some settings. 2013. http://webcache.googleusercontent.com/search?q=cache:http://www.fda.gov/biologicsbloodvaccines/safetyavailability/ucm358271.htm.

69. Perner A, Haase N, Wetterslev J. Mortality in patients with hypovolemic shock treated with colloids or crystalloids. JAMA. 2014;311:1067.

70. James MFM, Michell WL, Joubert IA, et al. Resuscitation with hydroxyethyl starch improves renal function and lactate clearance in penetrating trauma in a randomized controlled study: the FIRST trial (fluids in resuscitation of severe trauma). Br J Anaesth. 2011;107:693–702.
71. Finfer S. Hydroxyethyl starch in patients with trauma. Br J Anaesth. 2012;108:159–60. Author reply 160–1
72. Jungheinrich C, Neff TA. Pharmacokinetics of hydroxyethyl starch. Clin Pharmacokinet. 2005;44:681–99.
73. Bellmann R, Feistritzer C, Wiedermann CJ. Effect of molecular weight and substitution on tissue uptake of hydroxyethyl starch: a meta-analysis of clinical studies. Clin Pharmacokinet. 2012;51:225–36.
74. Wiedermann CJ, Joannidis M. Accumulation of hydroxyethyl starch in human and animal tissues: a systematic review. Intensive Care Med. 2013;40(2):160–70.
75. EMA. PRAC recommends suspending marketing authorisations for infusion solutions containing hydroxyethyl-starch. 2013. http://www.ema.europa.eu/docs/en_GB/document_library/Press_release/2013/06/WC500144446.pdf.

Latest Evidence

23

Chiara Sartini, Nicolò Maimeri, and Alessandro Belletti

Contents

23.1   General Principles

The body of scientific evidence increases continuously. Every day, researchers project, start and publish new randomized controlled trials (RCTs). Unfortunately, these trials often fail to demonstrate a significant difference in mortality as discussed in Chap. 1.

From 2017 to date, among the multitude of papers published in peer-reviewed journals, some had significant effect on mortality and reinforced (while others denied) the evidence demonstrated in previous trials.

C. Sartini (✉) · N. Maimeri · A. Belletti
Department of Anesthesia and Intensive Care, IRCCS San Raffaele Hospital, Milan, Italy
e-mail: belletti.alessandro@hsr.it

© Springer Nature Switzerland AG 2021   219
G. Landoni et al. (eds.), *Reducing Mortality in Critically Ill Patients*,
https://doi.org/10.1007/978-3-030-71917-3_23

This chapter collects the last-minute evidence (published up to 2020) about interventions reducing mortality not discussed in the previous sections of this book. Though interesting, this evidence requires further studies to be confirmed.

23.2 Angiotensin II

Angiotensin II (ATII) binds angiotensin receptors (AT1 and AT2), part of the renin-angiotensin-aldosterone system (RAAS). This molecule is a short-acting vasopressor with potent direct vasoconstrictor effect both on arteries and veins. Moreover, ATII increases the secretion of antidiuretic hormone (ADH), adrenocorticotropin hormone (ACTH), and aldosterone [1]. The synthetic molecule is known to have direct effect on renal efferent arterioles, with an increase of glomerular perfusion pressure [2]. In 2017, a multicenter randomized controlled trial (mRCT) on the use of ATII in catecholamine-resistant vasodilatory shock, the ATHOS-3 trial, was published [3]. This trial failed to demonstrate a mortality benefit in the overall population, but a secondary post hoc analysis found a reduction in mortality in the subgroup of patients on renal replacement therapy (RRT). Indeed, 28-days mortality was lower in patients on RRT treated with ATII (as an adjunctive to norepinephrine treatment) than in placebo group (unadjusted hazard ratio 0.52; 95% CI 0.30–0.87, p value = 0.012) [4].

23.3 Bicarbonate

The use of bicarbonate in metabolic acidosis is controversial. Low pH can cause cellular dysfunction, so intravenous sodium bicarbonate administration, increasing pH, might be beneficial. On the other hand, potential side-effects are intracellular acidification due to the accumulation of carbon dioxide and the risk of hypocalcemia [5].

The BICAR-ICU trial, performed in 2018 in 26 intensive care units (ICUs), randomized 389 patients with severe metabolic acidemia (pH <7.2, bicarbonate <20 mmol/L, lactate >2 mmol/L, and normal carbon dioxide) to receive bicarbonate (in order to achieve a pH >7.3) or placebo. Bicarbonate had no effect on mortality in the overall population but demonstrated a benefit in patients with acute kidney injury (AKIN 2–3), with 46% of patients dying at day 28 in the bicarbonate group and 63% in the placebo group (p value =0.016) [6].

23.4 Airway Management in Cardiac Arrest

Advanced life support during resuscitation for cardiac arrest requires effective minute ventilation. In the out-of-hospital scenario, endotracheal intubation (ETI) might be challenging and it is not always performed by personnel with adequate training on airway management. Literature reports significant rates of unrecognized tube misplacement, need for multiple ETI attempts, and ETI insertion failure [7]. Thus, the use of a supraglottic device might be a valuable alternative.

An mRCT was performed in 2018, involving 27 emergency medical services [8]. More than 3000 patients were randomized to receive laryngeal tube (LT) insertion or ETI. Survival at 72 h was 18.3% and 15.4%, respectively (p value = 0.04), with a slight increase in the rate of aspiration pneumonia in LT group although not significant. The survival benefit was still present at hospital discharge (p value = 0.01).

23.5 Steroids in Acute Respiratory Distress Syndrome (ARDS) Including COVID-19 Patients

Glucocorticoids (steroids) have inhibitory effects on a broad range of immune responses and are efficacious in managing many of the acute disease manifestations of inflammatory and autoimmune disorders. The main field of research about steroids use in critically ill patients are septic shock and ARDS. Hydrocortisone in septic shock has been discussed in Chap. 10.

The use of steroids in pulmonary pathologies is a matter of debate since years.

The first RCT showing a mortality effect was a small mRCT performed in 1998 and enrolling 24 ARDS patients who had no improvement after 7 days of conventional treatment. Methylprednisolone (2 mg/kg/die for 32 days) demonstrated a survival benefit over placebo for in-hospital mortality [9]. A subsequent trial in 2006 found the opposite result, with increased mortality in patients who started methylprednisolone treatment after 14 days from ARDS onset [10].

In 2007, early administration (<72 h from onset) of methylprednisolone (1 mg/kg/die for 28 days) was tested in patients with severe ARDS. The study found a reduction of in-hospital mortality in the treatment group over placebo [11].

A recent task force suggested that methylprednisolone may be considered in patients with moderate-severe ARDS early (up to day 7 from onset) in a dose of 1 mg/kg/day and late (after day 6 from onset) in a dose of 2 mg/kg/day followed by slow tapering over 13 days [12].

In addition, two new trials investigating the effect of dexamethasone were performed in 2020. The first is an mRCT enrolling 277 patients with moderate-severe ARDS after 24 h from onset where patients received dexamethasone or placebo (20 mg/die for 5 days and 10 mg/die for the subsequent 5 days). At 60 days mortality was strongly reduced in treatment group as compared with placebo group (21% vs 36% respectively, p value = 0.004) [13].

The second trial is a preliminary report on the use of dexamethasone in hospitalized Coronavirus disease-19 (COVID-19) patients. Two thousand patients were randomized to receive dexamethasone (6 mg/die for 10 days) regardless of disease severity or placebo. Mortality at 28 days was reduced in the subgroup of patients with respiratory support receiving dexamethasone (either oxygen—23.3% vs 26.2% or mechanical ventilation—29.3% vs 41.4%) but not in the subgroup of patients not requiring oxygen, where there was a trend towards harm [14].

23.6   Tranexamic Acid

Tranexamic acid is an antifibrinolytic agent previously discussed in Chap. 14 as far as trauma setting is concerned.

In this section, two recent studies on the use of tranexamic acid in post-partum hemorrhage and intracerebral hemorrhage are discussed.

23.6.1 Tranexamic Acid in Post-Partum Hemorrhage

Primary post-partum hemorrhage is the leading cause of maternal death worldwide. Similar to trauma, early activation of fibrinolysis is also recorded after childbirth [15]. The WOMAN trial is a large double-blind mRCT involving 20,000 women after cesarean section or vaginal birth with primary PPH. Tranexamic acid (1 g bolus + 1 g in case of ongoing hemorrhage) reduced mortality for bleeding cause in treatment group compared to placebo (1.5% vs 1.9% respectively, p value = 0.045) [16].

23.6.2 Tranexamic Acid in Intracerebral Hemorrhage

After establishing the beneficial effect of tranexamic acid in trauma and post-partum hemorrhage, the results of another trial were published in 2018. TICH-2 was an mRCT enrolling patients with acute intracerebral hemorrhage within 8 h of stroke symptom onset. They were treated with tranexamic acid (1 g bolus + 1 g in 8 h continuous infusion) or placebo. At day 7, mortality was lower in treatment group (9% vs 11%, p value = 0.041) although this benefit was lost at 90 days. Tranexamic acid did not increase the number of venous thromboembolic or arterial occlusion events [17].

23.7   Point-of-Care Testing for Coagulation

Significant postoperative bleeding has to be expected in up to 10% of patients undergoing cardiac surgery, and it is associated with worse outcome [18]. Algorithm guided by point-of-care thrombelastometry (ROTEM®) might be associated with substantial benefits as they are capable to quickly identify potential coagulation disorders allowing specific treatment [19].

In 2018, a single center RCT (sRCT) enrolled 104 patients with significant blood loss after cardiac surgery. Patients were randomized to an ROTEM-guided strategy or a standard coagulation test strategy to correct hemostasis after arrival in ICU. Patients with long cardiopulmonary bypass time (> 115 min, 55 patients) showed reduced 5-years mortality when treated with an ROTEM-based approach (0% vs 15%, p value = 0.03) [20].

23.8   Thrombolytic Removal in Intraventricular Bleeding

Ventricular hemorrhage in the context of spontaneous intracranial bleeding is associated with devastating consequences. Acute obstructive hydrocephalus can develop and the injection of thrombolytic agents through an intraventricular catheter might ameliorate cerebrospinal fluid drainage and reduce neurotoxicity [21].

The CLEAR III trial is an mRCT conducted in 2017 where 500 patients were randomized to receive intraventricular alteplase (1 mg up to 12 doses in total) or placebo. Mortality was lower in patients treated with alteplase than with placebo (18% vs 29% respectively, p value = 0.006). Of note, functional outcome assessed by modified Rankin score (mRS) was worse in the treatment group [22].

23.9   Other Evidence

Minor evidence, not included in previous chapters of this book and not discussed above, are collected in Table 23.1. These evidence have been judged less important due to the quality of the study (i.e., sRCT, small population) or the topic itself. As for all other interventions discussed in this chapter, further evaluation of potential survival benefit is required.

Table 23.1 List of interventions reducing mortality published from 2017, not discussed in the present and previous chapters

Year	First author	Journal	Topic	Title
2017	Ceccato A	PLoS one	Infectious disease	Treatment with macrolides and glucocorticosteroids in severe community-acquired pneumonia: a post hoc exploratory analysis of a randomized controlled trial
2018	Welte T	Intensive care med		Efficacy and safety of trimodulin, a novel polyclonal antibody preparation, in patients with severe community-acquired pneumonia: a randomized, placebo-controlled, double-blind, multicenter, phase II trial (CIGMA study)
2019	Luyt CE	JAMA		Acyclovir for mechanically ventilated patients with herpes simplex virus oropharyngeal reactivation: a randomized clinical trial

(continued)

Table 23.1 (continued)

Year	First author	Journal	Topic	Title
2017	McAuley DF	Lancet Respir med	Acute respiratory distress syndrome	Keratinocyte growth factor for the treatment of the acute respiratory distress syndrome (KARE): a randomized, double-blind, placebo-controlled phase 2 trial
2019	Mahmoud A	JCVA		Streptokinase versus unfractionated heparin nebulization in patients with severe acute respiratory distress syndrome (ARDS): a randomized controlled trial with observational controls
2018	Calfee CS	Lancet Respir med		Acute respiratory distress syndrome subphenotypes and differential response to simvastatin: Secondary analysis of a randomized controlled trial
2017	Guidet B	JAMA	Health care management	Effect of systematic intensive care unit triage on long-term mortality among critically ill elderly patients in France: a randomized clinical trial
2017	Shimabukuro DW	BMJ open Respir res		Effect of a machine learning-based severe sepsis prediction algorithm on patient survival and hospital length of stay: a randomized clinical trial
2017	Ojima M	J intensive care		Hemodynamic effects of electrical muscle stimulation in the prophylaxis of deep vein thrombosis for intensive care unit patients: a randomized trial
2017	Bergamin FS	Crit care med	Transfusions	Liberal versus restrictive transfusion strategy in critically ill oncologic patients: The transfusion requirements in critically ill oncologic patients randomized controlled trial
2018	Cardenas JC	Blood Adv		Platelet transfusions improve hemostasis and survival in a substudy of the prospective, randomized PROPPR trial
2019	Gobatto A	Crit care		Transfusion requirements after head trauma: a randomized feasibility controlled trial

Table 23.1 (continued)

Year	First author	Journal	Topic	Title
2017	Schädler D	PLoS one	Hemofiltration and acute kidney injury	The effect of a novel extracorporeal cytokine hemoadsorption device on IL-6 elimination in septic patients: A randomized controlled trial
2018	You B	Critical care		Early application of continuous high-volume hemofiltration can reduce sepsis and improve the prognosis of patients with severe burns
2018	Pickkers P	NEJM		Effect of human recombinant alkaline phosphatase on 7-day creatinine clearance in patients with sepsis-associated acute kidney injury
2017	Andrews B	JAMA	Hemodynamic management	Effect of an early resuscitation protocol on in-hospital mortality among adults with sepsis and hypotension: a randomized clinical trial
2019	Noormandi A	Eur J Clin Pharmacol		Effect of magnesium supplementation on lactate clearance in critically ill patients with severe sepsis: a randomized clinical trial
2018	Lu Y	Pak J med Sci		Controlled blood pressure elevation and limited fluid resuscitation in the treatment of multiple injuries in combination with shock
2018	Arora V	Hepatology		Terlipressin is superior to noradrenaline in the management of acute kidney injury in acute on chronic liver failure
2017	Nabi T	Saudi J Gastroenterol	Liver	Role of N-acetylcysteine treatment in non-acetaminophen-induced acute liver failure: a prospective study
2019	Abdoli A	Bull Emerg trauma	Traumatic brain injury	Efficacy of simultaneous administration of nimodipine, progesterone, and magnesium sulfate in patients with severe traumatic brain injury: a randomized controlled trial

References

1. Basso N, Terragno NA. History about the discovery of the renin-angiotensin system. Hypertens. 2001;38(6):1246–9. https://doi.org/10.1161/hy1201.101214.
2. Wan L, Langenberg C, Bellomo R, May CN. Angiotensin II in experimental hyperdynamic sepsis. Crit Care. 2009;13(6):R190. https://doi.org/10.1186/cc8185.
3. Khanna A, English SW, Wang XS, et al. Angiotensin II for the treatment of vasodilatory shock. N Engl J Med. 2017;377(5):419–30. https://doi.org/10.1056/NEJMoa1704154.
4. Tumlin JA, Murugan R, Deane AM, et al. Outcomes in patients with vasodilatory shock and renal replacement therapy treated with intravenous angiotensin II. Crit Care Med. 2018;46(6):949–57. https://doi.org/10.1097/CCM.0000000000003092.
5. Berend K, de Vries APJ, Gans ROB. Physiological approach to assessment of acid-base disturbances. N Engl J Med. 2014;371(15):1434–45. https://doi.org/10.1056/NEJMra1003327.
6. Jaber S, Paugam C, Futier E, et al. Sodium bicarbonate therapy for patients with severe metabolic acidaemia in the intensive care unit (BICAR-ICU): a multicentre, open-label, randomised controlled, phase 3 trial. Lancet. 2018;392(10141):31–40. https://doi.org/10.1016/S0140-6736(18)31080-8.
7. Wang HE, Yealy DM. How many attempts are required to accomplish out-of-hospital endotracheal intubation? Acad Emerg Med Off J Soc Acad Emerg Med. 2006;13(4):372–7. https://doi.org/10.1197/j.aem.2005.11.001.
8. Andersen LW, Granfeldt A, Callaway CW, et al. Association between tracheal intubation during adult in-hospital cardiac arrest and survival. J Am Med Assoc. 2017;317(5):494–506. https://doi.org/10.1001/jama.2016.20165.
9. Meduri GU, Headley AS, Golden E, et al. Effect of prolonged methylprednisolone therapy in unresolving acute respiratory distress syndrome: a randomized controlled trial. J Am Med Assoc. 1998;280(2):159–65. https://doi.org/10.1001/jama.280.2.159.
10. Steinberg KP, Hudson LD, Goodman RB, et al. Efficacy and safety of corticosteroids for persistent acute respiratory distress syndrome. N Engl J Med. 2006;354(16):1671–84. https://doi.org/10.1056/NEJMoa051693.
11. Meduri GU, Golden E, Freire AX, et al. Methylprednisolone infusion in early severe ards: results of a randomized controlled trial. Chest. 2007;131(4):954–63. https://doi.org/10.1378/chest.06-2100.
12. Annane D, Pastores SM, Rochwerg B, et al. Correction to: guidelines for the diagnosis and management of critical illness-related corticosteroid insufficiency (CIRCI) in critically ill patients (part I): Society of Critical Care Medicine (SCCM) and European Society of Intensive Care Medicine (ESIC). Intensive Care Med. 2018;44(3):401–2. https://doi.org/10.1007/s00134-018-5071-6.
13. Villar J, Ferrando C, Martínez D, et al. Dexamethasone treatment for the acute respiratory distress syndrome: a multicentre, randomised controlled trial. Lancet Respir Med. 2020;8(3):267–76. https://doi.org/10.1016/S2213-2600(19)30417-5.
14. Horby P, Lim WS, Emberson JR, et al. Dexamethasone in hospitalized patients with Covid-19 - preliminary report. N Engl J Med. 2020; https://doi.org/10.1056/NEJMoa2021436.
15. Tunçalp O, Souza JP, Gülmezoglu M. New WHO recommendations on prevention and treatment of postpartum hemorrhage. Int J Gynaecol Obstet Off Organ Int Fed Gynaecol Obstet. 2013;123(3):254–6. https://doi.org/10.1016/j.ijgo.2013.06.024.
16. Shakur H, Roberts I, Fawole B, et al. Effect of early tranexamic acid administration on mortality, hysterectomy, and other morbidities in women with post-partum haemorrhage (WOMAN): an international, randomised, double-blind, placebo-controlled trial. Lancet. 2017;389(10084):2105–16. https://doi.org/10.1016/S0140-6736(17)30638-4.
17. Sprigg N, Flaherty K, Appleton JP, et al. Tranexamic acid for hyperacute primary IntraCerebral Haemorrhage (TICH-2): an international randomised, placebo-controlled, phase 3 superiority trial. Lancet. 2018;391(10135):2107–15. https://doi.org/10.1016/S0140-6736(18)31033-X.

18. Karkouti K, Wijeysundera DN, Yau TM, et al. The independent association of massive blood loss with mortality in cardiac surgery. Transfusion. 2004;44(10):1453–62. https://doi.org/10.1111/j.1537-2995.2004.04144.x.

19. Royston D, von Kier S. Reduced haemostatic factor transfusion using heparinase-modified thrombelastography during cardiopulmonary bypass. Br J Anaesth. 2001;86(4):575–8. https://doi.org/10.1093/bja/86.4.575.

20. Haensig M, Kempfert J, Kempfert PM, Girdauskas E, Borger MA, Lehmann S. Thrombelastometry guided blood-component therapy after cardiac surgery: a randomized study. BMC Anesthesiol. 2019;19(1):1–10. https://doi.org/10.1186/s12871-019-0875-7.

21. Gaberel T, Magheru C, Parienti J-J, Huttner HB, Vivien D, Emery E. Intraventricular fibrinolysis versus external ventricular drainage alone in intraventricular hemorrhage: a meta-analysis. Stroke. 2011;42(10):2776–81. https://doi.org/10.1161/STROKEAHA.111.615724.

22. Hanley DF, Lane K, McBee N, et al. Thrombolytic removal of intraventricular haemorrhage in treatment of severe stroke: results of the randomised, multicentre, multiregion, placebo-controlled CLEAR III trial. Lancet. 2017;389(10069):603–11. https://doi.org/10.1016/S0140-6736(16)32410-2.

Printed by Printforce, the Netherlands